WM
200
RUD

(3)

Serious Mental Illness

Serious Mental Illness

Person-Centered Approaches

Edited by

ABRAHAM RUDNICK, B.Med.Sc., M.D., M.Psych., Ph.D.,
C.P.R.P., F.R.C.P.C.

Associate Professor, Departments of Psychiatry and Philosophy
The University of Western Ontario, Canada

and

DAVID ROE, Ph.D.

Associate Professor, Department of Community Mental Health,
Faculty of Social Welfare and Health Related Sciences
University of Haifa, Israel

Foreword by

WILLIAM A. ANTHONY, Ph.D.

Executive Director, Center for Psychiatric Rehabilitation
Professor, Department of Rehabilitation Sciences
Sargent College of Health and Rehabilitation Sciences,
Boston University

Radcliffe Publishing
London • New York

Radcliffe Publishing Ltd
33–41 Dallington Street
London
EC1V 0BB
United Kingdom

www.radcliffepublishing.com

Electronic catalogue and worldwide online ordering facility.

British Library Cataloguing in Publication Data

A catalogue record for this book is available from the British Library.

ISBN-13: 978 184619 306 4

The paper used for the text pages of this book is FSC
certified. FSC (The Forest Stewardship Council)
is an international network to promote responsible
management of the world's forests.

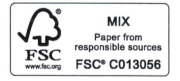

Typeset by KnowledgeWorks Global Ltd, Chennai, India
Printed and bound by TJI Digital, Padstow, Cornwall, UK

Contents

Series Editors' Introduction

A new clinical method, which has been developed during the 1980s and 1990s, has attempted to regain the balance between curing and caring. It is called the Patient-Centered Clinical Method and has been described and illustrated in the second edition of *Patient-Centered Medicine: transforming the clinical method.*[1] A third edition will be published next year. In the 2003 book, conceptual, educational and research issues were elucidated in detail. The patient-centered conceptual framework from that book is used as the structure for each book in the Series introduced here; it consists of six interactive components to be considered in every patient-practitioner interaction.

The first component is to assess the two modes of ill health: disease and illness. In addition to assessing the disease process, the clinician explores the patient's illness experience. Specifically, the practitioner considers how the patient feels about being ill, what the patient's ideas are about the illness, what impact the illness is having on the patient's functioning, and what he or she expects from the clinician.

The second component is an integration of the concepts of disease and illness with an understanding of the whole person. This includes an awareness of the patient's position in the life cycle and the proximal and distal contexts in which the person lives.

The third component of the method is the mutual task of finding common ground between the patient and the practitioner. This consists of three key areas: mutually defining the problem; mutually defining the goals of management/treatment; and mutually exploring the roles to be assumed by the patient and the practitioner.

The fourth component is to use each visit as an opportunity for prevention and health promotion. The fifth component takes into consideration that each encounter with the patient should be used to develop the helping relationship; the trust and respect that evolve in the relationship will have an impact on other components of the method. The sixth component requires that, throughout the process, the practitioner is realistic in terms of time, availability of resources and the role of collaborative teamwork in patient care.

However, there is a gap between the description of the clinical method and its application in practice. The series of books presented here attempts to bridge that gap. Written by international leaders in their respective fields, the series represents clinical explications of the patient-centered clinical method. Each volume deals with a common and challenging problem faced by practitioners. In each book, current thinking is organized in a similar way, reinforcing and illustrating the patient-centered clinical method. The common format begins with a description of the burden of illness, followed by chapters on the illness experience, the whole person, finding common ground, and the patient-practitioner relationship.

This book series is international, to date representing Norway, Canada, New Zealand, Australia, the U.S.A., England, Scotland and Israel. It is a testament to the universality of the values and concepts inherent in the patient-centered clinical method. We feel that an international definition of patient-centered practice is being established and is represented in this book series.

The vigor of any clinical method is proven in the extent to which it is applicable in the clinical setting. It is anticipated that this series will inform further development of the clinical method and move thinking forward in this important aspect of medicine.

Moira Stewart, Ph.D.
Judith Belle Brown, Ph.D.
Thomas R. Freeman, M.D., C.C.F.P.
April 2011

REFERENCE

1 Stewart M, Brown JB, Weston WW, *et al.*, editors. *Patient-Centered Medicine: transforming the clinical method*. 2nd ed. Oxford: Radcliffe Publishing; 2003.

Foreword

In the 1970s when I started talking and writing about helping people to choose their own goals, I was met with much resistance from the professional community. Comments were made such as: "people with severe mental illnesses don't know how to set goals," or, "they will set unrealistic goals", or "they will come up with destructive goals." In the early 1970s an important book such as *Serious Mental Illness: Person-Centered Approaches* could not even be envisioned, much less published. Discussions about "client-driven care" (as it was called then) did not occur in the mainstream mental health community. As a matter of fact, most of last century's written history of mental health care described a mental health system far removed from the idea of person-centered care. People with mental illnesses were not expected to recover; worse yet they were often dehumanized and devalued by both society and the treatment providers who were supposed to be helping. *Serious Mental Illness: Person-Centered Approaches* reflects a continued distancing from the outmoded and unsubstantiated belief that people with severe mental illnesses could not recover, and that they would respond positively only to goals and treatment plans chosen, designed and implemented by providers in order to prevent their further deterioration.

Serious Mental Illness: Person-Centered Approaches is certainly the first comprehensive text on person-centered approaches. But its value does not come from just being first; its value comes from the skillful and knowledgeable writing found in every section. The editors are to be congratulated for assembling experts able to write to the overarching theme of engaging people as people, regardless of their setting, context or label. In my experience, edited books often lack coherence; individual sections do not tie together nor relate directly to the main focus of the book. This is not the case in this edited book. The editors have recruited authors who bring their own personal expertise yet are familiar with person-centered approaches. With its well-thought-out organization and logical flow, *Serious Mental Illness: Person-Centered Approaches* reads like an authored text rather than an edited book.

Each chapter in *Serious Mental Illness: Person-Centered Approaches* is a treatise unto itself. Individual sections stand as the definitive work on person-centered approaches based on each author's own unique frame of reference. Even the historical sections are major contributions to the literature on person-centered approaches, such as Charland's analysis of how person-centered approaches are rooted in early 19th century moral treatment and Cross' description of Carl Rogers' relevance to person-centered approaches. A recurring theme in many of the sections is the critical nature of the relationship between the helper and the person with a serious mental illness. Repeatedly emphasized by most authors is the basic humanism of person-centered approaches, as evidenced in a variety of contexts.

I think readers of *Serious Mental Illness: Person-Centered Approaches* will have their favorite sections that they constantly reference as a valuable resource for their own work and which they refer to time and again. The breadth of this text is truly amazing. Anyone with an interest in the concept of person-centered approaches will discover new ideas in this book. Indeed, anyone with an interest in this sort of approach *has* to read this book. Not only is it the first such book on this topic, but it will serve as the gold standard in relation to person-centered approaches for years to come.

William A. Anthony, PhD.
Executive Director, Center for Psychiatric Rehabilitation
Professor, Department of Rehabilitation Sciences
Sargent College of Health and Rehabilitation Sciences, Boston University
April 2011

About the Editors

Rudnick, Abraham

Abraham (Rami) Rudnick, B.Med.Sc., M.D., M.Psych., Ph.D., C.P.R.P., F.R.C.P.C., received his M.D. from the Hebrew University, Jerusalem, and his Ph.D. in philosophy from Tel Aviv University, Israel. He completed a residency in psychiatry at the Tel Aviv Mental Health Center, a fellowship in psychiatry at the University of Toronto, and is a Certified Psychiatric Rehabilitation Practitioner from the International Association of Psychosocial Rehabilitation Services. He is an Associate Professor in the Departments of Psychiatry and Philosophy, the Chair of the Division of Social and Rural Psychiatry, the Director of the Extended Campus Program and the Clinical Director of the North of Superior Program, as well as the Head of the Canadian Unit of the International Network of the UNESCO (United Nations Educational, Scientific and Cultural Organization) Chair in Bioethics and the Bioethics Coordinator in the Department of Psychiatry, all at The University of Western Ontario. He is the Physician-Leader of the Psychosis Program at Regional Mental Health Care, St. Joseph's Health Care, London, Ontario, Canada. He was the chair of the research committee of the board of directors of the Ontario Chapter of Psychosocial Rehabilitation/ Réadaptation Psychosociale Canada, and he is a member of the board of directors and the chair of the research committee of Psychosocial Rehabilitation/Réadaptation Psychosociale Canada. His main research programs, on which he has published papers, book chapters and is currently editing books, address recovery and coping of individuals with serious mental illness such as schizophrenia and their person-centered care and psychiatric rehabilitation, as well as general and mental health care ethics. He has taught internationally, nationally and locally on psychiatric rehabilitation and on bioethics in academic, professional and public venues.

Roe, David

David Roe, Ph.D., is a licensed clinical psychologist and Professor and Chair of the Department of Community Mental Health, Faculty of Social Welfare and Health Sciences, University of Haifa, Israel. His research focuses on the psychosocial processes of recovery from serious mental illness and has been funded by several local and international sources, including the National Institute of Mental Health, The Israeli Ministry of Health, The Israel National Institute for Health Services Research and Health Policy, the Israeli National Insurance Institution and the Tauber and Rich foundations. Dr. Roe has published over 100 peer-reviewed journal and book chapters and serves on several editorial boards.

List of Contributors

Beattie, Nicole

Nicole L. Beattie, M.S., is a Research Assistant at the Roudebush VA Medical Center. Over the past seven years, she has been involved in the coordination of various studies, including metacognition, personal narrative, stigma and recovery in schizophrenia.

Charland, Louis

Louis C. Charland, Ph.D., is Professor in the Departments of Philosophy and Psychiatry at The University of Western Ontario in London, Ontario, Canada. He is the author of several articles on the history of moral treatment in psychiatry, and also co-translator, with Gordon Hickish and David Healy, of the first English translation of Philippe Pinel's Medico-Philosophical Treatise on Mental Alienation (Wiley-Blackwell, 2008). He has also published widely on the philosophy of psychiatry and the philosophy of emotion.

Coatsworth-Puspoky, Robin

Robin Coatsworth-Puspoky, M.Sc.N., is a Professor at Lambton College. She teaches in first year of the Practical Nursing Program. Robin's clinical area of expertise is geriatric mental health. She has held positions with the Regional Psychogeriatric Program and Regional Mental Health Care as a Clinical Nurse Specialist in Geriatric Psychiatry; and as a research assistant with the research project titled "Therapeutic Relationships: from hospital to community." She holds undergraduate degrees in sociology and nursing from The University of Western Ontario. She received her Master of Science in Nursing degree from The University of Western Ontario in 2001 with a specialty in nursing education. Her thesis research focused on exploring and comparing peer and nursing support relationships in mental health from the perspective of the persons receiving support. Her research interests include nurse-client relationships, geriatric mental health, knowledge translation and transcultural nursing.

Corrigan, Patrick

Patrick Corrigan, Psy.D., is an Associate Dean for Research at the Institute of Psychology, Illinois Institute of Technology in Chicago. For the past 25 years, he has worked to provide and research services for people with psychiatric disabilities.

About 15 years ago, his focus broadened to the stigma of mental illness. He has had support from the National Institute of Mental Health to develop and maintain the Chicago Consortium for Stigma Research for the past decade as its principal investigator. The Chicago Consortium for Stigma Research is a collection of more than a dozen researchers and advocates from academic and consumer groups in Northern Illinois. He has authored more than 250 papers and 10 books. He is also editor-in-chief for the American Journal of Psychiatric Rehabilitation.

Corring, Deborah

Deborah Corring, Ph.D., has worked in the mental health care field since 1972 as a clinician, an administrator and as a researcher. She has taught at the college and university level in both Canada and Australia and currently holds appointments at both the Department of Psychiatry and School of Occupational Therapy at The University of Western Ontario. She is also the Director of the Psychosis Program, Regional Mental Health Care London/St. Thomas, St. Joseph's Health Care London, Ontario, Canada.

Cross, Lara

Lara Elizabeth Cross, Ph.D. (c), is a doctoral student in counseling psychology at the University of Alberta and a Canadian Certified Counselor with the Canadian Counseling and Psychotherapy Association. She completed her master's studies in counseling psychology at the University of New Brunswick and her Honours Bachelor of Science in psychology at The University of Western Ontario, the latter with thesis supervision from Dr. Abraham Rudnick. Lara's undergraduate thesis focused on coping strategies of people with schizophrenia and cancer, whereas her master's thesis focused on positive psychology approaches concerning incarcerated youth with serious mental illness, which was supported by an internal university scholarship. Lara has served as a graduate student representative on the Canadian Psychological Association (CPA) committee for counseling psychology criteria for accreditation of pre- and post-doctoral internships, and she is currently the student representative for the counseling psychology section of the CPA. Lara completed her master's practicum at the University of New Brunswick's Counseling Services and regularly utilized a person-centered care approach when providing psychological care to university students.

Davidson, Larry

Larry Davidson, Ph.D., is a Professor of psychiatry and Director of the Program for Recovery and Community Health at the School of Medicine and Institution for Social and Policy Studies of Yale University. His work has focused on processes of recovery in serious mental illnesses and addictions, recovery as an integrating bridge between mental health and addiction and the treatment of individuals with co-occurring disorders, the effectiveness of peer-delivered services, and the development and evaluation of innovative recovery-oriented practices, as well as the facilitation of system transformation to the provision of recovery-oriented care.

Author of over 200 publications, he has recently published with colleagues a book titled *A Practical Guide to Recovery-Oriented Practice: tools for transforming mental health care*, and another book titled *The Roots of the Recovery Movement in Psychiatry: lessons learned*. His work has been influential both nationally and internationally in shaping the recovery agenda and in translating its implications for transforming mental health practice.

Desjardins, Nina

Nina Desjardins, M.D., was born in Saskatchewan. Her father was Cree, hailing from Muskeg Lake First Nation in Saskatchewan. After completing high school she was selected for the Page Programme in the House of Commons and studied Political Science at the University of Ottawa. She obtained her B.Sc. (Honors Biochemistry) from the University of Saskatchewan, her M.D. from the University of Alberta and completed her psychiatric residency at The University of Western Ontario. While at the University of Alberta she was a participant in the Aboriginal Health Careers Program, and her involvement in Aboriginal Mental Health continues to this day. She was recently a consultant psychiatrist to the London Assertive Community Treatment team and an Assistant Professor in the Department of Psychiatry at the Schulich School of Medicine and Dentistry at The University of Western Ontario.

Drake, Robert

Robert E. Drake, M.D., Ph.D., is the Andrew Thomson Professor of Psychiatry and Community and Family Medicine at Dartmouth Medical School and the Director of the Dartmouth Psychiatric Research Center. He was educated at Princeton, Duke, and Harvard Universities. At Dartmouth for over 25 years, he is currently Vice Chair and Director of Research in the Department of Psychiatry. He works as a community mental health physician and researcher. His research focuses on co-occurring disorders, vocational rehabilitation, health services research, and evidence-based practices. He has authored or co-authored 20 books and over 400 papers.

Fisman, Sandra

Sandra Fisman, M.D., is Professor and Chair of the Department of Psychiatry at the Schulich School of Medicine and Dentistry, The University of Western Ontario. Clinically she is a practicing child and adolescent psychiatrist and physician leader for a Tertiary Care Adolescent Program. Her research interests have included the impact of handicapped children on parents and siblings, epidemiology of eating disorders and preventive interventions in young adolescent women.

Forchuk, Cheryl

Cheryl Forchuk, Ph.D., is a Professor in the Labatt Family School of Nursing at The University of Western Ontario and a Professor in the Department of Psychiatry, Schulich School of Medicine and Dentistry. She is also an Assistant Director for the Lawson Health Research Institute, the research arm of the London hospitals. She received her Bachelor of Science in Nursing and her Bachelor of Arts degree in psychology from the University of Windsor. She attained her Master of Science in Nursing from the University of Toronto with a clinical specialty in mental health, and her Ph.D. is from the College of Nursing at Wayne State. Dr. Forchuk has published on many topics including housing, transitional discharge, therapeutic relationships, denial and sexuality. She has published a book through Sage on Hildegard Peplau's interpersonal theory of nursing. Currently, her research explores barriers and strategies for implementing best practices, the therapeutic aspects of the nurse-client relationship, inter-professional education, housing issues, and the transition from hospital to community. She is also a co-editor on a book titled *Homelessness, Housing and the Experiences of Mental Health Consumer-Survivors: finding truths creating change,* which is published by the Canadian Scholars Press.

Gill, Kenneth

Kenneth J. Gill, Ph.D., C.P.R.P., is Chair and Professor in the Department of Psychiatric Rehabilitation and Counseling Professions at the University of Medicine and Dentistry of New Jersey (School of Health-Related Professions). The first department of its nature in the country, it offers associate, bachelor's, master's and doctoral degrees in psychiatric rehabilitation as well as post-doctoral studies in psychiatric rehabilitation and a master's degree in rehabilitation counseling. He was one of the founders of the Certification Commission on Psychiatric Rehabilitation. Before coming to the University of Medicine and Dentistry of New Jersey in 1992, he worked for eight years in community mental health settings. A graduate of Columbia University (B.A., M.Phil., Ph.D.) and Marquette University (M.S.), his doctoral degree is in measurement, evaluation, and statistics. He is a co-author of the text *Psychiatric Rehabilitation,* an integrated introduction for the field, published in its 2nd edition by Elsevier in 2007. He is co-editor-in-chief of the *Psychiatric Rehabilitation Journal* and associate editor of the *American Journal of Psychiatric Rehabilitation.* He has been the recipient of a number of awards, including the United States Psychiatric Rehabilitation Association's John Beard and New Jersey's Mort Gati awards, both for career achievement in applying psychiatric rehabilitation principles. He serves on a number of governing and advisory boards of community mental health, professional organizations and housing services.

Gingerich, Susan

Susan Gingerich, M.S.W., is an independent trainer and consultant based in Philadelphia, Pennsylvania. She is the co-author of *Coping with Schizophrenia: a guide for families* (1994), *Social Skills Training for Schizophrenia: a step-by-step guide, second edition* (2004), *The Coping Skills Group: a session-by-session guide* (2005), and *The Complete Family Guide to Schizophrenia: helping your loved one get the most out of life* (2006), which received the 2007 Ken Book Award from the New York Metro Chapter of the National Alliance on Mental Illness. She also co-authored four chapters in William McFarlane's book, *Multifamily Groups in the Treatment of Severe Psychiatric Disorders.* She and Kim Mueser are the co-authors of *Illness Management and Recovery* (sometimes referred to as *Wellness Management and Recovery*), a program that helps individuals identify personally meaningful goals and learn strategies and skills that will help them achieve those goals.

Goldberg, Joel

Joel O. Goldberg, Ph.D., is Associate Professor and Director of Clinical Training at York University, Department of Psychology, York University and Associate Professor (part-time) for the Department of Psychiatry and Behavioural Neurosciences, McMaster University. For almost two decades, he was the Clinical Director of the Hamilton Program for Schizophrenia, a community-based psychiatric rehabilitation service. He was a co-author on the Canadian Psychiatric Association Working Group that developed the Clinical Practice Guidelines for Schizophrenia (both in 1998 and 2005). His research interests include: cognitive assessment, therapy and rehabilitation in schizophrenia and smoking cessation for people with serious mental illness.

Gritke, Jennifer

Jennifer Gritke, M.A., completed her Master of Arts degree in social anthropology from Dalhousie University and her Bachelor of Arts (Honours) from McMaster University. Her primary fields of interest include the health of marginalized populations, critical analysis of public health, and harm reduction. Her graduate thesis explored the media coverage on the debate over clean needle exchange programs in federal prisons in Canada. Currently, she is a research coordinator in London, Ontario.

Haslam, David

David Haslam, M.D., established the Mental Health Consultation and Evaluation in Primary-Care and Transition into Primary-Care Psychiatry collaborative (shared) care programs at Regional Mental Health Care London, Ontario. He is Assistant Professor at the Department of Psychiatry, Schulich School of Medicine and Dentistry, The University of Western Ontario. He is past Director of Postgraduate Education and continues to be active in teaching and training residents. He also holds a cross appointment with the Departments of Family Medicine and Epidemiology & Biostatistics. His area of publication and research focus is in collaborative mental health services and the study of translation of best evidence into practice. He has successfully collaborated on several projects and received funding from local, provincial and national envelopes. He is a sentinel reader for an online rating of evidence system and a peer reviewer for an online international journal of integrated care.

Hill, Bill

Bill Hill, M.S.W., is a social worker at Regional Mental Health Care London. He began working in the Mental Health field in nursing in 1982. Bill is a Haudenosaunee, or part of the "People of the Longhouse". He returned to school to complete a Social Service Worker diploma and continued on to the achievement of a bachelor's and then master's degrees in Social Work, along with a B.Ed., all First Nations specific. Since 1999, Bill has participated in curriculum development and teaching of the program: "Traditional Aboriginal Healing Methods - Native Community Worker" at the Anishinabek Education Institute. Bill strives to facilitate progressive communication and continuing education in his effort to bridge the gaps between traditional aboriginal health practices and standard medical care.

Karnieli-Miller, Orit

Orit Karnieli-Miller, PH.D., is an Assistant Professor in the Department of Community Mental Health and a fellow in the Concentration for Excellence in Patient-Professional Relationship in Health Care in University of Haifa, Israel. She recently finished a post-doctoral fellowship at the Indiana University School of Medicine and Regenstrief Institute for Health Care in Indianapolis. She earned her doctorate in social work at the University of Haifa, Israel. Her special emphases in teaching and research include qualitative research, health care provider-patient-caregiver communication, handling difficult conversations (breaking bad news), workers' professionalism, mental illness prevention and mental health promotion. She is a co-principle investigator on an Israeli Science Foundation grant focusing on diagnosis disclosure regarding Alzheimer Disease.

Keene, Melissa

Melissa Keene, M.D., is a Chicago native currently enrolled at Northwestern University Feinberg School of Medicine. She completed her Bachelor of Science degree in biology at the University of Wisconsin-Madison. She had the distinct pleasure of working with Prof. David Roe while studying and volunteering in Haifa, Israel. She has a particular interest in women's health and the unique psychosocial barriers women must overcome. She completed her medical doctorate degree in May 2010. In addition to her academic future, she hopes to volunteer in international settings throughout her career.

Lamoure, Joel

Joel Lamoure, B.Sc.PHM., is a mental health pharmacist at London Health Sciences Centre, Victoria Hospital. He also serves as an Assistant Professor and Assistant Director of Continuing Medical Education in the Department of Psychiatry at the Schulich School of Medicine and Dentistry, University of Western Ontario and Teaching Associate, Faculty of Pharmacy, University of Toronto. He recently became an accreditor with Accreditations Canada, specializing in medication management, infection control and mental health. He has won the Western Teaching Roll of Honour in Medicine, The University of Western Ontario Continuing Medical Education Award in Medicine and the University Of Toronto Teaching Award. He has published over 40 journal papers and consultant reviews on mental health medications and their impact on the patient. He writes as a psychopharmacotherapy expert for several national and international publications. He was awarded a fellowship in the American Society of Consultant Pharmacists (Geriatrics). His areas of interest and research include: medical conditions that overlap and augment the severity of psychiatric disorders and impacts of alternative treatments and psychopharmacology. He is an inductee in the Canadian Book of Who's Who and the International Book of Who's Who in Medicine.

Langford, Jane

Jane Langford, RN, has been employed with Regional Mental Health Care, London. Her education was obtained at Fanshawe College and King's University College in London, Ontario, as well as through various courses, workshops and projects. She obtained Certification in Psychiatric/Mental Health Nursing and has worked in a variety of nursing roles within the organization, including staff nurse and charge nurse in acute and tertiary in-patient care, and tertiary level out-patient care. She has been involved with the Collaborative/Shared Care Program, in both the Transition into Primary-Care Psychiatry and the Mental Health Consultation and Evaluation in Primary-Care capacities.

Lysaker, Paul

Paul H. Lysaker, PH.D., is a clinical psychologist at the Roudebush Virginia Medical Center and a Professor of clinical psychology in the Department of Psychiatry at the Indiana University School of Medicine. He has been involved in the practice of psychotherapy for adults with severe mental illness for over 20 years. His active research activities include ongoing studies of the links between metacognition, personal narrative and stigma with recovery based outcomes in schizophrenia.

Mazmanian, Dwight

Dwight Mazmanian, PH.D., completed his undergraduate degree at St. Mary's University and his M.A. and Ph.D. degrees (clinical psychology) at The University of Western Ontario. Much of his clinical training and subsequent clinical experience was obtained in facilities providing services to persons with serious mental illnesses. He is currently an Associate Professor of psychology at Lakehead University, Ontario, and a consultant psychologist at the Behavioural Sciences Centre of St. Joseph's Care Group. He teaches graduate courses on mood disorders, psychological assessment, and clinical psychopharmacology. His research interests include mood disorders, psychological assessment and the biological bases of affect, mood and social behavior.

McAuley, Lisa

Lisa McAuley, RN, graduated from the Mohawk College of Applied Arts and Technology. She has worked with the Regional Mental Health Care in London, Ontario, following two years of service in acute psychiatric care at Kitchener Waterloo General Hospital. Her experience as an inpatient staff charge nurse supported the change to outpatient case management clinician. She acquired Psychiatric/Mental Health Certification via the Canadian Nurses Association. She joined the Transition into

Primary-Care Psychiatry Research Project and continues her clinical work with clients in collaborative care with family physicians.

McCay, Elizabeth

Elizabeth McCay, RN, Ph.D., is Associate Director-Scholarly, Research and Creative Activities in the Daphne Cockwell School of Nursing at Ryerson University. Her research focuses on the study of vulnerable youth and mental illness, negative psychological consequences of illness on self-concept, and the development and evaluation of group interventions to promote healthy self-concepts and resilience. She has held a number of research grants as a principle investigator from national funding agencies related to mental health needs, emotional regulation and resilience in street-involved youth, self-concept and engulfment in first-episode schizophrenia, as well as the development and evaluation of interventions to promote healthy self-concepts and resilience. She is also Co-Director of the Centre for Health in At-Risk Populations at Ryerson University, whose aim is to identify and address clinical research questions related to promoting health in vulnerable individuals, families and communities. Her teaching interests include conceptualizations of health and illness across a broad range of clinical and vulnerable populations.

Mejia, Jose

Born in Mexico City, Jose Mejia, M.D., Ph.D., pursued his training as an M.D. (psychiatry) and received his M.Sc. in neuropsychology. He subsequently worked as an attending psychiatrist in the first super-maximum secure prison in Mexico. He immigrated to Canada to pursue a Ph.D. in human genetics, focusing on the study of the genetic basis of criminal and violent behaviors. He then took a fellowship in forensic psychiatry at Queen's University, Kingston Psychiatric Hospital and Kingston Penitentiary. Since then, he has been devoted to clinical practice, education and research in forensic psychiatry and genetics. He has also taken graduate studies in mental health law and management.

Mueser, Kim

Kim T. Mueser, Ph.D., is a clinical psychologist and a Professor in the Departments of Psychiatry and of Community and Family Medicine at the Dartmouth Medical School in Hanover, New Hampshire. His clinical and research interests include family psychoeducation, the treatment of co-occurring psychiatric and substance use disorders, psychiatric rehabilitation for serious mental illnesses, and the treatment of post-traumatic stress disorder. He has published extensively and given numerous lectures and workshops on psychiatric rehabilitation. His research has been supported by the National Institute of Mental Health, the National Institute on Drug Abuse, the Substance Abuse and Mental Health Administration, and the National Alliance for Research on Schizophrenia and Depression. He is the co-author of one text on family psychoeducation, *Behavioral Family Therapy for Psychiatric Disorders* (1999) and three books for families about mental illness: *Coping with Schizophrenia: a guide for families* (1994), *The Complete Family Guide to Schizophrenia* (2006), and

The Family Intervention Guide to Mental Illness (2007). Dr. Mueser is also the co-author of several other books, including: *Social Skills Training for Psychiatric Patients* (1989), *Integrated Treatment for Dual Disorders: a guide to effective practice* (2003), *Social Skills Training for Schizophrenia* (2004), *The Coping Skills Book: a session-by-session guide* (2005), *The Principles and Practice of Psychiatric Rehabilitation* (2008), and *Treatment of Posttraumatic Stress Disorder in Special Populations: a cognitive restructuring program* (2009). He can be reached at the Dartmouth Psychiatric Research Center, Main Building, 105 Pleasant St., Concord, NH, 03301; email: kim.t.mueser@dartmouth.edu.

Pratt, Carlos

Carlos W. Pratt, Ph.D., C.P.R.P., is a Professor and Director of the Ph.D. program in Psychiatric Rehabilitation, the Department of Psychiatric Rehabilitation and Counseling Professions in the School of Health Related Professions, University of Medicine and Dentistry of New Jersey. The Ph.D. program is the first to specifically offer the doctoral degree in psychiatric rehabilitation. He is the past President of the New Jersey Psychiatric Rehabilitation Association, a board member of Collaborative Support Programs of New Jersey, a state-wide consumer operated agency, and Vice President of the Board of Directors of Project Live Incorporated, Newark, NJ. He is first author of Psychiatric Rehabilitation (1999, 2006 Academic Press), the first comprehensive textbook on the subject. In addition to numerous conference presentations, he has authored articles in *American Journal of Psychiatric Rehabilitation*, *Psychiatric Rehabilitation Journal*, *Community Mental Health Journal*, *Psychiatric Rehabilitation Skills* and *Rehabilitation Education*.

O'Connell, Maria

Maria O'Connell, Ph.D., is an Assistant Professor in the Department of Psychiatry at the Yale University School of Medicine and Director of Research and Evaluation at the Yale Program for Recovery and Community Health. Her professional interests include program evaluation and design; conducting research on recovery-oriented topics including psychiatric advance directives, self-determination, recovery-oriented services, housing and other community-based programs; and providing consultation to programs on using evaluation tools to assess system and agency-level recovery indicators and translating the knowledge into changes in practice.

O'Reilly, Richard

Richard O'Reilly, M.D., is a psychiatrist who works in an Assertive Community Treatment team. He is a Professor of psychiatry at The University of Western Ontario and a Professor of mental health at the Northern Ontario School of Medicine. He is a member of the Schizophrenia Society of Ontario and works closely with a number of patient and family groups.

Rao, Jay

Jay Rao, M.D., is a specialist in developmental neuropsychiatry, having trained at the National Institute of Mental Health and Neuroscience in India. Subsequently he trained and worked as a senior clinical teacher and consultant in developmental disabilities at the University of Wales, UK. Currently he is an Associate Professor in the Department of Psychiatry, The University of Western Ontario. He consults widely, nationally and internationally. He has published research internationally and has won national awards for his work with the developmentally disabled and for his teaching. His current focus of research is in executive dysfunction and in developing multi-factor assessment tools. He is a member of the Royal College of Psychiatrists, UK, and a fellow of the College of Physicians and Surgeons of Canada.

Robilotta, Stephanie

Stephanie A. Robilotta, Ph.D. (c), is a doctoral candidate in the clinical-forensic psychology Ph.D. program at John Jay College of Criminal Justice, City University of New York. She received her Master's and Bachelor of Arts in forensic psychology at John Jay College of Criminal Justice. She has worked with children, adolescents and adults suffering from serious mental illness, particularly focusing on symptom and medication management, social functioning and housing options. Additionally, she has contributed to areas of research pertaining to the effects of coping strategies on psychological stability and recovery, and the development of therapeutic interventions that may enhance the community integration of adults with serious mental illness. Her primary areas of interest include housing conditions and services targeted towards the education of active coping styles and symptom management, and the impact these interventions may have on recovery.

Salyers, Michelle

Michelle P. Salyers, Ph.D., is co-director of the Assertive Community Treatment Center and Associate research Professor, Department of Psychology, Indiana University Purdue University Indianapolis. She is acting co-director of the Veterans Affairs Health Services Research and Development Center on Implementing Evidence-Based Practice, Roudebush Veterans Affairs Medical Center and a research scientist at Regenstrief Institute, Inc. She earned her doctorate in clinical rehabilitation psychology at Indiana University Purdue University Indianapolis. She completed her clinical internship at Dartmouth Medical School and was a National Association of State Mental Health Program Directors Research Institute post-doctoral fellow at the New Hampshire-Dartmouth Psychiatric Research Center. She is a mental health services researcher in the field of psychiatric rehabilitation, primarily focusing on implementing evidence-based practices. She has undertaken several federally funded research and implementation projects focusing on Assertive Community Treatment and illness management and recovery.

Sanghera, Parmjit

Parmjit Sanghera, Ph.D., is a clinical psychologist and currently holds a position at William Osler Health Centre in the mood and anxiety, psychosis and assessment units. She is also a consultant with Toronto Western Hospital, University Health Network, working in the area of chronic pain. Additionally, she works in private practice.

Sharma, Verinder

Verinder Sharma, M.D, is a medical graduate of Punjabi University, India, and completed his residency training in psychiatry at the University of Saskatchewan, Saskatoon. Currently, he is a psychiatrist with the mood and anxiety disorders program at the Regional Mental Health Care, London. He is also a Professor of psychiatry and has a cross-appointment to the Department of Obstetrics and Gynecology at The University of Western Ontario, London, Ontario. His clinical research interests include bipolar disorder, the effect of reproductive events on psychopathology, psychopharmacology and suicide.

Strasburger, Amy

Amy M. Strasburger, M.A., is a research program specialist at the Roudebush Veterans Affairs Medical Center. She has been involved in research and mental health therapy for adults with serious mental illness for over five years. Her active research activities include ongoing studies of the links between cognitive behavior therapy, mindfulness, metacognition, personal narrative and stigma with recovery based outcomes in schizophrenia.

Subramanian, Priya

Priya Subramanian, M.D., C.P.R.P., is a psychiatrist and Assistant Professor at The University of Western Ontario (Western), providing services at Regional Mental Health Care, a tertiary mental health center in London, Ontario. She obtained her undergraduate medical degree from Annamalai University, India, and completed her residency training in psychiatry in Bristol and Stoke-on-Trent, UK. She subsequently completed a clinical and research fellowship in psychiatric rehabilitation at Western. Throughout her training, Dr. Subramanian has been mentored by psychiatrists with excellent clinical skills and person-oriented approaches to mental health care. During her undergraduate training, she was a recipient of many prizes including some for sports and creative writing, and received the university's Silver Medal in Community Medicine. During her postgraduate training, she served as a resident representative and received prizes for research and service evaluation projects. She received a Trainee Award from the Department of Psychiatry, Western, in recognition of her work during her fellowship. Dr. Subramanian's clinical interest is the treatment and rehabilitation of individuals with severe psychiatric disabilities. Her research interests are in the areas of transcranial magnetic stimulation and psychiatric rehabilitation.

Swarbrick, Margaret

Margaret (Peggy) Swarbrick, Ph.D., O.T.R., C.P.R.P., is an Assistant Clinical Professor in the Department of Psychiatric Rehabilitation and Counseling Professions, University of Medicine and Dentistry of New Jersey and also the Director of the Institute for Wellness and Recovery Initiatives, Collaborative Support Programs of New Jersey (a large, statewide agency run by persons living with mental illness in collaboration with professionals). Her early personal life challenges and experiences in the mental health system led to a career focused on promoting wellness within the mental health system. She earned a doctorate in occupational therapy from New York University, and her dissertation research examined the relationship between social environment and member empowerment and satisfaction in peer-operated self-help centers. She completed a postdoctoral fellowship in advanced training and research at the National Institute on Disability and Rehabilitation Research (H133P050006), Department of Psychiatric Rehabilitation and Counseling Professions.

Takhar, Jatinder

Jatinder Takhar, M.D., is clinical team leader in collaborative (shared) care (transition into primary-care psychiatry/mental health consultation and evaluation in primary-care) at Regional Mental Health Care, London, Ontario, and Professor, Department of Psychiatry, Schulich School of Medicine and Dentistry, The University of Western Ontario. Her area of publication and interest include collaborative care model implementation, evaluation in collaborative care, early intervention and relapse prevention in individuals with serious mental illness. Other interests include how educational interventions can be designed, integrated and evaluated in conjunction with service delivery in collaborative care models for serious mental illness. She is active in teaching and training residents, medical students, other allied health care professionals and international medical graduates. She has taught undergraduate medical students within the context of the person-centered learning curriculum and has been involved in reviewing submissions to major psychiatric journals. She served as a continuing medical education director for four years with the Department of Psychiatry prior to assuming the role of Associate Dean in Continuing Medical Education at The University of Western Ontario.

Tondora, Janis

Janis Tondora, Psy.D., is an Assistant Clinical Professor in the Department of Psychiatry at the Yale University School of Medicine. Based at the Program for Recovery and Community Health, her professional interests focus on the design, implementation and evaluation of services that promote self-determination, recovery and community inclusion among individuals diagnosed with serious behavioral health disorders. She works closely with the Connecticut Department of Mental Health and Addiction Services and has coordinated a number of statewide training and consultation initiatives designed to promote the transfer of academic research into the public-sector behavioral health system. In recognition of her work, she has been invited to provide training and consultation to numerous states seeking to develop person-centered planning models and has been active as a steering committee member of the Substance Abuse and Mental Health Services Administration National Consensus-Building Initiative on person-centered care. She has shared her work with the field in numerous publications, including a recent book co-authored with several colleagues titled *A Practical Guide to Recovery-Oriented Practice: tools for transforming mental health care*.

Toto, Anna Marie

Anna Marie Toto, M.Ed., is a program coordinator at the University of Medicine and Dentistry of New Jersey, University Behavioral Healthcare. She has an extensive background in training, program development, curriculum design and in the implementation of education and community-based support/service models. Her clinical experience has included working with adolescents and adults with psychiatric, primary addiction and co-occurring disorders; family systems work, where she developed a passion and expertise in facilitating multi-family groups; substance abuse prevention; and wellness education programming. In addition, she has organized, led and consulted on statewide and national recovery and wellness initiatives, such as New Jersey's implementation of illness management and recovery and the National Partners for Excellence in Psychiatry: Neuroscience Treatment Team Partner Program, where she also co-authored "Solutions for Wellness" (2008) and other related journal articles. She has a compassion and steadfast commitment to the mental health community and to collaborative partnerships that help reduce stigma and raise the standard of awareness, service and care.

Vandevooren, Janice

Janice Vandevooren, M.Sc., completed her undergraduate degree in occupational therapy at The University of Western Ontario in 1985. She has since worked with individuals having serious and persistent mental illness in both hospital and community settings and has held various leadership roles within St. Joseph's Health Care, London. In 1999 she returned to The Western to complete a Master of Science degree. As a part-time Professor at The University of Western Ontario, she taught psychosocial rehabilitation for several years before taking on the position of Director of Forensic Psychiatry at Regional Mental Health Care, St. Thomas. She is a member of the Canadian College of Health Service Executives.

Verna, Marie

Marie D. Verna, B.A., works as a program support coordinator at University Behavioral Healthcare, New Jersey, where she supports the organization's efforts to include peer counselors in all programming and works to increase the consumer and family voice. When she first joined the organization, she worked for the Center for Excellence in Psychiatry as a senior training and consultation specialist, where she helped deliver the Neuroscience Treatment Team Partner Program wellness curriculum and provided consultation to organizations nationwide who were working on improving their wellness services. She was diagnosed with bipolar disorder and has devoted her professional career to improving the lives of people with mental illness through education and advocacy.

Vreeland, Betty

Betty Vreeland, M.Sc.N., A.P.R.N., is an advanced practice registered nurse at the University of Medicine and Dentistry of New Jersey, University Behavioral Health Care. She is also a Clinical Assistant Professor at the University of Medicine and Dentistry of New Jersey School of Nursing and in the university's Department of Psychiatry. She holds dual national board certification in psychiatric/mental health advanced practice nursing and adult health nursing. She has over 25 years of experience working in a variety of behavioral health and primary-care settings and is passionate about improving the health and well-being of people living with serious mental illness. She is an active researcher. Her areas of interest include psychoeducational interventions, integrating physical health into behavioral health care, wellness and healthy lifestyle choices. She has published over a dozen articles and book chapters in this specialty area as well as provided training to hundreds of behavioral health care organizations about how to bridge the gap between mental and physical health. She is also the co-author of two manualized wellness programs that were designed to inspire and assist people with serious mental illnesses to choose and live healthier lives.

Wilkniss, Sandra

Sandra Wilkniss, Ph.D., is Director of the Thresholds Institute, the research and training arm of Thresholds Psychiatric Rehabilitation Centers, and Adjunct Assistant Professor of Community and Family Medicine, Dartmouth Medical College. She has practiced and studied interventions for people with psychiatric disabilities; in services research in a community outreach context at Thresholds. She is a member of the Task Force on Serious Mental Illness with the American Psychological Association.

Williams, Jill

Jill Williams, M.D., is a Board-Certified addictions psychiatrist specializing in the treatment of tobacco and other addictions in mentally ill populations. She is an Associate Professor and Director of the Division of Addiction Psychiatry at the University of Medicine and Dentistry of New Jersey, Robert Wood Johnson Medical School, in the Department of Psychiatry. She also holds faculty appointments with the University of Medicine and Dentistry of New Jersey, School of Public Health Tobacco Dependence Program in New Brunswick and the Cancer Institute of New Jersey. She conducts research on smokers with serious mental illness including schizophrenia and bipolar disorder and was the recipient of a National Institute on Drug Abuse Mentored Patient-Oriented Research Career Development Award. Her research examines differences in nicotine intake, cigarette puffing and nicotine craving in individuals with schizophrenia hoping that that these discoveries will lead to better treatments in the future. She has received research funding from the National Institute on Drug Abuse, the National Institute of Mental Health, State of New Jersey, and the American Legacy Foundation. She lectures extensively on changing mental systems to incorporate tobacco dependence treatment and works with consumers to increase their knowledge about tobacco illness and the hope of treatment. She has participated in several important national and state initiatives related to tobacco and mental health and is the author of numerous peer-reviewed research papers. She is the co-founder and Medical Director of CHOICES, a consumer-driven initiative that provides outreach to smokers with mental illness in the community via mental health peer counselors (*see* www.njchoices.org). She also serves on the State of New Jersey Health Information Technology Commission Board.

Yanos, Philip

Philip T. Yanos, Ph.D., is an Associate Professor in psychology at the John Jay College of Criminal Justice, City University of New York. He received a doctorate in clinical psychology from St. John's University and completed a post-doctoral fellowship in mental health services research at Rutgers University's Institute for Health. Prior to coming to John Jay, he was a faculty member in the Department of Psychiatry of University of Medicine and Dentistry of New Jersey, New Jersey Medical School. He is committed to studying issues related to the recovery and successful community integration of persons with serious mental illness, to further the development of systems and interventions that can maximize opportunities for recovery. His specific areas of interest include the impact of active coping and other psychological variables on social functioning, the impact of housing on community integration and the impact of internalized stigma on recovery.

Acknowledgments

This book could not have been written without the extensive collaboration of all those involved. We thank all the authors who persevered with us and the research staff who assisted us, particularly Laura Wood, Jennifer Gritke, Shannon Rider, Ian Gallant, Sylvia Tessler-Lozowick and Shani Bril Barniv, the book series editors Moira Stewart, Judith Brown and Tom Freeman as well as their administrative staff, Andrea Burt, and the staff at Radcliffe – Michael Hawkes, Gillian Nineham and Jamie Etherington. We thank our families, friends and colleagues for their support. Last but most important, we thank all people with serious mental illness who have inspired us to propose and produce this book, and we hope that it will facilitate their person-centered care.

List of Abbreviations

AA	Alcoholics Anonymous
ACCESS	Access to Community Care and Effective Services and Support
ACT	Assertive Community Treatment
ADHD	attention-deficit hyperactivity disorder
APA	American Psychiatric Association
AMHS	Area Mental Health Services
BDI	Beck Depression Inventory
BMI	body mass index
CanMEDS	Canadian Medical Education Directives for Specialists
CBPR	community-based participatory research
CBT	cognitive behavioral therapy
CCMHI	Canadian Collaborative Mental Health Initiative
CLIPP	Consultation-Liaison in Primary-Care Psychiatry
CMHS	Center for Mental Health Services
COSP	Consumer Operated Service Program
CPA	Canadian Psychological Association
CPRP	certified psychiatric rehabilitation practitioner
DBSA	Depression and Bipolar Support Alliance
DSM	Diagnostic and Statistical Manual of Mental Disorders
DUC	drug use control
EBP	evidence-based practice
ECT	electroconvulsive therapy
EE	expressed emotion
FGA	first-generation antipsychotic
GAF	Global Assessment of Functioning

ICD	International Statistical Classification of Diseases and Related Health Problems
IMR	illness management and recovery
IPS	Individual Placement and Support
NAMI	National Alliance on Mental Illness
NASMHPD	National Association of State Mental Health Program Director
NCR	not criminally responsible
NEAR	Neuropsychological Educational Approach to Remediation
NIDA	National Institute on Drug Abuse
NIMH	National Institute of Mental Health
ORB	Ontario Review Board
PANSS	positive and negative syndrome scale
PAR	Participatory Action Research
PCA	person-centered assessment
PCC	person-centered care
PCCM	patient-centered clinical method
PSR	psychiatric/psychosocial rehabilitation
QI	quality improvement
rTMS	repetitive Transcranial Magnetic Stimulation
SAMHSA	Substance Abuse and Mental Health Services Administration
SCID	Structured Clinical Interview for DSM Disorders
SCL-90-R	Symptom CheckList-90-Revised
SDM	shared decision making
SE	Supported Employment
SFW	Solutions for Wellness
SGA	second-generation antipsychotic
SMI	serious mental illness
SMR	standardized mortality ratio
STAND	Scale to Assess Narrative Development
SSI	Supplementary Security Income
SUD	substance use disorder
TAG	Threshold Assessment Grid
TIA	transient ischemic attack
TIPP	Transition into Primary-Care Psychiatry Program

TMS   Transcranial Magnetic Stimulation
VNS   vagus nerve stimulation
WAIS   Wechsler Adult Intelligence Scale
WHO   World Health Organization
WRAP   Wellness Recovery Action Plan

Introduction: background and overview

Abraham Rudnick and David Roe

In the last half century there has been much progress in classifying and treating serious mental illness (SMI) such as schizophrenia and bipolar disorder, yet it is still not known how to cure or to prevent them. The disruptive impact of the signs and symptoms of the illness on the afflicted person's well-being and independent functioning, along with the troublesome impact of these impairments on the way the person with SMI is treated by others and experiences himself or herself, often leave people with SMI considerably disadvantaged. Specifically, they often suffer from poverty, are subject to stigma and discrimination, and are left with few social or recreational outlets and opportunities to acquire valued social roles within their community.

Despite these considerable barriers, the growing emphasis on psychiatric (also termed psychosocial) rehabilitation (PSR), and more recently on recovery, has engendered new hope. PSR focuses on helping people with SMI develop skills and access appropriate resources and supports that can facilitate their ability to articulate and pursue their personal goals. Recovery-oriented services, which include PSR as well as other types of service, aim at seeking, achieving and maintaining valued social roles and a personally meaningful life despite and beyond the limitations and challenges of the SMI. Recovery differs from cure as it does not require remission of symptoms or alleviation of other impairments.

Key to recovery-oriented services are approaches that put the person at the center of the service, i.e. as the main consideration of the service. Such person-centered approaches are individualized and contextualized to the person's environmental settings. Person-centered approaches are important in order to provide care and support that is respectful to the recipient of care, effective and welcomed by that person. Person-centered approaches in relation to people with SMI face distinct challenges, such as some providers' disbelief in the ability of people with SMI to recover, the tension between disorder-related versus society-focused conceptualizations and the limitations on autonomy of some individuals with SMI.

This book is the first comprehensive text to be published about person-centered approaches to people with SMI. It encompasses a range of theoretical views and empirical findings in relation to various aspects of person-centered care (PCC) and support for people with SMI, such as assessment, treatment, rehabilitation, self-help, policy-making, education and research. As such, this book is expected to serve providers, policymakers, educators, researchers, and – last but not least – people with SMI and their significant others. The book's subtitle highlights persons rather than patients, in order to emphasize a person-first approach rather than a strictly biomedical approach to the provision of health care for people with SMI. Wherever possible, the terms service users and providers are used, rather than more traditional terms such as patients, clients, consumers, clinicians, and professionals. The book follows, to a large extent, the organization of previous books in this book series; where it diverges from that, this is based on a strong rationale, such as adding a chapter on relevant academic activities due to health care becoming more evidence-based of late.

The first chapter of the book addresses the framework of person-centered approaches to people with SMI – conceptually, morally and historically. Section 1.1, *Foundations and Ethics of Person-Centered Approaches to Individuals with Serious Mental Illness*, argues that not all dimensions or aspects of PCC for people with SMI have to be present in order for care to be person-centered, and it outlines ethical principles and ethical challenges of PCC for individuals with SMI. Section 1.2.1, *Moral Treatment in the Eighteenth and Nineteenth Centuries*, presents moral treatment as a form of humane "psychological" therapy for people with mental illness that emerged towards the latter half of the eighteenth century and which enjoyed a golden age until the first quarter of the nineteenth century, when it gradually fell into disrepute as it was forced to abandon its person-centered ideals due to increasingly large, difficult-to-treat populations. Section 1.2.2, *Rogerian and Related Psychotherapies in the Twentieth Century*, argues that PCC has roots within psychological care, dating back to the 1940s to humanistic psychologist Carl Rogers, and that Rogers applied the core concepts of PCC when providing psychological care to a wide variety of service users, including those with SMI.

The second chapter of the book addresses the magnitude of the problem (related to SMI), specifically the two central sets of disorders – major mood disorders and schizophrenia-related disorders – that comprise SMI, narrowly defined. Section 2.1, *Mood Disorders: major depressive disorder and bipolar disorders*, describes the classification, diagnosis, epidemiology, course, outcome, postulated etiology and risk factors related to bipolar disorder and major depressive disorder. Section 2.2, *Schizophrenia-Spectrum Disorders: schizophrenia and schizoaffective disorder*, presents a similar type of description for schizophrenia and schizoaffective disorder.

The third chapter of the book addresses the person's experience of the illness. Section 3.1, *The Lived Experience: narratives through the lens of wellness*, explores the "lived experience" of people with SMI and their narratives. The section encourages providers to better understand how to help persons living with mental illness (service users) to share their lived experience through the lens of wellness. Section 3.2, *The Relationship between the Person with a Serious Mental Illness and His or Her Disorder*, attempts to shed light on the complex relation between the sense of self of persons with SMI and their SMI (or sense of it). The section discusses some of the implications of this relation for PCC.

The fourth chapter of the book addresses the context of the person, referring to family, culture, environment and systems of care. Section 4.1, *Collaborating with Families of People with Serious Mental Illness*, argues that family collaboration plays an important role in maximizing the social support that service users with SMI receive from (and give to) their loved ones. The section presents common elements of effective family collaboration. Section 4.2, *Trans-Cultural Issues in Person-Centered Care for People with Serious Mental Illness*, addresses cross-cultural aspects related to persons with SMI, particularly to aboriginal individuals and communities in Canada. The section argues for cultural safety as well as sensitivity, and demonstrates the need for providers and others to be informed and skilled in relation to cultural issues of individuals from diverse cultural backgrounds. Section 4.3, *Environmental Interventions in Relation to People with Serious Mental Illness*, argues for and illustrates the effects of the environment on persons with SMI, focusing on three environmental areas which are amenable to intervention: housing, public stigma and the financing of services. Interventions related to each of these areas are described and discussed in light of principles of PCC. Section 4.4, *Mental Health Systems and Policy in Relation to People with Serious Mental Illness*, argues that PCC should consider the person in the context of numerous systems and illustrates that the mental health care organization is one such system that can have policies that either support or undermine PCC. The section also addresses policy and law in relation to PCC.

The fifth chapter of the book addresses the person-centered relationship between the person with the SMI and the service provider, as well as special populations. Section 5.1, *Therapeutic Relationships with People with Serious Mental Illness*, argues that PCC is not possible without establishing and maintaining therapeutic relationships, that this is particularly important in mental health settings since persons with SMI may have difficulty establishing trusting relationships. The section argues that consideration of both the service provider and the service user is essential for understanding therapeutic relationships. Section 5.2, *Clinical Communication with Persons who have Serious Mental Illness*, argues that clinical communication has amassed a large body of research, but is just recently being examined in relation to people with SMI. The section argues that given the considerable impact that communication can have on health outcomes, and the centrality of good communication to PCC, there should be a focus on clinical communication with people who have SMI. Section 5.3, *Shared/Collaborative Care for People with Serious Mental Illness*, claims that there are limited data and experience in relation to collaborative or shared (mental and primary) health care for people with SMI and describes some programs that focus on collaboration in mental health care delivery for persons with SMI. The section includes clinical application of the person-centered concept through examples and real-life experiences in delivering services through collaborative care. Section 5.4.1, *Person-Centered Approaches for Adolescents with Serious Mental Illness*, reviews multiple considerations that contribute to the need for a pragmatic approach to successful PCC in relation to adolescents with SMI. These considerations include, among others, the phase of adolescent development. Section 5.4.2, *Dual Diagnosis: an individualized approach*, claims that dual diagnosis (the Canadian term for the common co-occurrence of psychiatric disorders in developmentally disabled individuals) is common in the population of the developmentally disabled, and that diagnosis of mental illness, including SMI, is a challenge in these individuals. The section emphasizes the importance of understanding the individual with dual diagnosis and his or her unique vulnerabilities, so that care can be individualized, resulting in effective PCC for this population. Section 5.4.3, *Serious Mental Illness: person-centered approaches in forensic psychiatry*, focuses on the application of person-centered approaches for individuals with SMI who have come in conflict with the law and, as a result, find themselves being cared for in a forensic mental health care setting. The section argues and illustrates that it is possible to combine the demands of the justice system with PCC for this forensic population. Section 5.4.4, *Treatment of Co-Occurring Substance Use Disorders using Shared Decision-Making and Electronic Decision-Support Systems*, claims that substance use disorders are common for people with SMI, and that many of the adverse outcomes related to SMI, such as relapse, homelessness and incarceration, are strongly associated with substance use disorders. The section briefly considers the "chronic" disease management model and offers guidelines for current mental health services in relation to people with such co-occurring disorders, including use of electronic systems.

The sixth chapter of the book addresses person-centered management (of the SMI) and finding common ground (with the person who has SMI). Section 6.1, *Person-Centered Assessment of People with Serious Mental Illness*, argues for person-centered assessment (PCA) as an important component of PCC, as it is one of the important first steps in the development of a PCC plan, and notes that there is limited systematic information in the literature regarding this important component. The section focuses on how various approaches and procedures can be utilized in a PCA, and challenges providers face when conducting a PCA with persons with SMI. Section 6.2, *Person-Centered Approaches to Psychopharmacology for People with Serious Mental Illness*, addresses psychotropic medications as well as other biological interventions such as electroconvulsive therapy in relation to PCC for people with SMI. The section also addresses adherence to (or concordance with) medications and capacity to consent to or refuse treatment. Section 6.3, *Person-Centered Individual Psychotherapy for Adults with Serious Mental Illness*, explores one way of conceptualizing a person-centered approach to individual psychotherapy for and with persons with SMI. The section focuses on the subjective experience of a diminished sense of self and how to try and improve that experience, and suggests principles and outcome assessment in relation to such a psychotherapy. Section 6.4, *Cognitive and Psychiatric Rehabilitation: person-centered ingredients for success*, illustrates the contribution of PCC-oriented cognitive and PSR interventions to the improvement of functioning and quality of life of people with SMI. The section highlights three key elements that center on the person and that are thought to contribute to success of these interventions: readiness, cognitive remediation and peer support.

The seventh chapter of the book addresses person-centered prevention and health promotion for people with SMI. Section 7.1, *Cultivating Physical Health and Wellness Utilizing a Person-Centered Approach*, argues that there is a large gap between physical and mental health services, which has led to an excess of medical morbidity and mortality among people with SMI. The section points to wellness resources and tools that can improve the physical wellness of people with SMI. Section 7.2, *Self-Help and Peer-Operated Services*, addresses types of self-help groups and peer-operated services deemed person-centered. The section illustrates that there is a growing body of literature illustrating the beneficial aspects of both self-help groups and peer-operated services for people with mental illnesses, including SMI.

The eighth chapter of the book addresses constraints on PCC for people with SMI. Section 8.1, *Some Sober Reflections on Person-Centered Care* argues that although PCC has benefits, treating and caring for individuals who have an SMI is a complex undertaking and it is unlikely that one approach will be the best in all circumstances. The chapter argues for and describes some situations where a person-centered approach to people with SMI may not be appropriate.

The ninth chapter of the book addresses academic activities related to PCC for people with SMI. Section 9.1, *Implications of Serious Mental Illness for Evidence-Based Practices*, addresses evidence-based practice and emerging practices in relation to PCC for SMI, including potential tensions between evidence-based practice and PCC. The section also considers the role of community-based participatory research (CBPR) in further development of evidence-based PCC practices. Section 9.2, *Educating Service Providers and Researchers in Person-Centered Principles Related to Serious Mental Illness*, discusses the education of practitioners and researchers in the competencies necessary to provide PCC to adults with SMI. This discussion is guided by principles of PSR.

The tenth chapter concludes the book. Section 10.1, *Making Sure the Person is Involved in Person-Centered Care* argues that there remains a lack of clarity in relation to what is PCC for individuals with SMI and related matters. The chapter describes a number of overarching principles to guide the development and evaluation of person-centered approaches to care planning and service delivery for people with SMI, and a set of criteria by which to judge the degree to which a care plan for a person with SMI is person-centered.

CHAPTER 1

Framework

This (first) chapter of the book addresses foundational or conceptual, as well as ethical and historical, underpinnings of PCC for people with SMI. Such a framework is helpful in order to try to understand the pertinent driving principles and fundamental challenges, as well as how and from what PCC for people with SMI developed, so that a deep and broad understanding of PCC for people with SMI can emerge. This chapter grounds the latter parts of the book in such an attempted understanding and prepares the way for a discussion of different aspects of PCC for people with SMI in the other chapters of the book. These chapters are structured according to the structure of the Patient-Centered Clinical Method (PCCM), which is the backbone of the book series to which this book belongs. The PCCM is briefly described in Section 1.1, *Foundations and Ethics of Person-Centered Approaches to Individuals with Serious Mental Illness*, as are some other person-centered approaches. As in other sections and chapters of this book, the aim is to present a pluralistic yet critically minded discussion of PCC for people with SMI.

Section 1.1 presents PCC as a multi-dimensional construct. The section argues that not all dimensions or aspects of PCC for people with SMI have to be present in order for care to be person-centered and outlines ethical principles and ethical challenges of PCC for individuals with SMI. Section 1.2.1, *Moral Treatment in the Eighteenth and Nineteenth Centuries*, presents moral treatment as a form of humane "psychological" therapy – and hence perhaps the closest at that time to PCC – that emerged towards the latter half of the eighteenth century and which enjoyed a golden age until the first quarter of the nineteenth century; it then gradually fell into disrepute as it was forced to abandon its person-centered ideals due to increasingly large difficult-to-treat populations. Section 1.2.2, *Rogerian and Related Psychotherapies in the Twentieth Century*, argues that PCC has roots within psychological care, dating back to the 1940s to humanistic psychologist Carl Rogers, and that Rogers applied the core concepts of PCC when providing psychological care to a wide variety of service users, including those with SMI.

1.1 Foundations and Ethics of Person-Centered Approaches to Individuals with Serious Mental Illness

Abraham Rudnick and David Roe

INTRODUCTION

PCC is widely considered a cornerstone of contemporary mental health services for people with SMI such as schizophrenia. This is clearly illustrated in psychiatric rehabilitation, which focuses on assisting individuals with SMI to enhance and maintain their living skills and supports so as to achieve their goals,[1] using evidence-based clinical and social interventions such as social skills training, supported employment (SE) and family psychoeducation.[2] Recovery-oriented services are part of a new vision of mental health care,[3] which is first and foremost person-centered. Recovery is viewed in this vision as both an outcome, which refers to reduction in symptom severity and increase in role functioning,[4] as well as a process, which refers to seeking and having a personally meaningful life and valued social roles.[5,6]

The foundational underpinnings of PCC and other person-centered approaches (such as self-help) for individuals with SMI have not been sufficiently analyzed in a systematic manner, e.g. in relation to the dimensions of PCC as a construct. Yet foundational understandings are arguably important for maturation of mental health care practice and research.[7] In addition, ethical aspects of PCC, including associated challenges such as legal issues, are still under considerable debate, e.g. in relation to individuals whose capacity to make decisions about their lives is impaired due to their mental illness. In this section, we conduct a conceptual analysis of foundations and ethics of PCC for individuals with SMI, based on writings about PCC in other populations and on writings about individuals with SMI. Conceptual analysis may be said to address the internal consistency within a concept and the mutual coherence between concepts.[8] As such, it is suitable for study of the concept and of the derived construct of PCC.

FOUNDATIONS OF PERSON-CENTERED CARE

Person-Centered Care as a Multi-Dimensional Construct

There is still much controversy about what PCC means; indeed, the related notion of (the personal process of) recovery of individuals with SMI, as described above, is currently so rife with diverse meanings that it is at risk of becoming meaningless if not clarified.[9] The meaning of PCC appears clearer when applied to other clinical populations. For instance, the PCCM approach, which was originally designed for a primary health care population, includes six interactive components of the person-centered process: 1. exploring both the disease and the illness experience (history, physical, lab and dimensions of illness – feelings, ideas, effects on function and expectations); 2. understanding the whole person (the person, the proximal context such as family, and the distal context such as culture); 3. finding common ground (problems and priorities, goals of treatment and/or management, and roles of service user and provider (physician); 4. incorporating prevention and health promotion (health enhancement, risk avoidance, risk reduction, early identification, and complication reduction); 5. enhancing the service user – provider relationship (compassion, power, healing, self-awareness, and transference and countertransference); 6. being realistic (time and timing, teambuilding and teamwork, and wise stewardship of resources).[10]

A thematic analysis of relevant centeredness (person-centeredness, patient-centeredness, client-centeredness, family-centeredness and relationship-centeredness) across health care contexts revealed 10 common themes: 1. respect for individuality and values; 2. meaning; 3. therapeutic alliance; 4. social context and relationships; 5. inclusive model of health and well-being; 6. expert lay knowledge; 7. shared responsibility; 8. communication; 9. autonomy; 10. professional as a person.[11] Analysis of PCC with particular focus on elderly populations has demonstrated four components (the VIPS model): 1. the absolute **V**alue of all human lives; 2. an **I**ndividualized approach, recognizing uniqueness; 3. an understanding of the world from the **P**erspective of the service user; 4. a **S**ocial environment that encourages well-being.[12]

PCC for individuals with SMI can be argued to be: *person-focused*, i.e. the person is the (intended) beneficiary of care; *person-driven*, i.e. the person decides on his or her care; *person-sensitive*, i.e. the person's particular needs are addressed; and *person-contextualized*, i.e. the person's history and current circumstances are considered in providing care. We suggest that these are different dimensions of the construct of PCC, which under some conditions may be complementary, yet under other conditions may be in conflict. In what follows, we elaborate on each dimension of PCC and note potential conflicts between these dimensions, in preparation for the discussion on ethics of PCC for individuals with SMI near the end of this section.

Person-Centered Care as Person-Focused

The person-focused dimension of PCC refers to the person as the (intended) beneficiary of care. PCC is explicitly aimed at the person with the health problem. More specifically, it is aimed at that person's benefit, such as alleviating a health problem, e.g. treating and hence curing pneumonia with antibiotics, or reducing a persistent health problem's disruptive impact, e.g. managing and hence stabilizing diabetes mellitus with a healthy lifestyle (in addition to medications if needed). In relation to people with SMI, PCC may sometimes alleviate the problem, such as in treatment for an acute episode of major depressive disorder, and at other times it may reduce the problem's disruptive impact, such as in management of schizophrenia.[13] Note that SMI sometimes defies the distinction between a problem that can be alleviated and a persistent problem that has disruptive impact which can be reduced. The clinical manifestations of SMI commonly recur, with remitting-relapsing and exacerbation patterns such as recurrent depressive or manic episodes in major mood disorders[14] and psychotic relapses in schizophrenia,[15] in addition to ongoing manifestations such as residual negative symptoms and neurocognitive impairments in schizophrenia.[16,17]

It may be considered a given that care aims at benefiting the individual with an SMI. Yet this is not always so, as in some cases care is provided to individuals with SMI in order to benefit others. This is particularly so in cases of involuntary commitment of individuals with SMI who pose an aggressive threat to others due to their SMI, such as in manic or psychotic episodes where an individual's delusions or hallucinations may lead him or her to act aggressively toward others. In such cases, the benefit of the individual with the SMI is considered of secondary importance, and although that individual commonly benefits by being protected from legal and other normative social consequences of his or her own aggression, in some cases such individuals are not thankful for such protection even after the fact. This characteristic of care for some individuals with SMI qualifies PCC in such cases, as will be discussed later in relation to ethics of PCC. Note that if person-focus is viewed as a continuous dimension, the question of health care benefit to the individual with the SMI versus to others (particularly those directly impacted by that individual's life and care, or lack of care), can be viewed as a matter of balance, i.e. more or less benefit to the individual with the SMI versus more or less benefit to others.[18] This matter of balance is not unique to SMI, as it is relevant to some other health conditions such as infectious diseases (particularly respiratory and sexually transmitted diseases, which are commonly reportable to public health authorities even without the infected individual's consent), but it may be more prominent and common in relation to SMI.

Person-Centered Care as Person-Driven

The person-driven dimension of PCC refers to the person as the decision-maker about his or her care. According to health care legislation in Western countries and in some other jurisdictions, individuals with health problems have the right to decide on their own care, including the right to refuse any care; this right is also grounded as a principle in contemporary health care ethics.[19] As the person-driven dimension of PCC addresses the person's decision (consent or refusal) in relation to health care, it seems that this dimension is not unique to PCC, at least as an expected norm in contemporary health care. Alternatively, or complementarily, this dimension of PCC may be the strongest influence of PCC on contemporary health care.

Personal choice in relation to health care assumes that the person is capable of making informed decisions about his or her health. Both health care legislation and health care ethics assume this capacity exists, but make provisions for the assessment of this capacity and for alternative decision making if a person is determined as incapable to decide on his or her own health care. Individuals with SMI are at times at risk of being incapable to decide about their mental health care,[20] because of impairments such as mania, severe depression, psychosis with lack of illness awareness (insight) and/or severe neurocognitive deficits, all of which can disrupt the relevant decision-making capacity in one or more ways.[21] This (occasionally temporary and sometimes permanent) characteristic of some individuals with SMI qualifies PCC in such cases, as will be discussed later in relation to ethics of PCC; still, approaches that develop treatment-related decision-making of individuals with SMI and support them by means of shared decision-making (SDM) have been developed lately.[22] Note that there are other populations with a similar type of risk, such as people with intellectual disabilities or dementia, which disrupt the relevant decisional making capacity when they are sufficiently severe,[20] as with people with other health conditions.[23]

Person-Centered Care as Person-Sensitive

The person-sensitive dimension of PCC refers to care as addressing particular needs of the person. Health care addresses health needs, as involved in prevention, treatment and rehabilitation. Needs are different from wishes or choices, as they consist of requirements that are necessary for a person to fulfill in order to survive (as pertain to basic needs) and thrive (as pertain to more advanced needs).[24] Basic health needs involve vital functions such as respiration and circulation. More advanced health needs involve more developed functions, such as ambulation and cognition. PCC brings into health care the recognition that addressing health needs may involve some of the most developed functions that are required for a person to thrive, such as envisioning one's desired future and social cognition.[25] The distinction between advanced health needs and other types of needs, such as needs related to a person's social welfare, is not necessarily absolute and may shift according to social conventions and resources available to the various care sectors.

Some people with SMI suffer from severely disrupted mental functions such as impaired affect, perception, and thinking; these are widely considered advanced health needs for which mental health care is helpful. Thus, the person-sensitive dimension of PCC is aligned with care for people with SMI. Yet these needs may not align with the choices of some individuals with SMI, nor may it be possible or feasible to address them, either because of lack of scientific or technological knowledge of how to do so or because of lack of resources to deliver relevant services. Such matters will be discussed later in relation to conflict between dimensions of PCC as related to ethics of PCC. Note that some of the mental health needs of people with SMI are only recently being recognized, such as existential needs[26] and needs related to social cognition impairments,[25] hence knowledge of the person-sensitive dimension is changing considerably of late.

Person-Centered Care as Person-Contextualized

The person-contextualized dimension of PCC refers to care as considering the person's history and current circumstances, i.e. context (both the present and the past leading to it, such as social historical developments leading to legislation and to societal attitudes toward people with SMI). A person's history refers to past events experienced by the person, health problems, family background, biopsychosocial development, education and work experience, culture, social and leisure involvement, religious and spiritual background, longstanding plans and more. A person's circumstances refer to his or her current living environments, i.e. residential, vocational, educational, social (family, friends and others), recreational, political, spiritual and more. History and circumstances can be viewed as both objective and subjective. That is, the actual occurrences and external conditions can be considered (as agreed or disagreed on by various observers), as well as the ways in which they are experienced and viewed by the person at a given moment and over time; the latter have a significant impact on the person's life,[27] sometimes more than the actual occurrences and external conditions. For instance, a person's chosen health care may be determined by his or her health beliefs,[28] which in turn are influenced by his or her endorsement or rejection of cultural and family practices with which he or she grew up.

People with SMI often experience occurrences and external conditions which are commonly challenging, such as poverty, trauma, coercion and more, both pre-morbidly and later, more so than the general population.[29] This is so because of family predisposition; commonly occurring disability after the onset of the SMI; and predominant social discrimination against people with SMI, among other factors. PCC addresses the history and circumstances of the person with an SMI, viewed objectively and subjectively, as well as the patterns of history and circumstances commonly occurring to and experienced by people with SMI as a group, thus addressing the past and the present as well as the likely (although malleable) future of the particular person. The history and circumstances of a person with SMI, viewed objectively and subjectively, such as in relation to culturally influenced health beliefs, may pose challenges to the benefit or choice of the person. Such matters will be discussed in the next part of this section in relation to conflict between dimensions of PCC as related to ethics of PCC.

ETHICS OF PERSON-CENTERED CARE

Ethics Principles of Health Care

Health care is rife with ethical challenges, as due to its involvement with human beings and their lives, it is value-laden, and some of the values involved come into conflict with each other in some health care situations, even when all the values involved are acceptable. Hence, many if not most or all ethical problems in health care can be simply characterized as conflicts of values in a given health care situation, where the values in conflict with each other are all acceptable to various parties involved, yet they cannot all be satisfied. There are various ethical theories that propose ways of resolving such ethical problems. The most established of these ethical theories are deontology (simply characterized as a theory of moral duties), consequentialism or utilitarianism (simply characterized as a theory of morally acceptable consequences of actions), and virtue theory (simply characterized as a theory of morally acceptable intentions). Some other ethical theories can be viewed as derived from these established theories, e.g. care ethics can be viewed as derived from consequentialism and virtue ethics in conjunction.[30] Yet other ethical theories may not be derived from these established theories, particularly those that view ethical dialogue – rather than predetermined values – as fundamental to ethics.[31] The most commonly used theory in contemporary health care ethics is principlism, which is partly derived from more general ethical theories, particularly from deontology and consequentialism; principlism addresses a few central values in health care, which it reframes as (ethical) principles, and attempts to balance them in various health care situations so as to resolve ethical problems that arise in those situations.[19]

The principles addressed by principlism are: **a**utonomy; **b**eneficence; **n**on-maleficence; and **j**ustice. Autonomy, also termed self-determination and broadly conceived as respect for persons, refers to the view that a person's health care decisions or choices should be respected, including refusal of care. Autonomy assumes that the person is free to make choices, hence it is qualified if the person is not fully free to make choices, either due to external constraints (such as coercion) or to internal constraints (such as lack of capacity to make such choices). Beneficence, conceived as consideration of the best interests of a person, refers to the view that health care should aim at benefiting individuals with health problems. Beneficence assumes that the person knows best what his or her best interests are, unless the person is not capable to make such decisions. Non-maleficence, termed since the Hippocratic Oath "(first) do no harm," refers to the view that health care should aim at preventing and not causing harm to individuals with health problems. Non-maleficence is commonly combined with beneficence in contemporary health care ethics, due to the realization that most if not all health care procedures may cause harm, so that a balance of least harm and most benefit is aimed for. Justice, conceived as fairness to all stakeholders involved in health care, refers to the view that health care to a person with a health problem should balance that person's interests with those of other impacted parties, due to limited health care resources (where different persons who all have health problems and are deserving of health care compete for health care resources), due to risks posed by a person with a health problem to other people (where a health care decision in relation to one person or group of people can impact on the health of other people, such as with highly infectious diseases), or due to other reasons.

It is argued that these principles are prioritized and balanced in different health care situations primarily by means of intuition and reasoned argument.[19] A typical example of such prioritizing and balancing in general health care ethics is in end-of-life situations, particularly in so-called medical futility situations, where a terminally ill person's family requests extraordinary (heroic) measures to prolong the person's life (which refers to beneficence), whereas the health care team prefers not to do that in order to reduce the person's suffering (which refers to non-maleficence) and in order to use their limited health care resources for the care of another person whose life may actually be saved (which refers to justice). In such situations, various strategies may assist in resolving the ethical problem, such as legislation, policies and dialogue, although the latter has been found to be most helpful in many situations;[19] note that full dialogue can be challenging with some individuals with SMI, due to their severe mental impairments, but there may be ways of accommodating them so that fruitful ethical dialogue can still occur.[32]

Ethical Challenges of Person-Centered Care for Individuals with Serious Mental Illness

Various dimensions of PCC may come into conflict with each other in certain health care situations where individuals with SMI are involved. When such conflict involves conflict of ethical principles, as it commonly does, the identification, prioritizing and balancing of the relevant principles can be helpful to determine how to approach PCC in these situations.

As mentioned above, the person-focused dimension of PCC for individuals with SMI (which refers to beneficence) may be in conflict with the interests of others (which refers to justice), e.g. when a person with schizophrenia acts aggressively towards others due to a (usually persecutory) delusion or imperative auditory hallucination. In such cases, coercion such as involuntary commitment of the person with the SMI may be justified in order to protect others from risk of grave harm (it would be more a matter of contention if the risk was of less serious harm). As a result, the person-focused dimension of PCC may be compromised, as coercion is not usually beneficial, at least to the person, e.g. involuntary commitment has been suggested to lead to post-traumatic stress disorder;[33] note that involuntary commitment of a person with SMI in order to protect others from harm may prevent legal proceedings against the person, which may be considered a benefit to the person, although some individuals with SMI dispute that and state that they prefer legal proceedings where they can be judged on par with other people who do not have an SMI rather than be committed to a hospital with less legal rights (although the right of legal appeal against involuntary commitment exists in many jurisdictions). Note that although the person-driven dimension may also be compromised in such cases, as it addresses personal choice (which refers to autonomy), and in such cases the person's choice to refuse mental health care in general and a psychiatric hospital admission in particular would be declined, the other dimensions of PCC are not necessarily compromised, i.e. the person-sensitive and the person-contextualized dimensions, as the person's health needs and the person's history and circumstances, respectively, can and should still be addressed.

The person-driven dimension of PCC can be compromised by another type of ethical situation. As mentioned above, SMI may consist of temporary or permanent impairments such as mania, severe depression, psychosis with lack of illness awareness (insight) and/or severe neurocognitive deficits, all of which can disrupt a person's health care related decision-making capacity in one or more ways. If such disruption of decision-making capacity occurs, then the person's choice is not fully free, due to these internal constraints, and the person cannot fully decide on his or her health care, in which case a surrogate decision maker is appointed who considers the best interest of the person (according to the person's previously capable decisions, if possible). Note that some approaches in PCC call for more freedom of choice for individuals with SMI whose relevant decision-making appears significantly disrupted.[34] A different relevant situation is when a service user waives his or her right to make health-related decisions and requests that others such as providers decide on those matters. Such a choice should usually be respected in the short-term, as part of respect for autonomy, while attempting in the longer-term to explore and address reasons for such a choice and to educate the service user on benefits of deciding for himself or herself, recognizing that in some cultures that is not sanctioned as much as it is in modern Western culture.[35]

The person-sensitive dimension of PCC (which refers to the person's needs, particularly to his or her health needs, hence to beneficence and non-maleficence) may be compromised by an ethical situation involving individuals with SMI, where it comes into conflict with the person-driven dimension of PCC, which refers to the person's health care choice, hence to autonomy.[18] This is illustrated in situations where the person with an SMI chooses to forego mental health care and other services, e.g. use of medication.[36] When such choices are made in a capable manner, the person's choice usually trumps, both according to principlist ethics as well as according to legislation in many jurisdictions. Yet when such choices are made in an incapable manner, e.g. due to a persecutory delusion that staying in housing will lead to persecutors finding and harming the person and his or her loved ones, the person's choices should be overridden, both according to principlist ethics as well as according to legislation in many jurisdictions, at least when these choices involve risk of serious harm to the person such as exposure to the elements in freezing winter conditions.[37]

The person-contextualized dimension of PCC (which refers to the person's history and circumstances, i.e. context, both as viewed by others and as experienced and viewed by the person, hence to autonomy, at least in relation to the person's health beliefs), may be compromised by an ethical situation involving individuals with SMI where it comes into conflict with the person-focused dimension of PCC (which refers to beneficence) or with the person-driven dimension of PCC (which refers to autonomy). The ethical conflict of the person-contextualized dimension of PCC with the person-focused dimension of PCC is similar to that illustrated in the above discussion on the conflict of the person-sensitive dimension of PCC with the person-driven dimension of PCC. The ethical conflict of the person-contextualized dimension of PCC with the person-driven dimension of PCC (subjectively viewed) is intriguing, as both dimensions refer to autonomy. Yet while the person-driven dimension refers to autonomy narrowly defined, i.e. to the person's actual choices, the person-contextualized dimension may refer to autonomy broadly defined, e.g. to the person's choice to give over his or her decision making to a significant other. These situations arise commonly in some non-Western cultures, such as in traditional Japanese culture, where a person's health care – and other – decisions are expected to be made by the family or by the community.[35] In such settings, more traditional individuals with SMI would defer to their family or to their community for their health care decisions, whereas less traditional individuals with SMI would prefer to make their own health care choices; knowledge of their culturally-related health beliefs would be helpful in order to determine which of the two relevant dimensions of PCC trumps in such situations. Note that Western culture has legislated such decision-making by proxy by means of the institution of power of attorney.

CONCLUSION

PCC can be characterized as a multi-dimensional construct, consisting (at least) of four dimensions: a person-focused dimension, which involves the ethical principle of beneficence; a person-driven dimension, which involves the ethical principle of autonomy (narrowly defined); a person-sensitive dimension, which involves the ethical principles of beneficence and non-maleficence; and a person-contextualized dimension, which involves the ethical principle of autonomy (broadly defined). These dimensions may come into ethical conflict with each other and with other ethical principles (primarily justice) in situations involving health care for some individuals with SMI, in which case a principlist approach, complemented by accommodating dialogue with all parties involved, may resolve the ethical problem satisfactorily. In cases where some dimensions of PCC for individuals with SMI may be compromised because of ethical (and legal) requirements, other dimensions of PCC may be upheld. Hence, PCC may still be helpful in such cases.

REFERENCES

1 Anthony WA, Cohen M, Farkas M, *et al. Psychiatric Rehabilitation. 2nd ed.* Boston: Center for Psychiatric Rehabilitation; 2002.

2 Corrigan PW, Mueser KT, Bond GR, *et al. Principles and Practice of Psychiatric Rehabilitation: an empirical approach.* New York, NY: Guilford; 2008.

3 Anthony WA, Huckshorn KA. *Principled Leadership in Mental Health Systems and Programs.* Boston: Center for Psychiatric Rehabilitation; 2008.

4 Liberman RP, Kopelowicz A. Recovery from schizophrenia: a concept in search of research. *Psychiatric Services.* 2005; **56**(6): 735–42.

5 Anthony WA. Recovery from mental illness: the guiding vision of the mental health service system in the 1990s. *Psychosocial Rehabilitation Journal.* 1993; **16**(4): 11–23.

6 Deegan PE. Recovery: the lived experience of rehabilitation. *Psychosocial Rehabilitation Journal.* 1988; **11**(4): 11–19.

7 Rudnick A. The molecular turn in psychiatry: a philosophical analysis. *J Med Philos.* 2002; **27**(3): 287–96.

8 Yehezkel G. A model of conceptual analysis. *Metaphilosophy.* 2005; **36**: 668–87.

9 Roe D, Rudnick A, Gill KJ. The concept of "being in recovery." *Psychiatric Rehabilitation Journal.* 2007; **30**(3): 171–3.

10 Stewart M, Brown JB, Weston WW, *et al. Patient-Centered Medicine: transforming the clinical method.* 2nd ed. Oxford: Radcliffe Medical Press; 2003.

11 Hughes JC, Bamford C, May C. Types of centredness in health care: themes and concepts. *Med Health Care and Philos.* 2008; **11**(4): 455–63.

12 Brooker D. What is person centred care? *Reviews in Clinical Gerontology.* 2004; **13**: 215–22.

13 Mueser KT, Corrigan PW, Hilton DW, *et al.* Illness management and recovery: a review of the research. *Psychiatr Serv.* 2002; **53**(10): 1272–84.

14 American Psychiatric Association. *Diagnostic and Statistical Manual of Mental Disorders, 4th Edition, Text-Revised (DSM-IV-TR).* Washington, DC: American Psychiatric Association; 2000.

15 Hafner H, van der Heiden W. Course and outcome. In: Mueser KT, Jeste DV, editors. *Clinical Handbook of Schizophrenia.* New York, NY: Guilford; 2008. pp. 100–13.

16 Savla GN, Moore DJ, Palmer BW. Cognitive functioning. In: Mueser, op. cit. pp. 91–9.

17 Vahia IV, Cohen CI. Psychopathology. In: Mueser, op. cit. pp. 82–90.

18 Roe D, Weishut DJN, Jaglom M. *et al.* Patients' and staff members' attitudes about the rights of hospitalized psychiatric patients. *Psychiatric Services.* 2002; **53**(1): 87–91.

19 Beauchamp TL, Childress JF. *Principles of Biomedical Ethics.* 5th ed. New York, NY: Oxford University Press; 2001.

20 Appelbaum PS, Grisso T. *Assessing Competence to Consent to Treatment: a guide for physicians and other health professionals.* New York, NY: Oxford; 1998.

21 Rudnick A. Depression and competence to refuse psychiatric treatment. *J Med Ethics.* 2002; **28**: 151–5.

22 Deegan PE, Drake RE. Shared decision making and medication management in the recovery process. *Psychiatr Serv.* 2006; **57**(11): 1636–9.

23 Cournos F. Do psychiatric patients need greater protection than medical patients when they consent to treatment? *Psychiatric Quarterly.* 1993; **64**(4): 319–29.

24 Thomson G. *Needs.* London, UK: Routledge & Kegan Paul; 1987.

25 Corrigan PW, Penn DL, editors. *Social Cognition and Schizophrenia.* Washington, DC: American Psychological Association; 2001.

26 Wagner LC, King M. Existential needs of people with psychotic disorders in Pôrto Alegre, Brazil. *Br J Psychiatry.* 2005; **186**: 141–5.

27 Lazarus RS, Folkman S. *Stress, appraisal and coping.* New York, NY: Springer, 1984.

28 Becker MH, Maiman LA. Sociobehavioral determinants of compliance with health and medical care recommendations. *Medical Care.* 1975; **13**: 10–24.

29 Warner R. *The Environment of Schizophrenia: innovations in practice, policy and communications.* London, UK: Brunner-Routledge; 2000.

30 Rudnick A. A meta-ethical critique of care ethics. *Theoretical Medicine and Bioethics.* 2001; **22**: 505–17.

31 Rudnick A. The ground of dialogical bioethics. *Health Care Anal.* 2002; **10**(4): 391–402.

32 Rudnick A. Processes and pitfalls of dialogical bioethics. *Health Care Anal.* 2007; **15**(2): 123–35.

33 Rosenberg SD, Mueser KT. Trauma and posttraumatic stress syndromes. In: Mueser, op. cit. pp. 447–58.

34 Freeth R. *Humanising Psychiatry and Mental Health Care: the challenge of the person-centred approach.* Oxford: Radcliffe Publishing; 2007.

35 Macklin R. *Against Relativism: cultural diversity and the search for ethical universals in medicine.* New York, NY: Oxford University Press; 1999.

36 Roe D, Goldblatt H, Vered Baloush-Kleinman V, *et al.* Why and how do people with a serious mental illness decide to stop taking their medication: exploring the subjective process of making and activating a choice. *Psychiatr Rehabil J.* 2009; **33**(1): 38–46.

37 Rudnick A. The goals of psychiatric rehabilitation: an ethical analysis. *Psychiatr Rehabil J.* 2002; **25**(3): 310–13.

1.2 Historical Antecedents of Contemporary Person-Centered Approaches to Serious Mental Illness

1.2.1 MORAL TREATMENT IN THE EIGHTEENTH AND NINETEENTH CENTURIES

Louis C. Charland

INTRODUCTION

Towards the end of the eighteenth century, a new approach to the care and treatment of the mentally ill called "moral treatment" began to appear across Europe. Major milestones in the history of this new treatment modality vary considerably in their historical antecedents and sociocultural determinants. Moral treatment itself often assumed quite different forms in the different jurisdictions where it was practiced. Neither was it uniformly adopted. In many cases, it figured as one among several more traditional treatment alternatives, against which it had to compete for scientific acceptability and public monies. This is therefore an area where one must be wary of generalizations. One must also be careful not to commit anachronisms, which are the uncritical insertion of contemporary beliefs and terms into historical evidence. Hence, I will use original terminology as much as possible, e.g. patients rather than service users. In this section, I will review some historical evidence about moral treatment and I will try to relate it to PCC as understood today.

Background

At times, moral treatment assumed the guise of a relatively strict behavioral therapy program built on simple rewards and punishments.[1] Other more cognitive forms focused on the inner struggles of patients as they were taught to cope with wayward passions and delusions.[2] Finally, many varieties of moral treatment resorted to manipulating features in the environment, such as diet, exercise and occupation.[3] So there were variations. Nonetheless, there are some broad preconditions that underlay the practice of moral treatment in many of the settings where it was practiced.

One important precondition of moral treatment is the view that the mentally ill are not totally devoid of reason and that, despite their illness, they are still human souls deserving of care and respect. This humanism stands in marked contrast to other prevailing views of madness of the time. According to one such view, the "mad" were thought to be like wild beasts devoid of reason that deserve to be brutally domesticated. Another view was that the mad are immoral sinners and degenerates, possibly even demonically possessed. The Enlightenment humanism on which moral treatment was based contrasted sharply with these earlier views. The "mad" were now persons with rights and feelings that deserved the same care and respect as other members of society. In some versions of moral treatment the humanity of the mentally ill lay in basic feelings of benevolence and other primitive affective capacities that somehow survived the "wreck of the intellect."[1] In other cases, simple Enlightenment-inspired humanism formed the basis of general political reforms that permitted the emergence of moral treatment.[3]

In general, adherents of moral treatment favored psychological interventions over physical ones though often the two approaches were conjoined. This emphasis on psychological rather than physical means of treatment is a second precondition of moral treatment. Most practitioners of moral treatment were in fact very skeptical about the value of existing physical treatments for the mentally ill, which they saw as harmful. Indeed, the discovery that moral treatment was a highly effective form of therapy was accompanied with the collateral discovery that existing physical treatments were often extremely harmful. This discovery that traditional physical treatments often caused harm to psychiatric patients – sometimes even to the point of making them incurable – represents the first official evidence-based recognition of iatrogenic harm in psychiatric care.

From the outset, moral treatment was patient-centered in an important sense. It was based on the premise that the mad were deserving of care and respect as individual persons. This philosophical premise was also reflected in clinical care, where each patient was treated as a separate individual case. This clinical focus on the individual patient is a third precondition of moral treatment. This new patient-centered clinical attitude represented a marked departure from the indiscriminate administration of multiple treatments to large masses of individuals, the standard of care at the time. Patients were typically housed and treated *en masse* with little attention to diagnosis and no follow-up or individualized treatment plan. In sharp contrast, moral treatment represents one of the first models of individual patient-centered clinical care in the history of psychiatry.

A complicating factor in assessing the contribution of moral treatment to the history of clinical care in psychiatry is that it had both compelling lay and medical versions. This raised serious questions about its integrity as a purely medical scientific intervention. That said, in its medical guise moral treatment reconciled two laudable goals that are often thought to be in opposition. It combined attention to the patient as a clinical object of study and research, while at the same time highlighting the importance of the patient as a human subject with an inalienable right to respect and kindness. There is an interesting irony to this dual commitment. For at the same time that medicine turned its clinical gaze onto the psychiatric patient as an object of research, to be studied according to the methods of the natural sciences, it also extolled the importance of that object as human subject, a spiritual being possessed of an inalienable right to kindness and respect. Modern psychiatry is still struggling to reconcile these two goals today.

Moral Treatment at York and the Salpêtrière

The English expression "moral treatment" has a rather interesting and eclectic history. It only really officially enters the English medical lexicon with the appearance of Samuel Tuke's publication of *Description of the Retreat*.[1] Samuel Tuke (1784–857) was an amateur Quaker medical scholar and grandson of the famous William Tuke (1732–822), the original founder of the York retreat for insane persons. This small hospice devoted to the care of the mentally ill first opened its doors in 1796. Its mission was initially to provide care and comfort to Quakers who suffered from SMI. In keeping with the Quaker pledge to offer care and charity to all living souls, that mandate soon expanded to include mentally ill patients of all stripes.

It was the suspicious death of a local Quaker at the nearby York Asylum that led William, a wealthy businessman, to create a safe haven where Quakers who were mentally ill could be cared for by their own. There they would be free from religious discrimination and treated in accordance with Quaker values. The small family establishment soon grew in size but never housed more than several dozen patients at a time. It also grew in fame, partly as a result of the popularity of Samuel's book, which was written to extol its laurels. To this day, the Retreat still provides care for the mentally ill and remains a site for medical pilgrims from all over the world.

Samuel Tuke uses the expression "moral treatment" to characterize the kind of treatment practiced at the Retreat in its early years. He borrows the expression from the French doctor Philippe Pinel (1745–826), who named his own approach to treatment "*traitement moral.*" There is much else in the *Description* that Samuel borrows from Pinel. Samuel's goal in writing his book was to present a medically palatable picture of the Retreat and its success to medical men, while at the same time praising its lay origins in the Quaker faith. Pinel's work provided an ideal framework with which to cast the achievements and practices of the Retreat in medical terms. And yet the Retreat never was a medical establishment in any accepted sense. William himself had no medical training. And the treatment practiced at the Retreat is best interpreted as a common-sense form of affective conditioning based on Quaker religious values.[4]

Although it relied entirely on charitable donations to finance its operations, the Retreat was economically self-sufficient in most other respects. It had a small farm attached to it and able patients were encouraged to work at farming and other domestic tasks. Patients and staff always ate together, like a family, and diversions and games were also encouraged in order to combat idleness, a vice Quakers considered inimical to a healthy mind and attitude. All of these developments make the Retreat an interesting experiment in the history of occupational therapy.

In searching for a medical model to make the Retreat and its innovations more medically palatable, Samuel chose to borrow from Philippe Pinel, whose celebrated *Traité medico-philosophique sur l'aliénation mentale ou la manie* was by then widely known and respected.[5] Shortly after the French revolution, the prestigious French doctor was appointed to head the largest mental hospital in France, the infamous Salpêtrière hospital for insane women in Paris. He remained there until his death several decades later, publishing, among other things, an expanded and much larger and revised edition of his original Traité, newly titled *Traité medico-philosophique sur l'aliénation mentale*.[2] This work, just recently translated into English for the first time, is perhaps the best clinical statement of moral treatment as a medical therapy.[6] Pinel was aware of William's innovations at the Retreat – the "English secret," he called it – and took great pains to distinguish his own medical therapy from the religious foundations of the Quaker model. Pinel in fact believed that religious worship and devotion were generally inimical to recovery from mental illness, and often one of its precipitating causes. Despite these differences between Pinel and Tuke, there remain important similarities between the moral treatment offered at the York Retreat and the *traitement morale* offered at the Salpêtrière. Both establishments were largely run according to the preconditions adumbrated above.

One major difference deserves special mention. This is size. Pinel's hospital housed hundreds of patients at any given time. And yet he claimed to practice moral treatment (*traitement moral*) as a patient-centered medical intervention. A small doctor to patient ratio was evidently not a precondition for moral treatment, at least according to Pinel. Not surprisingly, case notes and patient files indicate that Pinel was not only a meticulous and careful clinician, but also clearly indefatigable. What really counted was scrupulous and concentrated daily attention to the individual patient, an equally important characteristic of patient care at the Retreat. No doubt, Pinel was not alone in gathering and transcribing clinical logs. Nonetheless, the voluminous and very detailed descriptions he provides of his patients – their daily habits, diets, behaviors and treatment plans – provide indisputable proof that size was not an obstacle to individual patient-centered care in his hospital. Surprisingly, neither the overall size of patient populations, nor even high or low caregiver to patient ratios, appear to have been obstacles to the success of moral treatment. Both Samuel and Pinel provide outcome measures and other data as proof of the success of their respective establishments. And many leading historians concur that moral treatment was indeed very successful compared to other existing treatments of the time.

Meaning of "Moral"

Let us now turn to moral treatment itself. In what did it consist? And how are we to understand the term "moral" in this context? These are treacherous exegetical waters.

We have seen that moral treatment was built around a principle of respect for persons. Above all, everyone had to observe the Hippocratic imperative to "do no harm." Tuke speaks of the importance of "judicious kindness" towards patients. Pinel refers repeatedly to the "ways of gentleness" (*les voies de la douceur*) as a therapeutic imperative. Yet neither Pinel nor William was wary of imposing strict discipline in their establishments. Both also resorted to fear as a therapeutic instrument, although only within carefully circumscribed parameters. In both establishments, moral treatment also involved a strict paternalistic stance. It was thought that the doctor or healer had to have a position of "moral ascendancy" (*ascendant moral*) over the patient in order for treatment to be successful. The parental obligation to love and protect children, together with the responsibility to instill discipline and self-control, provides a compelling analogy for understanding this special brand of paternalism in moral treatment. Indeed, in this context, patient care and rehabilitation were often viewed on analogy with the education of children.

The term "moral" itself is highly problematic in these discussions and is responsible for a large number of misinterpretations and misappropriations of moral treatment.[4] The problems exist in both French and English and are invariably compounded in translation. There are several senses of the term "moral" ("*moral*") that can be discerned in Pinel's work. First, there is "*moral*" in the sense of "*le moral*," meaning what is psychological or mental ("*mentale*") as opposed to what is physical ("*physique*"). The other major sense of "*moral*" that Pinel uses has to do with ethics and "*la morale*." A third sense of the term "*moral*" is arguably involved in the reference to "moral faculties" ("*facultés morales*"). There is also a fourth possible sense; for example, when a reference is made to "moral affections" ("*affections morales*")*,* meaning affective posits like passions, emotions and feelings. Finally, fifth, in this context it is common to find the general expression "moral sciences" ("*sciences morales*"). No wonder there is such confusion! And note that most of these ambiguities also occur in English.

In general, the safest exegetical assumption is to suppose that "moral" in "moral treatment" refers to the therapeutic manipulation of psychological variables, sometimes extending to wider environmental factors that have a psychological impact, such as architecture, geographical location and even diet. What moral treatment is decidedly not, is physical. Thus, physical treatments such as the administration of tonics and opiates, as well as bloodletting, purgatives, emetics and other bodily interventions, do not count as "moral methods" ("*methods morales*"). However, such methods, as well as warm baths and cold showers, can on occasion figure in an overall treatment plan. And often they did, though to a very limited degree. In sum, the advent of moral treatment marks the beginning of a new, clinical, evidence-based psychotherapy, even though some of the interventions involved are more than merely "psychological" in a strict sense.

It is important to recognize that – Tuke aside – moral treatment is not tantamount to the philosophical therapy of the ancient Stoics, or others like them. It was for many of its medical proponents a medical therapy in the strictest sense of the word; certainly in the case of Pinel. The clinical character of the patient-centered care provided in moral treatment is fundamental to its importance in the history of patient-centered care in psychiatry. First, moral treatment was based on careful clinical observation of individual patients, who were then classified, lodged and treated, according to the reigning nosological categories of the time. Second, moral treatment was based on carefully maintained clinical daily logs that documented all aspects of patient life, including responses to ongoing treatment. Moral treatment was therefore evidence-based in a very important sense of the term; at least in Pinel's hospitals. Note that Pinel was also among the first to calculate treatment outcomes and relapse rates using the probability calculus, a pioneering innovation for which he typically fails to get due credit.

Moral Treatment in Other Regions

Moral treatment also arose in Italy and Germany around the same time that Tuke and Pinel were experimenting with their new therapies. In Germany, moral treatment is usually associated with the name of Johann Christian Reil (1759–813), who was also the first to introduce the word psychiatry (*"psychiatrie"*) into the medical lexicon. Reil's chief work on this topic, which is titled *Rhapsodien über die Anwendung der psychischen Curmethode auf Geisteszerrüttungen*, is based on very different philosophical and scientific assumptions than those of Pinel.[7] Yet the emphasis on "moral," or psychic (*"psychischen"*), methods is central here, as it is in Pinel. There is also the same pervasive humanism and hope that is present in Tuke and Pinel.

In the case of Italy, the most famous proponent of moral treatment is undoubtedly Vincenzo Chiarugi (1759–820). His major work in the area is titled *Della pazzia in genere, e in specie tratto medico-analitico con una centuria di osservazioni*.[3] Chiarugi's concern with the care and well-being of the mentally ill is reminiscent of the other major proponents of moral treatment we have considered. There is no doubt that Pinel considered Chiarugi an important rival, and he wasted no time in deriding the Florentine doctor's achievements. On the other hand, Pinel was apparently totally unaware of Reil and his work.

In addition to these German and Italian examples of moral treatment there are other precedents in Spain.[8] Moral treatment eventually found its way to America, where the lessons of Tuke and Pinel proved an inspiration to many practitioners concerned with the care of the mentally ill.[9] The name of Benjamin Rush (1745–813) is often associated with the early beginnings of moral treatment in America, although some of his own treatment innovations – like the tranquilizing chair – arguably did not conform to its ideals.[10]

CONCLUSION: REMEMBERING MORAL TREATMENT

In discussing the history of moral treatment and its contributions to patient-centered care one must be careful to specify which particular period of the history of moral treatment one is referring to. This is because the early success of moral treatment bears no resemblance to its lamentable fate in later years. Indeed, from the middle of the nineteenth century onwards, moral treatment started to collapse under the pressure of its own popularity, crushed by increasing patient populations and diminishing resources.[11] It eventually became a bitter and sad caricature of its original self; a travesty of its earlier ideals and clinical excellence. In a tragic irony of history, moral treatment turned into a repugnant sin against its own original mission of individualized clinical care. All that was left was a blurred, anonymous and furtive impersonal shadow as the object of institutional management.

REFERENCES

1 Tuke S. *Description of the Retreat*. London: Process Press; 1813.
2 Pinel P. *Traité médico-philosophique sur l'aliénation mentale, 2ᵉ. éd., entièrement refondu et très augmenté*. Paris: Brosson; 1809.
3 Chiarugi V. *Della pazzia in genere, e in specie tratto medico-analitico con una centuria di osservazioni*. Florence: Luigi Carlieri; pp. 1793–4.

4 Charland LC. Benevolent treatment: moral treatment at the York retreat. *Hist Psychiatry.* 2007; **18**(1): 61–80.

5 Pinel, op. cit.

6 Hickish G, Healy D, Charland LC, translators. *Medico-Philosophical Treatise on Mental Alienation.* 2nd ed., entirely reworked and expanded (1809). Oxford: Wiley-Blackwell; 2008.

7 Reil JC. *Rhapsodien uber die Anwendung der psychischen Kurmethode auf Geisteszerruttungen.* Halle: Curtsche Buchhandlung; 1803.

8 Herreda-Torres MP, Brea Riverio M, Martinez-Piedrola RM. Origen de la terapia ocupacional en Espāna. *Rev Neurol.* 2007; **45**(11): 695–8.

9 Goodheart LB. *Mad Yankees: the Hartford retreat for the insane and nineteenth century psychiatry.* Amherst and Boston, MA: University of Massachusetts Press; 2003.

10 Whitaker R. *Mad in America: bad science, bad medicine, and the enduring mistreatment of the mentally ill.* Cambridge, MA: Perseus Books; 2002.

11 Scull, A. *The Most Solitary of Afflictions: madness and society in Britain 1700–1900.* New Haven, CT: Yale University Press; 1993.

1.2.2 ROGERIAN AND RELATED PSYCHOTHERAPIES IN THE TWENTIETH CENTURY

Lara Cross

INTRODUCTION

This section will outline the development of PCC in the work of Carl Rogers, a leader in PCC in 20th century psychological care. Topics discussed are the evolution of PCC (including service user populations addressed and outcomes demonstrated), the psychological care process, core qualities of PCC service providers, and current contributions and applications of PCC.

PCC is not a new approach to client care. Its fundamental tenets were articulated by humanistic psychologist Carl Rogers in the late 1930s as person-centered therapy, or Rogerian psychotherapy. PCC has its roots in humanistic psychology, a historical movement in the field of psychology, which offered alternative views of human nature to psychoanalysis and behaviorism. Rogers' basic assumptions that service users are fundamentally good, in control of making changes, and that growth is enhanced by the service provider/service user relationship have challenged traditional psychoanalytical and behaviorist psychological care perspectives.[1] Despite Rogers' death in 1987, many mental health care service providers continue to acknowledge and integrate PCC in their work with service users. Rogers' reputation for revolutionizing the psychological care practice and defining PCC has made him one of the most influential psychological care providers in the past century.[2] His impact on psychological care is still felt today, as PCC continues to be at the forefront of caring practice, continually evolving and incorporating new research and areas of application.

Evolution of Person-Centered Care

PCC has evolved in name, style and service user application since its conception in the late 1930s. According to Bozarth, Zimring, and Tausch,[3] there are four key periods of the development of PCC:

Period one: frustration with traditionalist models of care (1930s and 1940s)
In 1942, Carl Rogers published *Counseling and Psychotherapy: newer concepts in practice,* which described his new approach to care – a nondirective style.[4] Nondirective service providers focus on establishing an accepting and caring atmosphere for the service user. This is achieved by reflecting and clarifying the service user's feelings to help the service user gain a better understanding of his or her emotions and unconscious beliefs. This caring framework was very radical for its time since it purported an alternative to the well-established approaches of psychoanalysis and behaviorism. Rogers rejected the assumption that the service provider is in charge

of care and challenged the appropriateness of rigorously practiced caring techniques such as direction, teaching, advice and interpretation. Rogers felt diagnostic procedures were overused, inaccurate and not representative of various cultural and ethnic groups and thus, Rogers was cautious when utilizing such techniques with service users.

In this time period, Rogers utilized his non-directive approach with children coping with SMI and regularly documented successful outcomes of the PCC approach to care when working with these populations.[5] Rogers also published various case studies with adults with SMI to document the service user's experience with the PCC approach. A famous case was that of Herbert Bryan, a service user with a traditional "neurotic" diagnosis who sought the PCC approach since he was not responsive to other forms of care.[6] Rogers detailed a series of eight interviews with this service user and showed how Mr. Bryan benefited from the PCC approach to care.[7]

Period Two: Phenomenological Emphasis (1950s)

Moreover, the second period of PCC development began in 1951 when Rogers published *Client-Centered Therapy: its current practice, implications and theory* and renamed his approach "client-centered therapy" to emphasize the service user rather than the nondirective methods.[8] This period was characterized by a shift from the classification of the service user's feelings to the phenomenological world of the service user; the service user's own experiences, called the phenomenal field. Rogers believed to truly help service users become fully functional in their lives, it is necessary to understand the service user from their own subjective frame of reference. Furthermore, Rogers' 1959 paper titled *A Theory of Therapy, Personality, and Interpersonal Relationships, as Developed in the Client-Centered Framework* further refined the phenomenal field.[9] As humans develop, a portion of the phenomenal field becomes "the self," which are traits and characteristics the individual perceives are unique to him or herself. It is the relationships with others and the environment that shapes the development of the self and people are born with a desire to grow, learn and enhance themselves. This inborn motivation is called the actualizing tendency, which is inherently positive as it continues the growth and development of the self. The goal of psychological care is to help people become increasingly autonomous and achieve self-actualization.

Rogers continued publishing case studies to illustrate care outcomes of adults with SMI. Rogers also documented how the PCC approach is appropriate and helpful for individuals with personality disorders, such as that of Mrs. Oak, who experienced positive outcomes with the PCC approach to care.[10] Development also continued on Rogers' PCC approach with children with SMI through refinement and further research on play therapy, which traditionally encompassed a psychoanalytic perspective. Research illustrated the importance of the child's experience throughout care and positive outcomes through the PCC approach.[11] In addition, group care began to be utilized with a wide variety of service users, such as individuals with anxiety and individuals with schizophrenia.[12]

Period Three: Necessary and Sufficient Conditions of Care (1960s and 1970s)
This period was marked by an extensive increase in research on the client-centered approach, particularly with individuals with schizophrenia.[13] Rogers and associates were interested in determining what was necessary for progress in psychological care, and the service user/service provider relationship was extensively studied as an important caring component that leads to the service user's personality change.[14] Rogers was the first to initiate the empirical study of the psychological care process.[15] In 1957, Rogers published *The Necessary and Sufficient Conditions of Therapeutic Personality Change* and proposed that specific therapeutic conditions are necessary in order to determine service user growth.[16] To build upon this research, Rogers published *On Becoming a Person* in 1961 and *Person to Person: the problem of being human* in 1967 with Barry Stevens, which described how the service provider's goal is to help people become the person they truly are.[17,18] This important book also documented refinements of the PCC approach when working with individuals with schizophrenia and included unique insight on how to apply PCC with individuals living with this SMI. These influential works emphasized how the service user has to be willing to be a part of new experiences and to trust him- or herself throughout this process.

Period Four: Broadening Applications and Person-Centered Development (1980s–1990s)
Considerable development, application and expansion of the client-centered approach into different industries began in the early 1980s into the 1990s. There was growth and application of PCC in group counseling,[19,20] art therapy,[21] children and play therapy,[22] perceptual psychology,[23] education,[24] nursing,[25] gender studies,[26] conflict resolution,[27,28] and cross-cultural relations.[29] Because Rogers' approach was so easily and successfully applicable to a wide range of areas and people, the theory became known as the person-centered approach. Rogers published *A Way of Being* in 1980, where he discussed the necessary growth of research and applications of PCC in a wide variety of areas.[30]

The Psychological Care Process

PCC focuses on the constructive side of human nature. PCC embodies the philosophy that humans are trustworthy, resourceful, capable of self-understanding and self direction, able to make constructive changes and able to live effective and productive lives.[31] In PCC, the role of the service provider, service user and service provider/service user relationship are important components of the caring experience.

The Service Provider's Role in Person-Centered Care

The uniqueness of PCC is the service provider's attitude and way of being that is important, not the use of specialized techniques or demands placed on the service user. It is this inherent real and supportive attitude that helps facilitate change in service users more so than any technique, theory or specialized knowledge.[32] The service provider keeps all content open and accessible to service users; they do not keep their knowledge a secret. The person-centered service provider uses themselves as an instrument of change by relating on a personal level, without the use of a rigidly defined provider role. This view of service user's self-healing and control is a contrast to such care as psychodynamic and behavioral, which advocates that service provider techniques are responsible for service user change and views knowledge and understanding of the service user's frame of reference as occurring externally to the service user's experiential world.[33] Instead of viewing the service user as requiring diagnosis and care, the service provider meets the service user on his or her own experiential level with an attitude of genuine caring, understanding, respect and support. This requires the service provider to be true to oneself and present in the moment with the service user.[34] When the service provider embodies these characteristics, the service user feels more comfortable to explore areas of his or her life that were possibly denied or distorted prior to care. Relating and believing in the service user's inherent ability to make changes in their life creates a supportive and encouraging environment for personal growth. It is crucial the service provider is emotionally present and genuine in the relationship with the service user in order to establish trust. This genuinely authentic demeanor demonstrated by the service provider is known as congruence. If service provider congruence is not fully established in the relationship with the service user, it will negatively affect the caring process.[35]

The Service User's Experience Throughout Care

People live their lives in a natural progression towards self-actualization. Rogers[36] described people who are becoming actualized as sharing four characteristics: 1. openness to experience; 2. trust in themselves; 3. an internal source of evaluation; and 4. a willingness to continue growing. People structure their sense of self through conditions of worth, which are personal internal values that are influenced by others.[37] A positive condition of worth is articulated when an individual's self-experience is sought out because it increases the individual's self-regard. Likewise, when self-experience is avoided because it is less worthy of self-regard, this is characteristic of a negative condition of worth.[38] Experiences that are congruent with one's conditions of worth are perceived accurately; however, concerns that are incongruent are often perceived as threatening and their meaning is often distorted or denied. This can cause people to feel vulnerable, helpless, powerless, and feel ineffective in their lives. It is in this state of incongruence that many service users seek care.[39]

Through the dynamic of the service provider/service user relationship, service users enter a safe place where they can speak freely about their feelings without judgment. As service users feel understood and respected by the provider, they are able to become less defensive, which leaves them more open to experience. Service users gradually begin to understand the discrepancy between their self-concept and their ideal self-concept and move towards acceptance of who they are rather than distortion of reality. Service users learn new ways of becoming true to themselves and become more trusting in that the actualizing tendency will move them towards positive growth.[40]

The Service Provider/Service User Relationship

In 1957, Rogers discussed elements of personality change based on the service provider/service user relationship.[41] Rogers purported that for constructive personality change to occur during care, six conditions are necessary to exist and continue over a period of time:

1 two persons are in psychological contact
2 the first, whom we shall term the service user, is in a state of incongruence, being vulnerable or anxious
3 the second person, whom we shall term the service provider, is congruent or integrated in the relationship
4 the provider experiences unconditional positive regard for the service user
5 the provider experiences an empathic understanding of the service user's internal frame of reference and endeavors to communicate this experience to the service user
6 the service user understands and experiences the provider's empathetic understanding and unconditional positive regard throughout care.

These conditions are all that are necessary and sufficient for service user growth to occur, and they do not vary among service users.[42]

Another important aspect of the service provider/service user relationship is that of a shared journey. Both the service provider and service user reveal themselves on a human level and participate in a growing experience. The service provider acts as a guide for the service user throughout this journey since he or she is more psychologically mature.[43] However, the dichotomy between the service provider and service user's emotional maturity is not meant to segregate these individuals, but rather, both experience a different level of growth throughout care. Both must be congruent within the relationship. The service provider/service user journey broadens the horizons of the service provider and deepens each one's own sense of well-being and personal discovery.[44,45,46]

Core Qualities of Person-Centered Care

The following subsections discuss the three core caring components unique to person-centered service providers.[47]

Congruence/Genuineness

This core component implies that service providers are present and integrated in the care they are providing to the service user. This is often illustrated by the service provider's ability to match their expressions with experiences, openly express feelings, thoughts, reactions and attitudes with the service user. Being real and authentic is an important aspect of congruence. The service provider is a model because when the service user experiences how the service provider is listening and accepting of their concerns, they will learn to listen acceptingly of themselves. Being authentic also includes elements of self-disclosure; however, self-disclosure should be used as appropriate. Many service providers will use self-disclosure simply because they feel it is good for the service user, and this would be considered incongruent. Self-disclosure is appropriate and helpful for the service user only when the service provider feels truly moved and inspired to share.

Rogers emphasizes that service providers are human too, so congruence does not necessitate a service provider be fully self-actualized.[48] Congruence exists on a continuum, rather than on an all-or-nothing scale. There are times when a service provider will feel one way and act another towards a service user. Nevertheless, as long as service providers are committed to being congruent in their relationships with service users, trust will form and the caring process will unfold.

Unconditional Positive Regard

Unconditional positive regard is a deep caring attitude for the service user and the service user's concerns that is free of any judgment. The emphasis is the service user as valued and respected by the service provider regardless of the service user's thoughts, feelings, and behaviors; there are no stipulations on his or her acceptance by the service provider. For example, this attitude is often expressed as "I accept you as you are" (unconditional positive regard) rather than "I will accept you when …" (conditional positive regard). This attitude is extremely important for facilitating service user self-actualization, because the service user needs to feel free to express thoughts and feelings without risking loss of their service provider's acceptance. It is important to note that service provider acceptance does not necessitate approval of all behavior. Acceptance is the service provider's recognition that service users have the right to their own thoughts and feelings, but the service provider does not have to share these views for care to be effective. The service provider simply needs to actively demonstrate that regardless of the service user's beliefs and values, he or she is accepted and valued. By accepting the service user as a whole person, the service user is now able to learn to accept the self awareness experiences that occur as a part of self-discovery.

Accurate Empathetic Understanding

Along with the service provider/service user relationship, accurate empathy is considered a crux of PCC.[49,50] A goal for a person-centered service provider is to strive to understand the service user's subjective experiences. This is called empathy, not to be confused with sympathy or feeling sorry for the service user. The service provider feels and understands with the service user, as if the service provider were experiencing what the service user was experiencing. However, it is important for the service provider to keep his or her own separate identity – not to become lost in the service user's story. It is only when the service provider is able to fully understand the service user's world, while keeping his or her own identity separate, will constructive change occur for the service user.

The uniqueness of accurate empathetic understanding is the service provider's ability to not only feel the service user's feelings as if they were his or her own, but also reflecting deeper meaning and understanding to the service user regarding these feelings. This process requires the service provider to be real and present in the care he or she is providing and constantly checking in with the service user that his or her story has been understood. This helps the service user develop self-awareness. The service provider's use of language can help convey he or she has understood the service user from his or her own frame of reference. The use of "I" and "you" statements, such as "tell me how this feels for you" can help facilitate feelings and understanding and rapport.

Current Contributions and Applications of Person-Centered Care

PCC has inspired over 60 years of research on the service provider/service user relationship and outcomes of psychological care. Rogers desired to research the service provider/service user process, but required a model of scientific investigation that would allow him to analyze the subjective internal experiences of people. Rogers was the first to transcribe and critically analyze the care he provided service users as a form of data.[51] This was pioneering research, since previous research evaluated provider techniques and care outcomes.[52] Although this initially created controversy, Rogers' work continues to inspire service providers to examine their own caring style and relationships with service users. Particularly, Rogers' necessary and sufficient conditions for therapeutic personality change continue to be an area of exploration and refinement,[53,54,55] as well as empathy and the importance of the service provider/service user relationship.[56,57,58]

Moreover, PCC is continually evolving and practiced all over the world. Its fundamental tenets have attracted different researchers and service providers to examine and apply PCC with a wide variety of individuals, couples, families and groups.[59] Further developments of PCC continue with power and gender issues,[60,61] cultural counseling,[62,63,64] business,[65] conflict resolution,[66] interpersonal communication,[67] and cooperative student-centered learning in schools.[68] Rogers believed regardless of the service user's concern, PCC will be effective when the service user is able to feel supported and a part of the care process.[69]

CONCLUSION

Rogers' contributions to the field of PCC are important for developing a phenomenological approach to understanding people, which emerged as a third viewpoint that counterbalanced traditionalist views offered by psychoanalysis and behaviorism. This wholly different perspective of the human condition has been profoundly felt all over the world. Rogers was committed to capturing the subjective phenomenon of being human. Through the qualities of congruence, unconditional positive regard, and accurate empathetic understanding PCC service providers are able to build a supportive and caring relationship with the service user, which helps them share feelings and experiences while becoming more self-actualized. The concepts of respect and treating the service user fairly and without judgment are fundamental components of providing effective PCC.[70] It is important to recognize Rogers did not intend PCC to be a closed system, but rather, have his theory be open to interpretation and refinement.[71] Current research has indeed done this, and hopefully research will continue to refine and discover new applications of PCC. PCC is truly a journey for service providers and users to discover what it truly means to be human.

REFERENCES

1 Tallman K, Bohart AC. The client as a common factor: clients as self-healers. In: Hubble MA, Duncan BL, Miller SD, editors. *The Heart and Soul as Change: what works in therapy.* Washington, DC: American Psychological Association; 1999. pp. 91–131.

2 Haggbloom SJ, Warnick R, Warnick JE, *et al.* The 100 most eminent psychologists of the 20th century. *Review of General Psychology.* 2002; **6**(2): 139–52.

3 Bozarth JD, Zimring FM, Tausch R. Client-centered therapy: The evolution of a revolution. In: Cain DJ, Seeman J, editors. *Humanistic Psychotherapies: handbook of research and practice.* Washington, DC: American Psychological Association; 2002. pp. 147–88.

4 Rogers CR. *Counseling and Psychotherapy: newer concepts in practice.* Boston, MA: Houghton Mifflin; 1942.

5 Rogers CR. *The Clinical Treatment of the Problem Child.* Cambridge, MA: The Riverside Press; 1939.

6 Rogers, 1942, op. cit.

7 Ibid.

8 Rogers CR. *Client-centered therapy: its current practice, implications, and theory.* Boston, MA: Houghton Mifflin; 1951.

9 Rogers CR. A theory of therapy, personality, and interpersonal relationships as developed in the client-centered framework. In: Koch S, editor. *Psychology: a study of Science.* New York, NY: McGraw Hill; 1959. pp. 184–256.

10 Rogers CR, Dymond RF, editors. *Psychotherapy and Personality Change: co-ordinated research studies in the client-centered approach.* Chicago, IL: The University of Chicago Press; 1954.

11 Rogers, 1951, op. cit.

12 Ibid.

13 Rogers CR. *The Therapeutic Relationship and its Impact: a study of psychotherapy with schizophrenics.* Madison, WI: The University of Wisconsin Press; 1967.

14 Ibid.

15 Goldfried MR. What has psychotherapy inherited from Carl Rogers? *Psychotherapy: theory, research, practice, training.* 2007; **44**(3): 249–52.

16 Rogers CR. The necessary and sufficient conditions of therapeutic personality change. *Journal of Consulting Psychology.* 1957; **21**(2): 95–103.

17 Rogers CR. *On Becoming a Person.* Boston, MA: Houghton Mifflin; 1961.

18 Rogers CR, Stevens B. *Person to Person: the problem of being human.* Moab, UT: Real People Press; 1967.

19 Berg RC, Landreth GL, Fall KA. *Group Counseling: concepts and procedures.* 3rd ed. New York, NY: Routledge/Taylor & Francis Group; 1998.

20 Rogers CR. *On Encounter Groups.* New York, NY: Harper and Row; 1970.

21 Rogers N. Person-centered expressive arts therapy. In: Rubin J, editor. *Approaches to Art Therapy: theory and technique.* 2nd ed. New York, NY: Brunner-Routledge; 2001.

22 Axline V. *Play Therapy.* New York, NY: Churchill Livingstone; 1989.

23 Combs AW. *Being and Becoming: a field approach to psychology.* New York, NY: Springer; 1999.

24 Combs AW, Miser AB, Whitaker KS. *On Becoming a School Leader: a person-centered challenge.* Washington, DC: Association for Supervision & Curriculum Development; 1999.

25 Lindberg JB, Hunter ML, Kruszewski AZ. *Introduction to Person-Centered Nursing.* Philadelphia, PA: Lippincott Williams & Wilkins; 1983.

26 Natiello P. The person-centered approach, collaborative power, and cultural transformation. *Person-Centered Review.* 1990; **5**(3): 268–86.

27 Combs, *Being and Becoming,* op. cit.

28 Rogers CR. *A Way of Being.* Boston, MA: Houghton Mifflin; 1980.

29 Sue DW, Sue D. *Counseling the Culturally Different: theory and practice.* 2nd ed. New York, NY: John Wiley & Sons; 1990.

30 Rogers, 1980, op. cit.

31 Rogers, 1961, op. cit.

32 Ibid.

33 Tallman, op. cit.

34 Rogers, 1959, op. cit.

35 Ibid.

36 Rogers, 1961, op. cit.

37 Rogers, 1959, op. cit.

38 Ibid.

39 Ibid.

40 Rogers, 1980, op. cit.

41 Rogers, 1957, op. cit.

42 Ibid.

43 Rogers, 1959, op. cit.

44 Ibid.

45 Rogers, 1957, op. cit.

46 Rogers, 1961, op. cit.

47 Rogers, 1951, op. cit.

48 Rogers, 1967, op. cit.

49 Ibid.

50 Clark AJ. *Empathy in Counseling and Psychotherapy: perspective and practices.* New York, NY: Routledge/Taylor & Francis Group; 2007.

51 Cain DJ. Person-centered therapy. In: Frew J, Spiegler MD, editors. *Contemporary Psychotherapies for a Diverse World.* Boston, MA: Lahaska Press; 2008. pp. 177–227.

52 Ibid.

53 Goldfried, op. cit.

54 Wachtel PL. Carl Rogers and the larger context of therapeutic thought. *Psychotherapy: theory, research, practice, training.* 2007; **44**(3): 279–84.

55 Watson JC. Reassessing Rogers' necessary and sufficient conditions of change. *Psychotherapy: theory, research, practice, training.* 2007; **44**(3): 268–73.

56 Clark, op. cit.

57 Watson, op. cit.

58 Brown LS. Empathy, genuineness – and the dynamics of power: a feminist responds to Rogers. *Psychotherapy: theory, research, practice, training.* 2007; **44**(3): 257–9.

59 Elliott R, Freire E. Classical person-centered and experiential perspectives on Rogers (1957). *Psychotherapy: theory, research, practice, training.* 2007; **44**(3): 285–8.

60 Brown, op. cit.

61 Natiello P. *The Person-Centered Approach: a passionate presence.* Ross-On-Wye, UK: Ross PCCS Books; 2001.

62 Gielen UP, Draguns JG, Fish JM, editors. *Principles of Multicultural Counseling and Therapy.* New York, NY: Routledge/Taylor & Francis Group; 2008.

63 Moore C, Mathews HF, editors. *The Psychology of Cultural Experience.* Oxford, UK: Cambridge University Press; 2001.

64 Murphy-Shigematsu S. *Multicultural Encounters: case narratives from a counseling practice.* New York, NY: Teachers College Press; 2002.

65 Hsu C, Pant S. *Innovative Planning for Electronic Commerce and Enterprises: a reference model.* New York, NY: Springer Publishing; 2000.

66 Jones TS, Brinkert R. *Conflict Coaching: Conflict management strategies and skills for the individual.* Thousand Oaks, CA: Sage Publications; 2007.

67 Baxter LA, Braithwaite DO. *Engaging Theories in Interpersonal Communication: multiple perspectives.* Thousand Oaks, CA: Sage Publications; 2008.

68 Gillies RM. *Cooperative Learning: integrating theory and practice.* Thousand Oaks, CA: Sage Publications; 2007.

69 Kirschenbaum H, Henderson VL. *The Carl Rogers Reader.* Boston, MA: Houghton Mifflin; 1989.

70 Watson, op. cit.

71 Kirschenbaum, op. cit.

CHAPTER 2

Magnitude of the Problem

This (second) chapter of the book presents clinical information on SMI, i.e. major mood disorders and schizophrenia-related disorders, in order to ground an understanding of approaches to PCC for people with SMI in current biopsychosocial clinical evidence. Such grounding is important for a feasible and practical PCC. For instance, it is important to recognize cognitive impairments that commonly afflict individuals with schizophrenia and which pose ethical and other challenges to PCC for these individuals, as discussed and illustrated in chapters 1 (Framework), 5 (The Person/Patient-Provider/Clinician Relationship) and 6 (Management and Finding Common Ground) of this book. It is also important to recognize opportunities that PCC raises for people with SMI, such as addressing stigma and other environmental as well as personal barriers, which impact on course and outcome of SMI, as discussed and illustrated in chapters 4 (Understanding the Context of the Individual) and 7 (Prevention and Health Promotion). Thus, some of the clinical facts presented in this chapter constrain PCC, yet PCC in its turn may transform clinical facts for the better if PCC for people with SMI is pursued systematically and persistently.

Section 2.1, *Mood Disorders: major depressive disorder and bipolar disorders*, describes the classification, diagnosis, epidemiology, course, outcome, postulated etiology and risk factors related to bipolar disorder and major depressive disorder. Section 2.2, *Schizophrenia-Spectrum Disorders: schizophrenia and schizoaffective disorder*, presents a similar type of description for schizophrenia and schizoaffective disorder.

2.1 Mood Disorders: major depressive disorder and bipolar disorders

Dwight Mazmanian and Verinder Sharma

INTRODUCTION

The major mood disorders are common and potentially incapacitating forms of SMI. The personal, interpersonal, social and economic costs of these disorders are immense. Major depression alone is currently a leading cause of disability, and it is expected to be the second leading cause of disability by the year 2020.[1] In this section we will present a brief overview of the classification and diagnosis of the major mood disorders, followed by a review of their prevalence, course and outcome. Finally, we will provide a brief review of risk factors and theories of etiology.

Classification and Diagnosis

Mood disorders are not recent social phenomena or cultural constructions. Early descriptions of the major types of mood abnormalities, depression and mania, and their presumed linkage, can be found in the writings of the ancient Greeks.[2] However, it was Kraepelin's work in the late 1800s and early 1900s that laid the foundations for our current understanding. As is well-known, Kraepelin was the first to distinguish dementia praecox (i.e. schizophrenia) from other psychotic (or potentially psychotic) disorders, such as mood disorders. Perhaps more importantly, he unified all major forms of recurrent mood disorders under the rubric of *manic-depressive illness*.[3] In this framework, recurrent episodes of depression, even in the absence of manic episodes, were considered a form of manic-depressive illness. All editions of the American Psychiatric Association's (APA) Diagnostic and Statistical Manual of Mental Disorders (DSM), up to and including the current edition (DSM-IV, Text Revision [TR]),[4] preserve Kraepelin's original distinction between schizophrenia and the major mood disorders. Since DSM-III, however, mood disorders have been divided into two distinct categories: bipolar disorders and unipolar disorders. As this is the most commonly-used classification system in North America, we will describe it in detail.

The DSM system is descriptive in nature and relies on concrete, observable criteria for diagnoses. Such an approach is relatively free of assumptions about etiology and theories of psychopathology. First, the diagnostic criteria for each type of mood episode are presented (i.e. major depressive, manic, mixed and hypomanic). An episode of major depression requires the presence of five or more of the following symptoms: depressed mood; loss of interest or pleasure in activities; change in weight (loss or gain) or appetite (increase or decrease); sleep disturbance (insomnia or hypersomnia); psychomotor agitation or retardation; fatigue or loss of energy; feelings of worthlessness or guilt; cognitive impairment (concentration problems, indecisiveness); or recurrent thoughts of death or suicidal ideation.[5] One of the symptoms must be *either* depressed mood *or* loss of interest or pleasure. The symptoms must be present for most of the day nearly every day during the same two-week period. The observed symptoms must also represent a distinct change from previous functioning and cause significant distress or impairment in functioning. Depression-like symptoms that are attributable to the direct physiological effects of substances (abusable substances or medication) or a general medical condition are not considered major depression. It is of interest to note that depressed mood per se (i.e., sadness or dysphoria), which is commonly believed to be the cardinal feature of depression, is not a required criterion for the diagnosis. Individuals who might be seriously depressed, but who are experiencing loss of interest or pleasure rather than depressed mood, can very often be missed and not receive appropriate treatment.

A manic episode requires a distinct period of elevated, expansive, or irritable mood for at least seven days (or a shorter period if the individual is admitted to hospital because of the mood change). During this same period, a minimum of three of the following symptoms must be present (or four if irritable mood only): "inflated self-esteem or grandiosity; decreased need for sleep; more talkative than usual or pressure of speech; flight of ideas or racing thoughts; distractibility; increased goal-directed activity, or excessive involvement in pleasurable activities that have a high potential for painful consequences".[6] The observed symptoms must cause significant impairment in functioning, or be severe enough to require hospitalization, or be accompanied by psychotic features. As is the case for an episode of depression, the observed symptoms of mania are not due to the direct physiological effects of substance or a general medical condition. A full manic episode is not something that is likely to be missed or overlooked by a mental health practitioner when it is occurring. It is possible to miss a prior manic episode when taking a history, however, as the service user may not be able to recall important aspects of the episode (perhaps due to state-dependent memory), or he or she might be too embarrassed or ashamed to report some of the behaviours – particularly those subsumed within the last criterion (e.g. sexual indiscretions, shopping sprees). Another difficulty arises when psychotic features are present during a manic episode. The immediate clinical presentation might be indistinguishable from a psychotic disorder such as paranoid schizophrenia.[7]

The third type of mood episode, mixed, requires that the diagnostic criteria be met for both a manic episode and a major depressive episode during the same seven-day period. The symptoms of mania and depression may alternate frequently. Historically, mixed states have also been described in terms of excited depressions, agitated depressions, mixed depressions, irritable-hostile depressions, or dysphoric manias,[8, 9] and many believe that the DSM-IV criteria may not capture all relevant aspects of this type of condition. As yet, there is no clear consensus on the exact terminology, nor is there consensus with respect to the various subtypes or variants of mixed states. However, there is a growing body of evidence suggesting that distinctions among the variants of mixed states might be important for understanding the underlying pathophysiology of mood disorders, predicting illness course or prognosis, and predicting response to treatment.[10, 11]

Hypomania is the fourth and last type of mood episode defined in DSM-IV. As the name suggests, hypomania is a less severe form of mania. The diagnostic criteria are essentially the same as those for mania, except that the required duration is only four days and the symptoms are *not* severe enough to cause marked impairment in functioning. In addition, a hypomanic episode does not usually necessitate hospitalization, and psychotic features are not present. Hypomania can, over the course of the episode, increase in severity and become a full manic episode. Because hypomanic episodes are "softer" or less severe than manic episodes, service users are less likely to have recognized them, and therefore less likely to report prior episodes when providing a history. Similarly, prior hypomanic episodes are frequently missed by service providers, which can result in misdiagnosis and, potentially, inappropriate treatment or treatment that is less than optimal (*see* Reference 12 for a review).

The type of initial episode and, when relevant, the types of subsequent episodes, determine the formal diagnosis and course specifiers. If one or more episodes of depression occur in the absence of a manic, mixed or hypomanic episode, the person is diagnosed with major depressive disorder, often called unipolar depression. If symptoms of depression have been present for two or more years, but the symptoms fail to meet the full criteria for an episode of major depression, a diagnosis of dysthymic disorder is given. Although it is not usually considered in the context of SMI, episodes of major depression may be superimposed on dysthymia subsequently. If the initial episode is manic, or if one or more episodes of major depression have occurred and there is a history of one or more manic or mixed episodes, the individual is diagnosed with bipolar I disorder. If one or more episodes of depression occur with a history of one or more hypomanic episodes, and if no manic or mixed episodes have ever occurred, the individual is diagnosed with bipolar II disorder. If a person experiences numerous periods with symptoms of hypomania and numerous periods with symptoms of depression over period of at least two years, but the symptoms do not meet the criteria for either hypomania or major depression, a diagnosis of cyclothymic disorder is given. As is the case with dysthymia, cyclothymia is not always considered in the context of SMIs. There is a 15–50% risk that someone with cyclothymia will eventually meet the criteria for a bipolar I or bipolar II disorder, however, so it warrants mention in this book.[13] Finally, there are diagnoses for mood disorders that are due to a general medical condition, substance-induced, or not otherwise specified.

The DSM also provides a wide range of "specifiers" to describe the current or most recent mood episode and longitudinal course in recurrent mood disorders. A mood episode can be mild, moderate, severe without psychotic features, severe with mood-congruent psychotic features, severe with mood-incongruent psychotic features, in partial remission, or in full remission. A mood episode can have catatonic features or post-partum onset. An episode of depression can be specified as chronic, or as having melancholic features or atypical features. For recurrent mood disorders, longitudinal course specifiers include "with full interepisode recovery" and "without full interepisode recovery."[14] Recurrent major depressive, bipolar I and bipolar II disorders may have a seasonal pattern specifier, and both bipolar I and bipolar II disorders may have a rapid-cycling specifier.

Using this classification system, what is commonly referred to as "postpartum depression" would be considered an episode of major depression with postpartum onset, and it could occur in the context of a major depressive disorder, a bipolar I disorder, or a bipolar II disorder. Similarly, what is commonly called "seasonal affective disorder" would be a major depressive disorder, recurrent, with seasonal pattern; or a bipolar I or II disorder, with seasonal pattern.

Although this system of classifying the mood disorders has been very useful, there are those who question this categorical approach and argue in favour of a dimensional approach, and those who question the categorical approach specifically with respect to mood disorders, particularly with respect to the validity of the bipolar-unipolar distinction in recurrent mood disorders, e.g. *see* References 15 and 16. There is also a growing body of empirical literature that directly challenges the current classification system for mood disorders. Many now argue that Kraepelin's original conceptualization of manic-depressive illness, which encompassed all forms of recurrent mood disorders, was correct. Akiskal and his colleagues speak of bipolar spectrum disorders with "hard" and "soft" phenotypes.[17] Goodwin and Jamison argue convincingly for a manic-depressive spectrum.[18] Although more research and "fine tuning" is required, a return to Kraepelin's unified formulation of manic-depressive illness, or an approach that is similar to this, might be seen in future editions of the DSM.

Occurrence, Course and Outcome

Mood disorders alone or in combination with other psychiatric conditions are among the most frequently occurring SMIs. According to DSM-IV, the lifetime risk for major depressive disorder is between 5% and 25%, with women having higher rates (10–25%) and men having lower rates (5–12%).[19] Epidemiological studies that have been conducted since 2000 have yielded lifetime prevalence rates ranging from 3–24% for major depressive disorder.[20] The DSM-IV reports lifetime prevalence rates of 0.4–1.6% for bipolar I disorder, and approximately 0.5% for bipolar II disorder. We mentioned earlier that it might be difficult to detect prior hypomanic episodes, so the *true* estimate for bipolar II disorders is likely to be higher than 0.5%. It is interesting to note that in several more recent studies using more sensitive instruments, the obtained prevalence rates for bipolar I or II disorders are higher than those reported in DSM-IV. Kessler *et al.* reported combined rates of 3.9%.[21] If one adopts a bipolar spectrum model, and if one permits the possibility of "subthreshold" hypomanic episodes that last for one to three days (as opposed to the four-day criterion DSM-IV), the estimated prevalence rates are even higher. Merikangas *et al.* reported a combined prevalence rate of 4.5% for bipolar spectrum disorders, i.e. bipolar I, bipolar II and subthreshold bipolar disorders.[22] In clinical populations, Piver *et al.* estimate that 70% of individuals with atypical depression, 50% of individuals referred to specialists with treatment-resistant depression, and 30% of individuals in primary care settings presenting with depressive or anxiety symptoms could potentially be experiencing bipolar spectrum disorders (*see also* Reference 23).[24]

It can be argued that episodes beget more episodes in mood disorders. If an individual experiences one episode of depression, there is at least a 60% chance that he or she will experience a second episode. About 70% of individuals who experience two episodes will experience a third, and 90% of individuals who experience three episodes will experience a fourth episode.[25] Individuals who experience a single manic episode have a 90% chance of experiencing future episodes, 5–10% of individuals who experience an initial episode of depression subsequently experience a manic episode,[26] and many more will experience hypomania or subthreshold hypomania.[27]

Kraepelin and others have argued that the serious recurrent mood disorders, i.e. manic-depressive illness, can be distinguished from schizophrenia on the basis of absence of cognitive impairment, and good or full inter-episode recovery. Recent evidence, however, calls these distinctions into question.[28,29,30] Many people with bipolar disorders or serious recurrent major depression experience some degree of cognitive impairment, which is present even during periods of euthymia. Many people do not experience full symptom remission between episodes, and the frequency and severity of episodes can often increase over time, leading to occupational impairment and other psychosocial difficulties. For these and other reasons, long-term functional outcomes for many people with major mood disorders might be poor.

Many people with mood disorders also have comorbid psychiatric conditions, either currently or in their lifetime. Anxiety disorders and substance-use disorders are the most common comorbid disorders in both major depressive disorders and bipolar disorders.[31,32] Completed suicide occurs in 10–15% of individuals with a major mood disorder,[33] and up to 44.5% of people with a bipolar disorder have made at least one suicide attempt.[34]

Risk Factors and Etiology

Gender is one of the most important risk factors for major depressive disorder. Women are more than twice as likely to experience major depression. Although the rates for bipolar disorders are approximately equal for men and women, women have much higher risk for the rapid-cycling variant and for mixed episodes. Family history is an important risk factor for both major depression and bipolar disorders. Having a first-degree relative with major depressive disorder increases the risk one and a half to three times. Having a first-degree relative with bipolar I disorder increases the risk of bipolar I, bipolar II and major depressive disorder. Other evidence suggests that there is an increased risk of alcohol abuse or dependence in first-degree relatives of individuals with major depressive disorder.[35] There is also evidence that negative life events, e.g. early loss events or abuse, or stressful life events in adulthood, may increase the risk of major depression.[36] In bipolar disorders, stressful life events are often associated with episode onset, particularly for initial or early episodes.[37] Work-related or stress-related sleep loss, or major reproductive events like childbirth, may play a very important – perhaps causal – role in episode onset.[38,39] The extent to which other forms of stressful life events are truly causal in the etiology of major depression or bipolar disorders, or causal in episode onset, remains open to question. Methodological problems limit the interpretability of many findings, and it is particularly difficult to establish the temporal antecedence of such putative causes. It is possible, for instance, that prodromal or subthreshold symptoms of depression could create interpersonal difficulties or relationship loss. Similarly, subthreshhold symptoms of mania could create a variety of life stresses, such as financial problems, trouble at work or relationship difficulties. Considerably more highly controlled longitudinal research is needed in this area.

Despite over a century of research, we still do not know the exact causes of either major depressive disorder or bipolar disorders. There has been no shortage of theories, however, particularly in the case of major depressive disorder. Many theories of major depressive disorder have met with only partial success, i.e. these theories are useful descriptively, but not etiologically. Although fewer theories have been proposed for bipolar disorders, a number have proven very useful, e.g. *see* Reference 40. Perhaps the most important work on the causes of bipolar disorders over the last 10 years has been in genetics and neurodevelopment.[41,42,43] There is growing evidence that the distinction between schizophrenia and bipolar disorder might not be as firm as was originally thought. The two disorders appear to have a common genetic basis. Additional genes and factors affecting neurodevelopment may alter, i.e. increase, the risk of schizophrenia for certain individuals.

CONCLUSION

We have presented a broad overview of the major mood disorders. They are quite properly considered forms of SMI, and they present some practical and philosophical challenges to those working from a person-centered approach. On the other hand, person-centered approaches may provide a fundamental basis for accurate assessment and effective treatment.

Authors' Note: we wish to thank Missy Teatero for her helpful comments and suggestions.

REFERENCES

1 Murray C, Lopez A. Alternative projections of mortality and disability by cause, 1990–2020: Global Burden of Disease Study. *Lancet.* 1997; **349**(9064): 1498–504.
2 Goodwin FK, Jamison KR. *Manic-Depressive Illness: bipolar disorders and recurrent depression.* 2nd ed. New York, NY: Oxford University Press; 2007.

3 Kraepelin E. *Manic-Depressive Insanity and Paranoia.* Edinburgh: E. & S. Livingstone; 1921.

4 American Psychiatric Association. *Diagnostic and Statistical Manual of Mental Disorders, 4th Edition, Text-Revised (DSM-IV-TR).* Washington, DC: American Psychiatric Association; 2000.

5 Ibid, p. 456.

6 American Psychiatric Association, op. cit, p. 362.

7 Goodwin, 2007, op. cit.

8 Ibid.

9 Kraepelin, op. cit.

10 Benazzi F, Koukopoulos A, Akiskal HS. Toward a validation of a new definition of agitated depression as a bipolar mixed state (mixed depression). Eur Psychiatry. 2004; 19(2): 85–90.

11 Maj M, Pirozzi R, Magliano L, *et al.* Agitated depression in bipolar I disorder: prevalence, phenomenology, and outcome. *Am J Psychiatry.* 2003; 160(12): 2134–40.

12 Piver A, Yatham L, Lam R. Bipolar spectrum disorders: new perspectives. *Can Fam Physician.* 2002; 48; 896–904.

13 American Psychiatric Association, op. cit.

14 Ibid, p. 425.

15 Goodwin, 2007, op. cit.

16 Widiger T, Samuel D. Diagnostic categories or dimensions? A question for the Diagnostic and Statistical Manual of Mental Disorders – Fifth Edition. *J Abnorm Psychol.* 2005; 114(4): 494–504.

17 Akiskal H. Validating "hard" and "soft" phenotypes within the bipolar spectrum: continuity or discontinuity? *J Affect Disord.* 2003; 73(1): 1–5.

18 Goodwin, 2007, op. cit.

19 Ibid, p. 372.

20 Goodwin R, Jacobi F, Bittner A, *el al.* Epidemiology of mood disorders. In: Stein DJ, Kupfer DJ, Schatzberg AF, editors. *Textbook of Mood Disorders.* Washington, DC: American Psychiatric Publishing; 2006. pp. 33–54.

21 Kessler R, Berglund P, Demler O, *et al.* Lifetime prevalence and age-of-onset distributions of *DSM-IV* disorders in the National Comorbidity Survey Replication. *Arch Gen Psychiatry.* 2005; 62(6): 593–602.

22 Merikangas K, Akiskal H, Angst J, *et al.* Lifetime and 12-month prevalence of bipolar spectrum disorder in the National Comorbidity Survey Replication. *Arch Gen Psychiatry.* 2007; 64(5): 543–52.

23 Sharma V, Khan M, Smith A. A closer look at treatment resistant depression: is it due to a bipolar diathesis? *J Affect Disord.* 2005; 4(2–3): 251–7.

24 Piver, op. cit.

25 American Psychiatric Association, op. cit.

26 Ibid.

27 Piver, op. cit.

28 Green MF. Cognitive impairment and functional outcome in schizophrenia and bipolar disorder. *J Clin Psychiatry.* 2006; 67(Suppl. 9: 3–8): discussion 36–42.

29 Mur M, Portella M, Martinez-Aran A, *et al.* Long-term stability of cognitive impairment in bipolar disorder: a 2-year follow-up study of lithium-treated euthymic bipolar patients. *J Clin Psychiatry.* 2008; 69(5): 712–19.

30 Hammar A, Lund A, Hugdahl K. Long-lasting cognitive impairment in unipolar major depression: a 6-month follow-up study. *Psychiatric Res.* 2003; **118**(2): 189–96.

31 Goodwin, 2007, op. cit.

32 Goodwin, 2006, op. cit.

33 American Psychiatric Association, op. cit.

34 Goodwin, 2007, op. cit.

35 American Psychiatric Association, op. cit.

36 Goodwin, 2006, op. cit.

37 Goodwin, 2007, op. cit.

38 Ibid.

39 Sharma V, Mazmanian D. Sleep loss and postpartum psychosis. *Bipolar Disord.* 2003; **5**(2): 98–105.

40 Post RM. Transduction of psychosocial stress into the neurobiology of recurrent affective disorder. *Am J Psychiatry.* 1992; **149**(8): 999–1010.

41 Ferreira M, O'Donovan MC, Meng Y, *et al.* Collaborative genome-wide association analysis supports a role for ANK3 and CACNA1C in bipolar disorder. *Nat Genet.* 2008; **40**(9): 1056–8.

42 Murray RM, Sham P, Van Os J, *et al.* A developmental model for similarities and dissimilarities between schizophrenia and bipolar disorder. *Schizophrenia Research.* 2004; **71**(2); 405–16.

43 O'Donovan MC, Craddock N, Norton N, *et al.* Identification of loci associated with schizophrenia by genome-wide association and follow-up. *Nat Genet.* 2008; **40**(9): 1053–5.

2.2 Schizophrenia-Spectrum Disorders: schizophrenia and schizoaffective disorder

Priya Subramanian

INTRODUCTION

Schizophrenia-spectrum disorders are common and arguably the most serious and enduring of mental illnesses, with schizophrenia taking a place among the 10 most disabling disorders in the world.[1] This section will review the epidemiology, current etiological theories, diagnosis, course and outcome of schizophrenia and highlight schizoaffective disorders as a spectrum in the continuum between mood disorders and schizophrenia.

Classification and Diagnosis

Although the term itself is only 100 years old, having been first coined by Eugen Bleuler in 1908, descriptions of schizophrenia can be found in writings as early as in Mesopotamia in the 3rd millennium BC and in ancient India, Greece and Rome.[2] In modern history, it was Emil Kraepelin who first described schizophrenia in 1887 and distinguished between *dementia praecox*, which was later termed schizophrenia, and *manic depressive psychosis*, although he later recanted this distinction.[3] Sadly, this period in history has also been fraught with examples of mistreatment of the mentally ill, not least those diagnosed with schizophrenia being subject to death on the grounds of eugenics.[4]

Kurt Schneider described symptoms of *first rank* that purportedly distinguish schizophrenia from other mental illnesses.[5] These include audible thoughts, voices heard arguing, voices heard commenting on one's actions, experience of influences on the body, thought withdrawal, thought insertion, thought diffusion and delusional perception. Although their specificity to schizophrenia has been reviewed recently with an inconclusive outcome,[6] many of these symptoms have been incorporated into the two current major classification systems, the World Health Organization's (WHO) International Statistical Classification of Diseases and Related Health Problems (ICD 10)[7] and the DSM IV-TR.[8] Both systems classify and categorize the disorder based on observable phenomena and reports by the individual and/or significant others.

The DSM IV-TR requires three criteria to be met in order to satisfy a diagnosis of schizophrenia. First, at least two of the following need to be present: delusions, hallucinations, disorganized speech, grossly disorganized or catatonic behavior and negative symptoms. Second, there must be social and occupational decline compared to pre-morbid functioning, for a significant period of time since the onset of illness. Third, the disturbance should persist for a minimum of six months, which can include prodromal changes.

The ICD 10 also lists similar criteria for the diagnosis of schizophrenia. Of note, while the duration of at least one month specified for the presence of symptoms appears to be significantly different from that in the DSM IV-TR, it is to be noted that this period is only for specific symptoms listed as major criteria and excludes prodromal changes. Both classification systems clarify that a diagnosis of schizophrenia should not be made in the presence of dominant manic or depressive symptoms, overt brain disease and states of intoxication or withdrawal. Based on the presentation (*see* below), the disorder can be further classified under the following subtypes. In the DSM IV, these subtypes are paranoid, disorganized, catatonic, undifferentiated or residual.[9] The ICD 10 contains two other subtypes, simple schizophrenia and post-schizophrenic depression.[10]

As per the DSM IV-TR criteria, both criteria for mood disorder as well schizophrenia need to be met to satisfy a diagnosis of schizoaffective disorder. However, psychotic symptoms should be present without affective symptoms for at least two weeks for the diagnosis to be made. While schizophrenia, schizoaffective and mood disorders have been considered part of a spectrum, in clinical practice there is often varying overlap between mood and psychotic symptoms within a diagnostic category of schizoaffective disorder. It has been argued therefore, that schizoaffective disorder is in itself a spectrum, and a dimensional approach to understanding this spectrum has been proposed as more accommodating of the relevant clinical complexity of presentations.[11]

Occurrence, Course and Outcome

The incidence of schizophrenia when narrowly defined varies between 7.7 and 43 per 100,000. It is slightly more common in men and in those born or living in urban environments.[12] The lifetime prevalence of schizophrenia is traditionally quoted as 0.5–1%. A more recent review suggested a similar value of four per 1000.[13]

The varied presentations in schizophrenia are often described as clusters of symptoms. Positive symptoms, such as hallucinations, delusions and disorganized thinking; and negative symptoms, such as avolition, alogia, anhedonia and apathy, characterize schizophrenia.[14] Other less-known common presentations include affective symptoms, such as depression and mania, motor symptoms, such as catatonic agitation or stupor, and cognitive impairments, such as deficits in attention, working memory, planning and organization. Studies on social cognition in individuals with schizophrenia have shown deficits in the "Theory of Mind,"[15] the ability to reflect upon one's own and other persons' mental states.[16] More recently, researchers have taken a renewed interest in the cognitive-perceptive "basic symptoms" of schizophrenia, defined as subclinical disturbances in drive, affect, thinking, speech, perception, motor action, central vegetative functions and stress tolerance.[17,18] Recognition of these symptoms has been identified as a means of addressing early detection, treatment adherence, remission and relapse prevention.[19]

Although many hypotheses have been propounded to explain the etiology of schizophrenia, this is perhaps best understood through a multi-factorial causation

model that incorporates biological, psychological and social predisposing, precipitating, protective and perpetuating factors.

Biological explanations aim to model schizophrenia as a neurological disease
and attempt to reduce societal and self stigma in the process. Genetic studies have
identified many susceptibility loci and candidate genes, only a few of which have
been replicated consistently. In a recent review of genetic linkage studies, dyso-
brevin binding protein (DTNBP1) and neuregulin (NRG1) have been strongly
implicated as susceptibility loci, and the evidence implicating catechol-o-methyl
transferase (COMT), regulator of G protein signalling-4 (RGS4), gene30/gene72
and D-amino acid oxidase (DAO/DAAO) as promising but not yet compelling
findings.[20] Genetic factors alone are neither necessary nor sufficient to produce
schizophrenia, and interplay between genes and the environment is believed to be
a better explanatory model. Complications during pregnancy and childbirth remain
one of the best-replicated risk factors for schizophrenia but the nature and strength
of the association are unclear.[21] Viral exposure of the fetus to influenza and toxo-
plasmosis, malnutrition[22,23] and vitamin D deficiency[24] in the prenatal period have
been postulated in the pathogenesis of schizophrenia.

Neurotransmitter imbalance theories identify serotonin, gamma-aminobutyric
acid (GABA), glutamate, acetylcholine and perhaps the most popular and well-
researched thus far, dopamine, as causative factors. The dopamine hypothesis postulates that an excess of dopamine in the sub-cortical regions is associated with positive
symptoms and a deficit of dopamine in the cortical regions with negative symptoms
and cognitive impairments.[25] This hypothesis has its basis in three key observations:
first, drugs that stimulate dopamine activity in the sub-cortical regions can mimic
symptoms of schizophrenia; second, dopamine antagonist can reduce these symptoms; and third, dopamine depletion in the cortex has shown to induce cognitive
deficits. (For a more detailed review of the dopamine hypothesis, *see* Reference 26.)

The neuro-developmental model of schizophrenia integrates findings related
to post-mortem neural abnormalities in cell migration, cell proliferation, axonal
outgrowth, myelination, synaptogenesis and apoptosis with structural and functional imaging evidence.[27] An alternative neurodegenerative model has also been
proposed[28] but has been critiqued[29] because in addition to lack of evidence for cell
death, there has also been a lack of evidence from longitudinal studies for decline
in cognitive function in most individuals with schizophrenia.

Psychoanalytic theory postulates a weakness or deficiency in ego-strength and
ego-functioning[30,31] in individuals with schizophrenia affecting areas such as reality
testing, personal adequacy and vitality, moral posture and emotional spontaneity.[32]
There is, as yet, no evidence for such psychodynamic factors as causative. Cognitive
models postulate that pre-existing beliefs and ongoing appraisals of experiences are
crucial for the development and persistence of positive symptoms of psychosis, and
that stress triggers particular emotional and cognitive changes, resulting in anomalies of conscious experience.[33] Both anomalies from deficits in moment-by-moment
integration of new input with stored memories[34] and anomalies in self-monitoring[35]
have been hypothesized.

Substance use disorders (SUDs) are a frequent co-morbid finding in individuals with schizophrenia, with nearly 50% having a lifetime history of SUDs, not including nicotine and caffeine.[36] Brain dopaminergic pathways have been thought to be a common underlying mediator for both SUDs and schizophrenia. The effect of the underlying neuropathology of schizophrenia on neuronal circuitry mediating drug reward and reinforcement may contribute to the increased vulnerability of these individuals to substance use.[37] It has also been noted that individuals with schizophrenia have as much as a 40% chance of worsening or induced psychotic symptoms as compared to 0% in healthy controls after a single exposure to amphetamine, supporting the suggestion that a direct relationship exists between dopamine release and psychosis.[38] In a recent meta-analysis by Koskinen *et al.* of cannabis use disorder in schizophrenia, as much as 25% of the sample had this diagnosis.[39] Furthermore, it was more common in males, in younger age and in first episode psychosis. Cannabis use has been associated with an increased risk of psychotic disorders, but a causal link has not yet been strongly established.[40] Although it has been suggested that cannabis use in individuals with schizophrenia may be related to its pharmacologically beneficial effects in the mediation of stress,[41] a recent Cochrane database review found insufficient evidence to support or refute the use of cannabis or cannabinoid compounds for individuals with schizophrenia.[42] Nicotine addiction is another commonly observed phenomenon in individuals with schizophrenia, and it has been postulated that this is related to a deficiency in the numbers and functioning of nicotinic receptors. Self-medication with nicotine may be a response to the improved cognitive function that is shown to occur with nicotine.[43]

Psychosocial factors that have been postulated and studied as etiological in schizophrenia include childhood trauma, high negative expressed emotion (EE) and migration. Childhood trauma has been linked to schizophrenia, although the evidence for this link being causative is controversial.[44] High negative EE, that is, high levels of criticism, emotional over-involvement, or hostility within the familial environment has been shown to be associated with a higher risk of relapse of schizophrenia.[45] It is also known that immigrants have a higher risk of developing schizophrenia, and this association is not explained by diagnostic bias or selective migration, which suggests it may be related to the psychological and social stresses of moving to a foreign environment.[46] Schizophrenia is increasingly conceptualized through a stress-vulnerability model: a combination of underlying genetic susceptibility and environmental influences that determines who develops the disorder.

Traditionally, schizophrenia has been thought to be a chronically relapsing illness. This earlier conceptualization has been replaced in recent years by a more optimistic view, based on a number of rigorous, longitudinal studies conducted around the world that found the long-term outcome of schizophrenia was heterogeneous, with 46–68% achieving significant improvement and often even full recovery across time.[47] Operational criteria for a positive course has varied and includes a focus on symptom remission with an emphasis on the duration and intensity of symptoms;[48] and functional recovery,[49] which focuses on form of productive activity such as work and school, self-care and community living and social-leisure functioning.

Finally, there has also been a focus on recovery as a subjective experience,[50,51] with an emphasis on hope and sustaining a positive identity despite the illness.

A relevant study in the area of outcome in individuals with schizophrenia is that by Harrow and Jobe.[52] In this study, two cohorts, one with a DSM-III diagnosis of schizophrenia and one without were assessed at admission and two years, four and a half years, seven and a half years, 10 years, 15 years and 20 years after hospital discharge. Nearly 40% of the individuals in the schizophrenia cohort were not on antipsychotic medication at the 15-year follow-up period. In the same follow-up period, 5% of individuals on antipsychotic medication and 40% of those not on antipsychotic medication met criteria for recovery, operationally defined as the absence of positive and negative symptoms throughout the follow-up year and adequate psychosocial functioning. The subgroup of those not on antipsychotic medication at 15-year follow-up were different in terms of having a significant internal locus of control, higher self-esteem and better prognostic factors at initial assessment (poor prognostic factors assessed prospectively in this study included no acute onset, no precipitating stress at index, poor work and social adjustment before index, no preoccupation with death, the absence of depressive symptoms, no confusion, no guilt, being unmarried and blunted affect). The authors suggest that a subgroup of individuals with schizophrenia who have good prognostic features, better pre-morbid developmental achievements and more favorable personality characteristics are more likely to stay off antipsychotic medication and be in recovery for a prolonged period. Interestingly, only just over half of those in the schizophrenia cohort had chronic or frequent delusional activity over the 20-year period, and over 25% of individuals had no delusional activity at any of the six follow-up periods.[53] Other positive prognostic factors not highlighted above include a short duration of untreated psychosis,[54] female gender[55] and lack of mood incongruence.

In the five-year follow-up point of the Danish OPUS trial, 45% of the study sample had no psychotic or negative symptoms.[56] Recovery, defined as no psychotic or negative symptoms, living independently, working or studying, was reached in 17% of individuals at two years and improved to 18% at five-year follow-up,[57] which is in accordance with previous studies[58,59] and provides evidence for the hypothesis that the course of the illness reaches a plateau after a period of time. However, the authors indicate the need for longer-term follow-up data before drawing firm conclusions about when this occurs.[60] Other outcome studies have shown that symptom remission is achieved in 25–30% of individuals with schizophrenia.

Helldin and colleagues recently published data from their longitudinal study of 242 individuals with schizophrenia, 38% of whom met criteria for cross-sectional remission.[61] The average follow-up duration in this study was five and a half years, and remission was defined as not scoring more than "mild" on eight items related to core symptoms of schizophrenia in the positive and negative syndrome scale (PANSS). Individuals who achieved cross-sectional remission required fewer subsequent specialized outpatient visits, inpatient hospitalization stays and need for sheltered living compared those who did not achieve remission.

Additional factors that play a key role in functional outcomes for individuals with schizophrenia are disempowerment and internalized stigma. Disempowerment can be viewed as a reduced sense of mastery over one's own life or also as an external locus of control. Internalized stigma may be due to one's acceptance of the stereotyped roles of a mentally ill person. Both these can contribute to worsened functional outcomes in individuals with schizophrenia.[62] Recent studies in schizophrenia suggest that external factors can affect cognitive stigma stress appraisal. Improvement in societal stigma can therefore influence internalized stigma and rejection sensitivity and may therefore determine outcome.[63]

It has been consistently reported that there is an excess of mortality in individuals with schizophrenia, and this can be attributed to both natural causes such as co-morbid somatic problems and unnatural causes such as suicide. A recent meta-analysis by Saha *et al.*[64] estimated that individuals with schizophrenia have a standardized mortality ratio (SMR) of 2.5; that is, compared to the general population those with schizophrenia have a two-and-a-half times higher rate of dying. Interestingly, the SMR is lowest in countries that are least developed and highest in those with most economic development. Warner, in his recent review, postulates that this may be due to a combination of increased rates of recovery and inclusive social conditions such as family support in the developing world.[65] The universality of improved recovery in the developing world as compared to the developed world has been criticized by other researches (for a detailed review, *see* Reference 66).

Saha also revealed that suicide was up to 12 times greater, although the risk was no different between males and females.[67] Suicide is more common in the initial stages of the schizophrenia, and a recent meta-analysis estimated its lifetime risk as 4.9%, which is lower than the 10% risk traditionally reported.[68] However, suicide is clustered in younger individuals and during the onset of schizophrenia with its risk reducing as the illness progresses. The rate of violent behavior is somewhat higher than in the general population, but this is only for violent physical behavior and not for violent sexual behavior.[69] Moreover, this can be predicted by factors such as co-morbid substance misuse,[70,71] non-adherence with treatment,[72] hostility and lack of insight.[73]

Although work has been traditionally believed to be a contributory stressor that worsens clinical outcomes for individuals for schizophrenia, this is not supported by research findings. In fact, being engaged in paid employment has been shown to increase empowerment and meaning, and promote recovery.[74] Employment outcomes such as rate of employment, time to obtaining the first work placement and duration of employment in individuals with schizophrenia are improved significantly with the Individual Placement and Support (IPS) model of SE.[75]

CONCLUSION

In summary, schizophrenia is a commonly occurring SMI with many candidate hypotheses about its etiology, pathogenesis and pathophysiology. It may form one end of a spectrum of mental illnesses that have affective and psychotic symptoms. Its course and outcome are varied, but the evidence supports the view that a large proportion of individuals with schizophrenia attain recovery, and a considerable proportion of individuals attain remission, with or without antipsychotic medication. Some prognostic indicators may predict which individuals are likely to have better functional outcomes, although prognosis itself can be improved by non-clinical interventions such as reducing stigma, increasing empowerment and assisting individuals in identifying, securing and maintain meaningful employment. This makes schizophrenia a truly complex and challenging, yet promising, area of research and clinical practice, complicated further by the need to provide care in a person-centered, empowering manner.

REFERENCES

1 World Health Organization. *World Health Report 2001 – Mental Health: new understanding, new hope.* Geneva: World Health Organization; 2001.
2 Jeste DV, del Carmen R, Lohr JB, *et al.* Did schizophrenia exist before the eighteenth century? *Compr Psychiatry.* 1985; **26**(6), 493–503.
3 Greene T. The Kraepelinian dichotomy: the twin pillars crumbling? *Hist Psychiatry.* 2007; **18**(3), 361–79.
4 Lifton RJ. *The Nazi Doctors: medical killing and the psychology of genocide.* New York, NY: Basic Books Inc; 2000.
5 Schneider K. *Clinical Psychopathology.* New York, NY: Grune & Stratton; 1959.
6 Nordgaard J, Arnfred SM, Handest P, *et al.* The diagnostic status of first rank symptoms. *Schizophr Bull.* 2008; **34**(1): 137–54.
7 World Health Organization. *The ICD-10 Classification of Mental and Behavioral Disorder.* Geneva: World Health Organization; 1992.
8 American Psychiatric Association. Schizophrenia. *Diagnostic and Statistical Manual of Mental Disorders, 4th Edition, Text-Revised (DSM-IV-TR).* Washington, DC: American Psychiatric Association; 2000.
9 Ibid.
10 World Health Organization, op. cit.
11 Peralta V, Cuesta M. Exploring the borders of the schizoaffective spectrum: a categorical and dimensional approach. *J Affect Disord.* 2008; **108**: 71–86.
12 McGrath JJ. (2006). Variations in the incidence of schizophrenia: data versus dogma. *Schizophr Bull.* 2006; **32**(1): 195–7.
13 McGrath J, Saha S, Chant D, *et al.* Schizophrenia: a concise overview of incidence, prevalence, and mortality. *Epidemiol Rev.* 2008; **30**: 67–76.
14 American Psychiatric Association, op. cit.
15 Ang GK, Pridmore S. Theory of mind and psychiatry: an introduction. *Australas Psychiatry.* 2009; **17**(2): 117–22.
16 Frith U, Frith CD. Development and neurophysiology of mentalizing. *Philos Trans R Soc Lond B Biol Sci.* 2003; **358**: 459–73.
17 Gross G. The 'basic' symptoms of schizophrenia. *Br J Psychiatry.* 1989; **7**(Suppl.): 21–5.
18 Huber G, Gross G. The concept of basic symptoms in schizophrenic and schizoaffective psychoses. *Recenti Prog Med.* 1989; **80**: 646–52.
19 Schultze-Lutter F. Subjective symptoms of schizophrenia in research and the clinic: the basic symptom concept. *Schizophr Bull.* 2009; **35**(1): 5–8.

20 O'Donovan MC, Williams NM, Owen MJ. Recent advances in the genetics of schizophrenia. *Hum Mol Genet.* 2003; **12**(Review Issue 2): R125–33.

21 Clarke MC, Harley M, Cannon M. The role of obstetric events in schizophrenia. *Schizophr Bull.* 2006; **32**(1): 3–8.

22 Susser E, Neugebauer R, Hoek HW, *et al.* Schizophrenia after prenatal famine: further evidence. *Arch Gen Psychiatry.* 1996; **53**: 25–31.

23 Xu M-Q, Sun W-S, Liu B-X, *et al.* Prenatal malnutrition and adult schizophrenia: further evidence from the 1959–1961 Chinese famine. *Schizophr Bull.* 2009; **35**(3): 568–76.

24 Kinney DK, Teixeira P, Hsu D, *et al.* Relation of schizophrenia prevalence to latitude, climate, fish consumption, infant mortality, and skin color: a role for prenatal vitamin d deficiency and infections? *Schizophr Bull.* 2009; **35**(3): 582–95.

25 Davis KL, Kahn RS, Ko G, *et al.* Dopamine in schizophrenia: a review and reconceptualization. *Am J Psychiatry.* 1991; **148**: 1474–86.

26 Abi-Dargham A. Do we still believe in the dopamine hypothesis? New data bring new evidence. *Int J Neuropsychopharmacol.* 2004; **7**(Suppl. 1): S1–5.

27 Fatemi SH, Folsom TD. The neurodevelopmental hypothesis of schizophrenia, revisited. *Schizophr Bull.* 2009; **35**(3): 528–48.

28 Lieberman JA. Is schizophrenia a neurodegenerative disorder? A clinical and neurobiological perspective. *Biol Psychiatry.* 1999; **46**(6): 729–39.

29 Weinberger DR, McClure RK. Neurotoxicity, neuroplasticity, and magnetic resonance imaging morphometry: what is happening in the schizophrenic brain? *Arch Gen Psychiatry.* 2002; **59**: 553–8.

30 Federn P. *Ego Psychology and the Psychoses.* Weiss E, editor. New York, NY: Basic Books; 1952.

31 Roazen P. *Brother Animal.* New York, NY: Knopf; 1969.

32 Bellak L, Hurvich M, Gediman H. *Ego Functions in Schizophrenics, Neurotics, and Normals.* New York, NY: Wiley; 1973.

33 Garety PA, Bebbington P, Fowler D, *et al.* Implications for neurobiological research of cognitive models of psychosis: a theoretical paper. *Psychol Med.* 2007; **37**(10): 1377–91.

34 Hemsley DR. The schizophrenic experience: taken out of context? *Schizophr Bull.* 2005; **31**: 43–53.

35 Frith C. The neural basis of hallucinations and delusions. *C R Biol.* 2005; **328**: 169–75.

36 Swofford CD, Scheller-Gilkey G, Miller AH, *et al.* Double jeopardy: schizophrenia and substance use. *Am J Drug Alcohol Abuse.* 2000; **26**: 343–53.

37 Chambers RA, Krystal JH, Self DW. A neurobiological basis for substance abuse comorbidity in schizophrenia. *Biol Psychiatry.* 2001; **50**: 71–83.

38 Abi-Dargham, op. cit.

39 Koskinen J, Löhönen J, Koponen H, *et al.* Rate of cannabis use disorders in clinical samples of patients with schizophrenia: a meta-analysis. *Schizophr Bull.* Epub 22 April 2009; **36**(6): 1115–30. Available at: http://schizophreniabulletin.oxfordjournals.org/cgi/reprint/sbp031 (accessed 30 April 2011).

40 Hall W, Degenhardt L. Cannabis use and the risk of developing a psychotic disorder. *World Psychiatry.* 2008; **7**(2): 68–71.

41 Koskinen, op. cit.

42 Rathbone J, Variend H, Mehta H. Cannabis and schizophrenia. *Cochrane Database of Systematic Reviews.* 2008; (3): Article CD004837.

43 Rezvani AH, Levin ED. Cognitive effects of nicotine. *Biol Psychiatry.* 2001; **49**(3): 258–67.

44 Morgan C, Fisher H. Environmental factors in schizophrenia: childhood trauma – a critical review. *Schizophr Bull.* 2007; **33**(1): 3–10.

45 Butzlaff RL, Hooley JM. Expressed emotion and psychiatric relapse. *Arch Gen Psychiatry.* 1998; **55**(6): 547–52.

46 Cantor-Graae E, Selten J-P. Schizophrenia and migration: a meta-analysis and review. *Am J Psychiatry.* 2005; **162**: 12–24.

47 Ciompi L, Harding CM, Lehtinen K. Deep concern. *Schizophr Bull.* 2010; **36**(3): 437–9.

48 Andreasen NC, Carpenter WT, Kane JM, *et al.* Remission in schizophrenia: proposed criteria and rationale for consensus. *Am J Psychiatry*; 2005: **162**: 441–9.

49 Harvey PD, Bellack AS. Toward a terminology for functional recovery in schizophrenia: is functional remission a viable concept? *Schizophr Bull.* 2009; **35**: 300–6.

50 Anthony WA. Recovery from mental illness: the guiding vision of the mental health service system in the 1990s. *Psychosoc Rehabil J.* 1993; **16**(4): 11–23.

51 Deegan PE. Recovery: the lived experience of rehabilitation. *Psychosoc Rehabil J.* 1988; **9**(4): 11–19.

52 Harrow M, Jobe TH. Factors involved in outcome and recovery in schizophrenia patients not on antipsychotic medications: a 15-year multi-follow-up study. *J Nerv Ment Dis.* 2007; **195**(5): 406–14.

53 Harrow M, Jobe TH. How frequent is chronic multiyear delusional activity and recovery in schizophrenia: a 20-year multi-follow-up. *Schizophr Bull.* Epub 2008 Jul 9; **36**(1): 192–204. Available at: http://schizophreniabulletin.oxfordjournals.org/cgi/reprint/sbn074 (accessed 30 April 2011).

54 Perkins DO, Gu H, Boteva K. Relationship between duration of untreated psychosis and outcome in first-episode schizophrenia: a critical review and meta-analysis. *Am J Psychiatry.* 2005; **162**: 1785–804.

55 Grossman LS, Harrow M, Rosen C, *et al.* Sex differences in schizophrenia and other psychotic disorders: a 20-year longitudinal study of psychosis and recovery. *Compr Psychiatry.* 2008; **49**(6): 523–9.

56 Bertelsen M, Jeppesen P, Petersen L, *et al.* Course of illness in a sample of 265 patients with first-episode psychosis – five-year follow-up of the Danish OPUS trial. *Schizophrenia Res.* 2009; **107**: 173–8.

57 Ibid.

58 Harrison G, Hopper K, Craig T, *et al.* Recovery from psychotic illness: a 15- and 25-year international follow-up study. *Br J Psychiatry.* 2001; **178**(6): 506–17.

59 Jobe TH, Harrow M. Long-term outcome of patients with schizophrenia: a review. *Can J Psychiatry.* 2005; **50**(14): 892–900.

60 Grossman, op. cit.

61 Helldin L, Kane JM, Hjärthag F, Norlander T. The importance of cross-sectional remission in schizophrenia for long-term outcome: a clinical prospective study. *Schizophr Res.* 2009 Nov; **115**(1): 67–73. Epub 2009 Aug 8.

62 Warner R. Recovery from schizophrenia and the recovery model. *Curr Opin Psychiatry.* 2009; **22**(4): 374–80.

63 Rüsch N, Corrigan PW, Wassel A, *et al.* A stress-coping model of mental illness stigma: I. predictors of cognitive stress appraisal. *Schizophr Res.* 2009; **110**(1–3): 59–64.

64 Saha S, Chant D, McGrath J. A systematic review of mortality in schizophrenia: is the differential mortality gap worsening over time? *Arch Gen Psychiatry.* 2007; **64**(10): 1123–31.

65 Warner, op. cit.

66 Ibid.

67 Saha, op. cit.

68 Palmer BA, Pankratz VS, Bostwick JM. The lifetime risk of suicide in schizophrenia: a re-examination. *Arch Gen Psychiatry*. 2005; **62**(3): 247–53.

69 Soyka M, Graz C, Bottlender R, *et al*. Clinical correlates of later violence and criminal offences in schizophrenia. *Schizophr Res*. 2007; **94**: 89–98.

70 Swanson J, Estroff S, Swartz M, *et al*. Violence and severe mental disorder in clinical and community populations: the effects of psychotic symptoms, comorbidity, and lack of treatment. *Psychiatry*. 1997; **60**(1): 1–22.

71 Soyka M. Substance misuse, psychiatric disorder and violent and disturbed behaviour. *Brit J Psychiatry*. 2000; **176**: 345–50.

72 Arango C, Calcedo BA, Gonzalez S, *et al*. Violence in inpatients with schizophrenia: a prospective study. *Schizophr Bull*. 1999; **25**(3): 493–503.

73 Soyka, op. cit.

74 Dunn EC, Wewiorski NJ, Rogers ES. The meaning and importance of employment to people in recovery from serious mental illness: results of a qualitative study. *Psychiatr Rehabil J*. 2008; **32**: 59–62.

75 Bond GR. An update on randomized controlled trials of evidence-based supported employment. *Psychiatr Rehabil J*. 2008; **31**: 280–90.

CHAPTER 3

The Person's Experience of the Illness

This (third) chapter of the book presents aspects of the viewpoint of the person with SMI, who is of primary importance in PCC. This viewpoint is of course multiple, as in practice if not by definition each person (with or without SMI) has a distinct viewpoint, both in relation to PCC as well as other care in general. Thus, the issues addressed in this chapter of the book inform and inspire all other chapters of the book, and set example standards of PCC for the remaining chapters of the book.

Section 3.1, *The Lived Experience: narratives through the lens of wellness*, explores the "lived experience" of people with SMI and their narratives. The section encourages providers to better understand how to help persons with mental illness (service users) to share their lived experience through the lens of wellness. Section 3.2, *The Relationship between the Person with a Serious Mental Illness and His or Her Disorder*, attempts to shed light on the complex relation between the sense of self of persons with SMI and their SMI (or sense of it). The section discusses some of the implications of this relation for PCC.

3.1 The Lived Experience: narratives through the lens of wellness

Margaret Swarbrick

INTRODUCTION

There is a renewed hope and optimism regarding the prospect of living with a mental illness. There is a growing recognition that much can be learned from the personal accounts of these individuals. Personal struggles, challenges and triumphs of persons living with mental illness have influenced mental health practice in terms of the design, delivery and evaluation of services. Professional publications such as the *Psychiatric Rehabilitation Journal, Psychiatric Services,* and *Schizophrenia Bulletin* now include first-person accounts as part of their regular range of reading options. In recent years there has been a growing number of personal accounts of the lived experience that seem to offer useful information to move the mental health field towards a recovery orientation.[1,2] In addition, qualitative research approaches that explore the lived experience provide rich data to better understand factors, interactions, interventions and environments that can foster recovery.[3,4,5,6] Based on my personal and professional experiences, I believe that *narratives* of the lived experience offer important information that can make a tremendous impact on relationships, services and ultimately outcomes.

This section will demonstrate the "lived experience" and encourage providers to better understand how to help persons living with mental illness (service users) to share their lived experience through the lens of wellness. This section will demonstrate how illness and recovery are perceived, or experienced, by an individual, and how providers can skillfully explore the "lived experience" to better design and deliver services. This section is divided into: Experience Defined; Illness and Stigma; Beyond a Diagnosis and Label; Narratives from the Lens of Wellness; Voices of Recovery; and Suggestions for Providers and Organizations.

Experience Defined

The first-hand lived experience can provide insightful lessons for service users and their supporters. The term "experience" comprises knowledge of, skill in, or observation of some one thing or some event gained through involvement in or exposure to that thing or event. With regard to the experience of mental illness, exposure and involvement are gained by virtue of having experienced mental health challenges and having been diagnosed with a mental disorder; and, subsequently, experience comes from coping with the signs, symptoms and resulting sequelae of that disorder. This includes stigma and dealing with the service system itself, as is also addressed in other sections in this book, such as Section 4.3, *Environmental Interventions in Relation to People with Serious Mental Illness,* (including in relation to stigma) and Section 4.4, *Mental Health Systems and Policy in Relation to People with Serious Mental Illness*. Knowledge that is based on experience is sometimes called "empirical knowledge," or "*a posteriori* knowledge." Someone who has considerable experience in a certain field generally earns the reputation as an expert in that field. Peer providers or prosumers[7] are specialized positions that recognize the lived experience as a key qualification.

Based on these definitions, the experience of living with and managing a mental illness and accessing services or treatment is considered a special knowledge or skill. An individual with this experience has an expertise in terms of living with and managing their illness. From the recovery perspective, the experience yields a special proficiency that cannot be found in someone who does not have this kind of first-hand experience. This viewpoint of the individual as the expert is quite different from the traditional medical model of treatment, which tends to view the provider as the expert. One could say that service provision is a meeting of experts, i.e. of clinical experts with experts who have lived experience.[8] Exploring the lived experience can be very valuable, and can help to understand how to be more helpful in assisting people as they move toward their recovery goals. However, it is important to remember that personal experience is subject to an individual's *perception* and *interpretation* of their own circumstances. Certain experiences of living with mental illness and its associated challenges can often be likened to the term "crisis," which can be a turning point that can lead to a better or worse outcome. In terms of life crisis, during a time of chaos and instability it may be considered a turning point. Others may deal with a crisis by regarding it as an opportunity that leads to personal growth and positive change. Their individual "experience" is determined by their personal *interpretations* of their circumstance. Therefore, when working with service users, it is important to tune into their *perceptual set of experiences* that have dictated how they deal with their illness, and how they are (or are not) moving toward personal recovery and wellness.

Disorder and Stigma

The lived experience is typically shared solely from the lens of disorder. Disorder is defined as a poor state of health. Mental disorder is a label for a category of diseases that include affective and emotional stability, and impact behavioral and cognitive functions. It sometimes is difficult for people who are labeled with a mental disorder to accept the idea of living indefinitely with what has been labeled a serious health problem. There are many disturbing signs, symptoms and resulting sequelae that service users encounter. In addition, service users are social beings. Society neither accurately understands mental disorders, nor does it portray mental disorders in a positive manner. And we wonder why people do not readily accept the mental disorder labels bestowed upon them. Furthermore, a variety of studies support the conclusion that stigma plays a role in delaying seeking care for mental disorder and in reducing adherence to prescribed medications and other treatments.[9,10,11,12]

Service users often experience stigmatization and/or marginalization. Too often persons living with mental illness are told that they should never work because they have a disorder that is chronic and disabling. This and many other messages of "gloom and doom" can lead to experiences of poverty, social isolation, inadequate access to quality health care, and many more negative consequences. It is important to recognize that these experiences can alter the trajectory of an individual's life, which could result in many losses: educational opportunities, employment, financial self-sufficiency, support, intimate relationships, and opportunities to use innate talents and skills.

Stigma associated with a diagnosis of a mental disorder can have a significant influence on the lived experience. Stigma can lead to discrimination, and people may experience personal losses (as above). People may feel as though they do not have the opportunity to pursue valued social roles, such as student, worker, family member and citizen, which can also be very devastating.

Service users may internalize stigma and experience a diminished sense of self and diminished sense of self-efficacy. *Self-stigma* is the prejudice that people with mental illness turn against themselves. Self-stigma can be destructive. It leads to shame and guilt, and other negative self-talk that can be a significant barrier to recovery. The person may feel and act as though they have lost their previous identities (roles such as student, worker or parent), and instead come to believe the stigmatizing views often held by other society members (for example, that service users can't get better, work or have a full life). There has been such a focus on examining the impact of self-stigma.[13,14]

For many people with SMI, daily life revolves around attending medical appointments, thus the individual may feel like he or she is solely in the patient role. This can be quite limiting in terms of one's identity and sense of self. A key aspect of recovery is helping a service user to examine his or her sense of self, therefore providers can play an important role in helping people with SMI to identify and maintain valued social roles. It is important to help service users pursue valued social roles (such as student, employee, member of the community or family member) that may be impacted by the illness experience. Age of onset is a very important factor when attempting to understand the lived experience. When someone is diagnosed at a younger age (adolescence to young adulthood), that person may experience losses (not finishing school, not becoming employed, not being able to live independently, etc.). Others who, prior to onset of the illness, completed school, became gainfully employed, and/or were able to become financially independent could lose these successes. This may be perceived as more devastating than the diagnosis. In either situation, it is important to appreciate what losses they encountered, and to understand how they adjusted to those losses of unfulfilled hopes or how they may become engulfed by the overwhelming barriers and challenges. Personal experience accumulates over a period of time. If a person spends most of his or her life in a patient role, receiving services through in- or outpatient day treatment programs, for example, that person's experience may be vastly different from someone who had the opportunity and support to graduate from a program in a time-limited period and was able to move forward toward personal recovery goals. If the person has received the prognosis of gloom and doom it may be very difficult, yet not impossible, for them to set and achieve recovery goals.

People in the self-help and peer support community may reject diagnostic labels. Some prefer to discuss having "mental health problems," or more comfortably disclose "learning difficulties" in school or work settings. Some cling to the idea that their symptoms are viral in origin, e.g. caused by Lyme disease. Some more readily disclose SUDs than Axis I psychiatric disorders. It is clear to this writer that many of these individuals do not want to associate themselves with the diagnoses disclosed by people around them that have led to unfulfilled and unproductive lives.

Beyond Diagnoses and Labels

Some people have a very difficult time understanding how the mental illness (disorder) "label" applies to them. Many people have been incorrectly diagnosed and/or labeled over the years. These individuals may not agree with the label (or, in some situations, multiple labels) that have been ascribed to them. Some providers and family members label these individuals as "in denial" of their diagnosis. It is important to note that people with mental illness are often given multiple diagnoses, and the labels given are not always consistent between providers. Psychiatric diagnosis is subjective; that is, despite inter-rater reliability, human observations rather than objective scales are used to establish specific diagnoses. It is also longitudinal; that is, a person's diagnosis can change over time due to diagnostic subjectivity and due to the emergence or recognition of additional symptoms. This can be confusing, and many people find such ambiguity distressing. From the lived experience perspective, for a person to take responsibility for his or her personal wellness it may *not* require that he or she openly admit that he or she has a diagnosis such as schizophrenia or bipolar disorder. Rather, it is important for the person to understand that he or she has some difficulties he or she wants to deal with and has the desire to make some positive changes in his or her life. Continuing to emphasize that the person has schizophrenia, or any other diagnostic categories, will continue to reinforce self-stigma and can be very damaging. Our role as providers is to help people manage difficulties and help them to make positive changes. We must learn to identify and guard against messages, practices and policies that may demoralize people, reinforce despair, engender unnecessary dependence and prolong disability.[15]

A concrete example of the impact of the focus on diagnosis is seen in obtaining public benefits and their accompanying medical benefit programs. Faced with no income, limited prospects, a backlog of hospital bills, and the need to fill expensive prescriptions, many people file for these benefits. Urging and helping people to file for benefits becomes a standard practice in our mental health care system. The benefit programs require that a person willingly attest to, and provide documentation of, a total or significant disability. People keep themselves totally unemployed and focused on disability during the often lengthy appeals process. By the time they have been granted their benefits, and then sent documentation about the programs designed to help them resume employment, many people have become resigned to a disability label. Some estimates say that as few as 1% of people who get on Supplementary Security Income (SSI) in the U.S. due to a psychiatric disability eventually get off the benefit program. Although this is an American fact, the situation is similar in many other countries, including in countries with different welfare systems, such as Canada and Israel.

First Person Recovery Narratives from the Lens of Wellness

First person recovery narratives are important resources that can help us refocus our thinking beyond the disorder and deficit perspective.[16] First person narratives serve as strong testimonies to the existence of inherent strengths of people who face the challenges of mental illness.[17] These accounts document the lived experience of managing and surviving the multiple challenges and barriers associated with the illness experience. Recovery narratives are important resources that should be transmitted to staff and persons served in every treatment setting.[18] Recovery narratives can engender hope,[19] and these accounts amplify the message that a positive life is attainable. In recent years, there has been a greater focus on examining the *lived experience from the lens of wellness*.[20] There has been some research on the notion of resilience and the lessons to be learned from the recovery experiences of persons living with mental illness.[21] Instead of focusing solely on the disorder, there is a focus on wellness (a holistic view of the person who is a multi-dimensional being, which includes intellectual, emotional, spiritual, physical, social, occupational and financial dimensions).

From a wellness perspective people learn to find meaning to their experiences and develop a sense of purpose that draws upon their personal strengths.[22,23] Using the crisis analogy, there is more of a focus on looking at the "opportunity" that the disorder brings. Service users are viewed as capable of assuming personal responsibility to learn and apply self-care skills and routines, which are important factors that can help the person achieve *wellness*. There are wonderful self-care and self-help resources that people access. Stress management and relaxation strategies can be useful to help a person deal with life's hassles and stress, which often exacerbate symptoms. Mary Ellen Copeland's *Wellness Recovery Action Plan* (*WRAP*) program is an excellent example and resource.[24,25]

As providers ascribing to a person-centered approach, we should work to forge a collaborative relationship by attempting to know the person through his or her own lens rather than the lens of labels ascribed by others. By taking the time to listen to persons we serve and seeking their understanding of their lived experience we may be able to develop better ways in which they can be personally and professionally supported.

As we get to know people, we so often learn that it is the issues related to treatment (medication side effects) and psychosocial stressors, especially poverty, that trouble them as much as or more than any specific psychiatric symptoms. People experience stigma when they do not have a valued role such as employee, parent or student. People experience financial stressors when they have insufficient incomes due to unemployment or underemployment, and "too much money at the end of the month." One young woman with a psychiatric disability whom this writer knows grew up in a middle class suburb and experiences great stigma when she needs to visit the food pantry due to "too much month left at the end of the money."

Example of a Wellness Narrative

Over 30 years ago I encountered the mental health system as an adolescent. Instead of spending my freshman year in high school, I received long-term inpatient and outpatient services. I was deeply distressed, depressed and my life was a mess. High school was a nightmare and a blur. I never fully integrated and struggled to graduate because I had no ambition for a career. My sense of future seemed bleak. I did not feel I could accomplish personal goals. I constantly wanted to return to the solace and safety of an institution. Through anger, frustration and anxiety, I developed a vision of trying to look at myself as a whole person. Initially, this kept me alive and now helps me live each day more fully.

I continue to acknowledge that I have some social and emotional vulnerabilities. I need to keep in check on a daily, weekly and annual basis. I have been able to focus on my own wellness (doing things such as swimming, pursuing educational goals, continually learning and most important being employed), which empower me to move forward to achieve personal goals – one step at a time. My mother helped me learn to resist my efforts to return to the hospital and helped me find my way into other types of institutions such as community college and work. I made slow and steady gains toward defining other roles I could pursue. I did work many less than minimum wage jobs and *work became an adaptive obsession* (I discovered that showing up for work was half the battle). *Work* challenged me to get out of my head, cast aside daily rituals, overcome constant self-doubt, and *do something for someone else*. *Work* also provided a financial reward, which helped me break away from my perceived control by others. *Work* empowers me to attain financial stability and not to be dependent on other people and society. *Accepting* that I have an emotional vulnerability was an important part of personal responsibility that led to better overall health. When I **stopped blaming** others and life's situations for the challenges I "perceived," life was less stressful and I was better able to handle stress, disappointments, and even successes.

Voices of Recovery

The Center for Psychiatric Rehabilitation at Boston University (the Center) first published *The Experience of Recovery*.[26] This was an anthology of stories and poems by people recounting their own recovery experiences. Recently, the Center published *Voices of Recovery*,[27] which is an updated and expanded version of *Experience of Recovery*. This publication offers the voices of lived experience. The first voice is a collection of accounts originally published in the "Coping With" column of *the Psychiatric Rehabilitation Journal* from 2000–2008.[28] In every issue of this journal, the "Coping With" column describes individuals' experiences of coping with mental illness and things leading them to their own personal recovery.

The second voice in this new publication is exhibited through a collection of "photovoice" projects. Photovoice is a process used in research, education, social change and policy. Cameras were provided to individuals with mental illness, and they used photovoice to describe their experiences. Short stories and messages are illustrated to explain the meaning behind the image from the photographer's point of view. Photovoice is a creative approach to help better understand the lived experience from first-hand accounts.

A 2010 review section on photovoice concluded that "photovoice appears to contribute to an enhanced understanding of community assets and needs and to empowerment."[29] When Thompson and colleagues (2008)[30] applied photovoice study to the experience of living with mental illness, their conclusions were almost a synopsis of this section: "Four major themes emerged: 1. Feeling misunderstood and invisible in the world; 2. Attempting to gain control and be safe through various actions and activities; 3. Making an ongoing effort to repair injured self-esteem; and 4. Using various coping skills."

CONCLUSION: SUGGESTIONS FOR PROVIDERS AND ORGANIZATIONS

Every service user needs to know that his or her lived experience is valuable. The intake process can include opportunities for people to discuss lessons learned and philosophy gained, rather than just a history of symptoms and treatments. Group and individual sessions can include discussions of journaling and writing exercises. Service users can be referred to speaker programs such as the National Alliance on Mental Illness (NAMI)'s *In Our Own Voice* program.[31] Providers and future providers could benefit from the opportunity to hear service users' lived experience and recovery stories as part of normal training programs.[32,33]

Service users, as well as others who have any involvement, e.g. colleagues, potential service users, family members, interacting practitioners, funders and the general community, deserve to know that lived experience provides valuable knowledge. This can be made a part of organizational action and culture through a variety of ways, such as incorporating narratives into written materials and public displays. A board of recovery quotes can be featured in the lobby. First-hand stories can be worked into annual reports. Public presentations by organizations should feature presentations by service users. This can eventually become a key part of organizational culture, and service users should be offered support and opportunities to share their experiences as part of their recovery journey. This is also highly consistent with the research on stigma reduction, which finds that first-hand accounts are highly effective at helping to dispel stigma.

The number-one way to incorporate service users' recovery stories and perspectives into an organization or practice is to maximize the inclusion of service users throughout the organizational structure, including in provider, evaluator and management roles. Employee and contractor positions that are not part of direct mental health service delivery (finance and accounting, pharmacy, quality assurance, transportation, marketing, etc.) should be offered to people who live with a mental illness whenever possible. Organizations can: 1. Make maximal use of service users as providers; 2. Provide those individuals with practical assistance and support in choosing, getting and keeping these roles inside or outside the organization; 3. Establish and sustain a culture where people in the workforce can value disclosing psychiatric histories; and 4. Work within their communities to develop and sustain sources of a service user workforce. At the same time, it is important to avoid tokenism, or to see service users relegated to menial roles. This will display a true commitment on the part of providers and organizations to embrace the value of lived experience. Employing people with SMI in a community mental health organization will be an important step towards combating stigma, increasing employment rates and helping to create opportunities to promote mental health recovery.

REFERENCES

1 Deegan PE. Recovery: the lived experience of rehabilitation. *Psychosocial Rehabilitation Journal.* 1988; **11**: 11–19.

2 McNamara S. *Voices of Recovery.* Boston, MA: Boston University Center for Psychiatric Rehabilitation; 2009.

3 Jacobson N. Experiencing recovery: a dimensional analysis of recovery narratives. *Psychiatr Rehabil J.* 2001; **24**(3): 248–55.

4 Spaniol L, Gagne C, Koehler M. Recovery from serious mental illness: what it is and how to assist people in recovery. *Continuum.* 1997; **4**(4): 3–15.

5 Spaniol L, Wewiorski NJ, Gagne C, *et al.* The process of recovery from schizophrenia. *International Review of Psychology.* 2002; **14**(4): 327–36.

6 Davidson L, Strauss JS. Sense of self in recovery from severe mental illness. *British Journal of Medical Psychology.* 1992; **65**: 131–45.

7 Manos E. Prosumers. *Psychiatr Rehabil J.* 1993; **16**(4): 117–20.

8 Slade M. *Personal recovery and mental illness: a guide for mental health professionals.* Cambridge: Cambridge University Press; 2009.

9 Cruz M, Pincus HA, Harman JS, *et al.* Barriers to care-seeking for depressed African Americans. *Int J Psychiatry Med.* 2004; **38**(1): 71–80.

10 Fung KM, Tsang HW, Corrigan PW. Self-stigma of people with schizophrenia as predictor of their adherence to psychosocial treatment. *Psychiatric Rehabilitation Journal.* 2008; **32**(2): 95–104.

11 Hudson TJ, Owen RR, Thrush CR, *et al.* A pilot study of barriers to medication adherence in schizophrenia. *J Clin Psychiatry.* 2004; **65**(2): 211–16.

12 Yang LH, Phelan JC, Link BG. Stigma and beliefs of efficacy towards traditional Chinese medicine and Western psychiatric treatment among Chinese-Americans. *Cultur Divers Ethnic Minor Psychol.* 2008; **14**(1): 10–18.

13 Corrigan PW, Wassel A. Understanding and influencing the stigma of mental illness. *J Psychosoc Nurs Ment Health Serv.* 2008; **46**(1): 42–8.

14 Rüsch N, Lieb K, Bohus M, *et al.* Self-stigma, empowerment, and perceived legitimacy of discrimination among women with mental illness. *Psychiatr Serv.* 2006; **57**(3): 399–402.

15 Ridgway P. Restorying psychiatric disability: learning from first person recovery narratives. *Psychiatr Rehabil J.* 2001; **24**(4): 335–42.

16 Ibid.

17 Ibid.

18 Ibid.

19 Deegan, op. cit.

20 Swarbrick M. A wellness approach. *Psychiatr Rehabil J.* 2006; **29**: 311–14.

21 Ridgway, op. cit.

22 Swarbrick, op. cit.

23 Swarbrick M. A wellness model for clients. *Mental Health Special Interest Section Quarterly.* 1997; **20**(3): 1–4.

24 Copeland ME. *Wellness recovery action plan.* Brattleboro, VT: Peach Press; 1997.

25 Copeland ME, Mead S. *Wellness recovery action plan & peer support: personal, group and program development.* West Dummerston, VT: Peach Press; 2004.

26 Spaniol L, Koehler M. *Experience of Recovery.* Boston, MA: Boston University Center for Psychiatric Rehabilitation; 1994.

27 McNamara, op. cit.

28 Ibid.

29 Catalani C, Minkler M. Photovoice: a review of the literature in health and public health. *Health Education & Behavior,* 2010; **37**(3): 424–51.

30 Thompson NC, Hunter EE, Murray L, *et al.* The experience of living with chronic mental illness: a photovoice study. *Perspectives in Psychiatric Care.* 2008; **44**(1): 14–24.

31 Wood AL, Wahl OF. Evaluating the effectiveness of a consumer-provided mental health recovery education presentation. *Psychiatr Rehabil J.* 2006; **30**(1): 46–53.

32 Barnes D, Carpenter J, Dickinson C. The outcomes of partnerships with mental health service users in interprofessional education: a case study. *Health Soc Care Community.* 2006; **14**(5): 426–35.

33 Bell JS, Johns R, Rose G, *et al.* A comparative study of consumer participation in mental health pharmacy education. *Ann Pharmacother.* 2006; **40**(10): 1759–65. Epub 2006 Sep 12.

3.2 The Relationship Between the Person with a Serious Mental Illness and His or Her Disorder

David Roe, Elizabeth McCay and Melissa Keene

INTRODUCTION

As modern medicine shifts towards more holistic and integrative models, the complex questions regarding the relation between the person and his or her disorder become all the more central. Historically, focus was on the medical model, which emphasized the disease process, reaching a valid diagnosis, understanding the etiology and predicting the prognosis. Gradually, however, as increasing evidence had shown that the person's experience of the disorder mediates its impact, and that the person's experience and response to the illness and its aftermath can actually have an impact upon its course,[1] it became apparent that it is necessary to replace these relatively simplistic, "clean" models for more "fuzzy" and complex ones. Person-centered approaches represent efforts to understand the person's experience and "use" it as a valued part of the ongoing dialogue between a service provider and user. This becomes particularly complicated within the context of mental illness, when it is the actual experience via perceptions and cognitions that is challenged by the illness.

In this section we will try to shed light on this complex relation and discuss some of its conceptual implications for person-centered practice. To do so we will briefly review: 1. How the disorder influences the person who is living with the disorder; 2. How the person perceives him or herself in relation to the disorder; and 3. How the person influences the disorder.

How Does the Disorder Influence the Person?

An SMI can be characterized by disturbances in multiple realms of a person's life, including biological, psychological, behavioral, interpersonal and social spheres.[2] Language and communication, content of thought, perception, affect, sense of self, volition, relationship to the external world and motor behavior are often typically affected. For example, in schizophrenic disorders, fundamental distortions of thought and perception often occur along with an inappropriate or decreased affect. These disturbances can alter the most basic human functions that give the person a sense of individuality, uniqueness and self-direction. A person may report that the most intimate thoughts and feelings seem to be known by others and explanatory delusions may develop as a result. Auditory hallucinations are common, as is the belief that common daily situations represent a special meaning intended solely for the individual.[3] It is also believed that metacognition, the capacity to think about one's own thinking, is compromised in schizophrenia. This inability to scrutinize one's thoughts and feelings may be a primary source of psychosocial impairment.[4] Such a decrease in self-reflection may lead persons to experience themselves as less of an actor in their own life,[5] thus further intensifying the challenges of coping with both the symptoms and the social context surrounding the illness.

Society places strong stigmatizing attitudes upon those with a SMI. At times, the person's identity is completely negated in the eyes of others. In this context, identity refers to the social category used by others to describe the individual.[6] For example, much of the general population believes individuals with an SMI cannot maintain employment, cannot make appropriate decisions about their own welfare, or may demonstrate increased levels of violence and disorderly conduct.[7] Because these attitudes tend to be widely accepted, it is exceedingly difficult for individuals with an SMI to ignore such perceptions. These stigmatized perceptions can be readily internalized by individuals, thus making it difficult to establish a sense of self that is distinct from the stigma of having an SMI.[8] The SMI label can diminish the individual's sense of self and subjectivity, challenging the most intimate aspects of one's inner world, such as one's thoughts, perceptions, feelings and reasoning.[9] Even worse, stigmatizing attitudes often produce a socially irresponsible platform in which individuals with an SMI are frequently abandoned to the illness instead of being nurtured to sustain or regain a coherent and continuous sense of self and ultimately a satisfactory quality of life (Stigma is addressed in more detail in 3.1 and 4.3).

Indeed, the lack of such "nurturing" contexts that hold the potential to help a person sustain or rebuild a sense of self or self agency to pursue self-identified goals is readily apparent. For example, persons with SMI often experience high unemployment. While low employment rates intrinsic to SMI cannot be solely attributed to social stigma, they certainly are representative of the cumulative effect of the social and economic pressures that individuals with SMI have to face.

In addition to coping with the external forces imposed by stigmatizing social attitudes and expectations, individuals must also cope with the risk of internalizing their illness and its negative connotation. The process by which stigma comes to be internalized has been termed "role-engulfment" and was originally described by Lally,[10] who defined engulfment as the process during which a person comes to accept the patient role as the primary definition of his or her self. Lally identified three stages of the engulfment process.[11] In the early stage, individuals deny and minimize their psychiatric problems, compare themselves with less fortunate individuals, and thus view themselves as better off than others. Important transitional events linking the early stage to the middle phase include the onset of major symptoms and repeated hospitalizations. In the middle stage, persons accept that they have psychiatric problems but minimize their potentially devastating implications and meaning by focusing primarily on the normality and commonality of mental illness. Transitional events leading to the final stage include hearing a diagnosis, applying for disability and resigning oneself to the permanence of the illness. In the final stage ("true" engulfment), an all-encompassing internalized definition of self as "mentally ill" is established. For example, a person at this stage who is asked to introduce or describe himself or herself might respond "a schizophrenic" or "a 34-year-old schizophrenic." This sort of response, which at least in some settings may not be rare, reflects having lost the sense of oneself as a person with multiple roles or identities. Instead, one has come to view himself or herself solely as an illness.

More recently the term "internalized stigma" has been used to describe the state in which a person displaces a previously held identity and replaces it with the internalized, negative views of SMI held by others in society. Pervasive negative cultural and social perceptions seem to have led to public disengagement and a general lack of understanding of persons with SMI, and in some cases, actual devaluation and rejection. The presence of these largely negative public attitudes can frequently have a dramatic impact on persons with SMI, so much so that persons with SMI have come to expect such rejection.[12] Recent studies have found internalized stigma to be relatively common among persons with SMI, with nearly one third of persons with SMI reporting high levels of internalized stigma.[13,14] There is substantial evidence that internalized stigma and related processes have profound negative effects upon both the objective and subjective components of recovery for persons with SMI that persist regardless of the severity of symptoms. Self-stigma and role engulfment have been found to be strongly negatively associated with hope, self-esteem and social functioning,[15] along with greater alienation and stereotype endorsement.[16] Individuals must then cope not only with the personal illness experience, but also the influence of SMI stigma on the societal structures in which they are involved.[17]

An examination of young people who are coping with an SMI early in the trajectory of the illness further illustrates the profound personal effect of the illness and its associated stigma. Despite the recent optimism regarding treatment for SMI, young people remain at profound risk for self-stigma and ultimately role engulfment. Propensity for engulfment is greatest when stigma is exceptionally strong and the individual's self-concept is not fully formed,[18] as is the case for young people living with SMI, who are developmentally in the throes of defining themselves and creating their future. The onset of an SMI, such as schizophrenia, frequently evokes a profound sense of loss, whereby images of a vibrant future, including occupational choice and a sustained relationship with a life partner are dramatically and suddenly lost.[19] This strong and overwhelming emotional response is frequently evoked by mere mention of a diagnosis such as schizophrenia. It has been observed that the secondary consequences of the disorder and its treatment frequently have long-lasting consequences for the individual, often surpassing the more immediate goal of treating acute symptoms.[20] For example, young people coping with perceived stigma associated with SMI may fear rejection and thus see their friends less frequently, ultimately resulting in social isolation. Increasing social isolation then impacts upon the individual's overall sense of self worth and self efficacy, which further limits opportunities to create new relationships and social connections necessary for future employment and an overall satisfying quality of life. For example, a young college student who suffers from a brief psychotic episode for which he was hospitalized may attempt to return to his previous routine but find that his peers look at him and treat him differently. They may fear him, avoid initiating contact and keep a distance from him. The painful sense of being rejected, particularly at such a time of crisis, is likely to reinforce isolation and loneliness, which further hinder opportunities to recover one's self-worth and quality of life.

How Does the Person Experience Him or Herself in Relation to the Disorder?

Persons with a psychiatric diagnosis perceive their disorder in a range of different ways. Those who appear to be unaware of their illness are considered to lack insight,[21,22,23] which appears to be quite common, particularly among those with schizophrenia, where it ranges between 50–80%.[24,25,26] Some have emphasized the neurophysiological basis for lack of insight, drawing an analogy with anosognosia, a neurological syndrome consisting of components of unawareness of the motor, sensory, cognitive, affective and interpersonal impairments and disabilities that are often the consequences of brain damage. This analogy implies that unawareness of mental illness is produced by the same subtle neurophysiological anomalies that give rise to the symptoms of the illness of which the person with the mental illness is frequently unaware.

An additional reason for why people may not be aware of their illness is that it has only been recently that the mental health system has begun to provide information and education about schizophrenia and its treatment. Thus, it was not reasonable to expect that individuals living with this SMI would be aware of the fact that they had a mental illness if they had not been provided with information about their illness in the first place. This would be similar to speculating that lack of insight is intrinsic to cancer, since people do not walk into their physician's office and report that they expect they might be growing a tumor. Without any advance education, and in the face of hundreds of years of stigma, people experiencing mental illness had little reason to guess that what was afflicting them was a psychiatric disorder.[27]

Even with such education, however, it is often difficult for individuals living with SMI to immediately embrace the SMI diagnosis. Ideally, the complex process involved in accepting this diagnosis should be viewed no differently than any other disease. Beyond the cognitive aspect of "knowing" whether one's internal experience is "consistent" with the given diagnostic label or not, there may be an emotional aspect whereby one prefers not to know that label. An individual with an end-stage malignancy may choose to deny his or her prognosis, just as an individual with am SMI may have difficulty accepting that he or she has a mental illness. Unfortunately, a double standard seems to exist where societal attitudes may limit peoples' capacity to fully accept and self-disclose their diagnosis. When individuals do not demonstrate sufficient insight, it is frequently blamed on the mental condition and not viewed as a common human response to illness and fragility, as is the case with other medical disorders. Furthermore, if a person offers an alternative narrative of his or her illness experience in comparison to the biomedical history, it is negated based on the presumption that it demonstrates lack of insight and validity.[28] Objective psychiatry tends to acknowledge insight only when it equates with the clinician's perspective. If the person agrees he or she is experiencing symptoms of SMI, this validates the allocated label. If the person does not agree with the diagnostic label of SMI, it is used as evidence that the person really is ill. With either response, the service user is trapped by the provider's diagnosis.

Persons may not want to discuss their diagnosis, as illness acceptance and dialogue about the disorder label may bring on emotions of hopelessness and low self-efficacy. Because the associated stigma may be demoralizing for service users, persons that actively reject the stereotypes of SMI and emphasize a unique self-identification separate from the disorder show the most favorable outcome,[29] consistent with engulfment theory.[30,31] Accordingly, decreased awareness of the social consequences associated with the label of mental illness has been found to be strongly correlated with less depressive symptomatology.[32] This lack of insight indicates that there is not one straightforward relationship between insight and mental disorder. It may vary between individuals, suggesting the need to separate the objective aspects of the disease from the subjective narrative experience of the illness.[33] Individualizing the illness experience will allow each service user to navigate his or her SMI and recovery process within the context of a personalized care plan. For example, a person who had experiences that were identified and labeled by a mental service provider as a psychotic symptom may not necessarily agree with this label. Even if the person was formally diagnosed and treated for a mental disorder based on the assessment of these symptoms, he or she may perceive them as experiences that are not necessarily pathological or a basis for diagnosing a disorder. Interestingly, in contrast to the traditional view that "acceptance" of or "insight into" having a disorder is necessary, or at least helpful, the described "meaning-making" efforts might be more helpful for some. Recent theoretical approaches focusing on first-hand experience as described in Section 3.1, *The Lived Experience: narratives through the lens of wellness*, and psychotherapies emphasizing subjective experience as described in section 6.3 *Person-Centered Individual Psychotherapy for Adults with Serious Mental Illness*, are important new developments in line with these recent conceptualizations.

How Does the Person Influence the Disorder?

In prior decades, severe mental illness was seen as a chronic condition with a poor prognosis. More recently, however, longitudinal research has shown that 45–65% of individuals meeting criteria for schizophrenia will significantly improve with time.[34] Medical and scientific advances in the treatment of schizophrenia have enabled the development of much more effective means to treat the disease, which helps to create a sense of hope that people with SMI can achieve healthy and satisfying lives.[35,36] Along with the recent advances in treatment for SMI, the recovery movement has initiated an important paradigm shift in the treatment of SMI, namely that people with severe SMI can grow and develop beyond the limits imposed by the disorder.[37] Hence it is necessary to establish new treatment strategies aligned with the current recovery paradigm to aid both the service user and provider in treating SMIs. One route of recovery that has shown significant promise utilizes the person's experience of the self in relation to the illness to navigate the journey. It is a person-centered approach with a strong emphasis placed on the underlying principle of self-determination. Through the use of the personal narrative, the individual can transition from being engulfed by the disorder and/or illness experience to being an active agent in his or her life story. The utilization of the narrative approach places value on the individual experience of SMI and puts a human face on that experience.[38] It serves as a useful framework to provide access to the process of change and recovery. For example, a person who attends psychotherapy similar to the approach described in Section 6.3, *Person-Centered Individual Psychotherapy for Adults with Serious Mental Illness*, will have the empowering opportunity to create his own personal narrative to make sense out of his experience, rather than struggling to passively accept explanations about his condition that can be presented by the service provider as scientific facts.

Every individual can produce an endless array of stories, all of which can be seen from various perspectives and none of which can earn the title of being necessarily the "correct" one, since there is no single story which is *the* "correct" one. Healthy and adaptive stories are ones that *change* over time as the narrator gains life experiences and also as he or she tells them to different people, and thus has the opportunity to negotiate, edit and rewrite the story.[39]

An important way in which the person influences the course of his or her disorder and paves a personal path towards recovery is through the process of negotiating its meaning and through "taking a stand," or in other words defining the self in relation to the disorder.[40] Through this process precedence is given to some experiences and not others; stories are subjective accounts and reflect a perspective that can shift viewpoints at any moment. Similarly, because stories are an individual's creation, they can and do change.[41]

In addition to the personal story, self-identity or self-concept, defined as the totality of thoughts and feelings about the self,[42] serves as a tool to negotiate continuity between one's internal and external environments. It is through the self that many of life's experiences, including those that pose challenges to the self, such as receiving a diagnosis of SMI, are perceived and ultimately responded to. In severe mental illness, a person's core identity and sense of self are clearly influenced over time. It is a major challenge for self-image. In order to facilitate the recovery process in SMI, the service user has to utilize his or her sense of self as a resourceful coping mechanism. Ultimately, the sense of self can provide a sense of continuity between who he or she was *prior* to illness onset and the person he or she becomes *after* illness onset. Ideally, the personal narrative is flexible enough to enable the individual to emerge with changes associated with living with an SMI, while also being able to maintain aspects of the self that are central to the self and not overtaken by the illness process, thus safeguarding the self from being engulfed by the illness.

This perspective is also consistent with the theoretical notion of recovery, which indicates that individuals living with SMI can simultaneously achieve competence while still coping with symptoms and dysfunction.[43]

While individuals with SMI may demonstrate variable cognitive impairments, they can simultaneously act as active agents involved in the process of meaning making. PSR is encouraged to utilize a person-centered approach, where the service user's personal values and needs are incorporated into the decision process. Service users tend to express a desire for greater participation in decisions about psychiatric care than they currently experience.[44] Active service user participation may increase satisfaction and treatment adherence and decrease symptom burden.[45] Through an interactive coping strategy, providers can work with service users to enhance living skills and environmental supports. Internalized stigma, lack of opportunities for self-determination, and the negative side effects of unemployment need to be addressed. This might be best accomplished when the provider facilitates coping by guiding the service user to focus on the growth of self as a personal meaning maker in his or her life. This can lead to the discovery of a more active sense of self with the realization of one's strengths and weaknesses and opportunities for change.[46]

The encouragement of a durable sense of self by the clinician replaces the previous focus on the patient role in disease-based models of treatment.[47] Instead, providers must know the service user and his or her history well enough to collaborate with him or her to identify beneficial outlets within the community. Value must be assigned to the knowledge gained from persons with SMI in navigating their own disease.[48] With the clinician's guidance, revised aspects of the self can then be put into action to effectively cope with SMI.

As such, new and innovative person-centered interventions for individuals recovering from SMI are needed to strengthen the self and to promote the process of recovery.[49] Optimal recovery can be enhanced through enabling the individual to explore the perceived meaning of the illness experience, reinforcing attempts to regain mastery and self-esteem, as well as confirming self attributes not necessarily associated with disorder.[50,51,52] Group interventions, such as the approach described by McCay *et al.*,[53,54] which seek to promote healthy self-concepts while mitigating the negative effects of internalized stigma, have been shown to minimize engulfment, increase hope and improve quality of life, compared to usual treatment in a group of young adults with first episode schizophrenia. This type of approach offers promise as a method that may contribute to a more satisfactory relationship between the person's sense of self and his or her disorder, and this can fully support the process of recovery.

CONCLUSION

Person-centered approaches are particularly challenging within the context of SMI. SMI is commonly characterized by symptoms that impair and compromise the core functioning of the person with whom the clinician strives to collaborate and work with (in a person-centered manner). Understanding the complex interactions between the person and the disorder may help shed light and better understand the complexity of the junction between the person and his or her disorder. It is suggested and recommended that a focus on narratives and metacognition can facilitate the person's recovery efforts and help transform her identity from one of being engulfed with the illness to becoming a separate and independent entity actively coping and growing. The person-centered clinician is one who can help facilitate this process and can recognize and support "personhood" – thus all this should lead to how the self/illness interactions actually help us practice PCC.

REFERENCES

1 Charmaz C. *Good days, bad days: the self and chronic illness.* New Brunswick, NJ: Rutgers University Press; 1993.

2 Africa B, Freudenreich O, Schwartz S. Schizophrenic disorders. In: Goldman H. *Review of General Psychiatry.* 5th ed. New York, NY: McGraw-Hill Companies; 2000.

3 World Health Organization. *The ICD-10 Classification of Mental and Behavioural Disorders: diagnostic criteria for research.* Geneva: World Health Organization; 1992.

4 Dimaggio G, Lysaker PH. *Metacognition and Severe Adult Mental Disorders: from basic research to treatment.* New York, NY: Brunner Routledge; 2010. pp. 233–46.

5 Lysaker JT, Lysaker PH. Being interrupted: the self and schizophrenia. *Journal of Speculative Philosophy.* 2005; **19**: 1–21.

6 Thoits PA. Self, identity, stress, and mental health. In: Aneshensel CS, Phelan JC. *Handbook of Sociology and Mental Health.* New York, NY: Kluwer; 1999. pp. 321–44.

7 Link BG, Phelan JC, Bresnahan M, *et al.* Public conceptions of mental illness: labels, causes, dangerousness, and social distance. *Am J Public Health.* 1999; **89**: 1328–33.

8 Corrigan PW, Watson AC. The paradox of self-stigma and mental illness. *Clin Psychol.* 2002; **9**: 35–53.

9 Roe D, Chopra M, Wagner B, *et al.* The emerging self in conceptualizing and treating mental illness. *J Psychosoc Nurs Ment Health Serv.* 2004; **42**(2): 1–8.

10 Lally SJ. Does being in here mean there is something wrong with me? *Schizophr Bull.* 1989; **15**(2): 253–65.

11 Ibid.

12 Roe, op. cit.

13 Ritsher JB, Phelan JC. Internalized stigma predicts erosion of morale among psychiatric outpatients. *Psychiatry Res.* 2004; **129**(3): 257–65.

14 McCay EA, Ryan K. Meeting the patient's emotional needs. In: Zipursky R, Schulz C. *The Early Stages of Schizophrenia.* Washington, DC: American Psychiatric Publishing; 2002. pp. 107–29.

15 McCay EA, Seeman MV. A scale to measure the impact of a schizophrenia illness on an individual's self-concept. *Arch Psychiatr Nurs.* 1998; **12**(1): 41–9.

16 Ritsher, op. cit.

17 Roe, op. cit.

18 Lally, op. cit.

19 McKay, 2002, op. cit.

20 McGorry PD. The concept of recovery and secondary prevention in psychotic disorders. *Aust N Z J Psychiatry*. 1992; **26**(1): 3–17.

21 David AS. Insight and psychosis. *Br J Psychiatry*. 1990; **156**: 798–808.

22 Lysaker PH, Bell MD, Bryson GJ, *et al*. Psychosocial function and insight in schizophrenia. *J Nerv Ment Dis*. 1998; **186**(7): 432–6.

23 Amador XF, Andreasen NC, Clark SC, *et al*. Awareness of illness in schizophrenia. *Arch Gen Psychiatry*. 1994; **51**(10): 826–36.

24 Amador XF, Kronengold H. Understanding and assessing insight. In: Amador XF, David A, editors. *Insight and Psychosis: awareness of illness in schizophrenia and related disorders*. Oxford: University Press; 2004. pp. 3–29.

25 Amador XF, Gorman JM, Strauss DH, *et al*. Awareness of illness in schizophrenia. *Schizophr Bull*. 1991; **17**(1): 113–32.

26 Lincoln TM, Lüllmann E, Rief W. Correlates and long-term consequences of poor insight in patients with schizophrenia: a systematic review. *Schizophr Bull*. 2007; **33**(6): 1324–42. Epub 2007 Feb 8.

27 Roe D, Davidson L. Self and narrative in schizophrenia: time to author a new story. *Med Humanit*. 2005; **31**: 89–94.

28 Estroff S. Subject/subjectivities in dispute: the poetics, politics, and performance of first-person narratives of people with schizophrenia. In: Jenkins JH, Barrett RG, editors. *Schizophrenia, Culture, and Subjectivity*. U.S.A.: Cambridge University Press; 2004. pp. 282–302.

29 O'Mahony PD. Psychiatric patient denial of mental illness as a normal process. *Br J Med Psychol*. 1982; **55**(Pt. 2): 109–18.

30 Lally, op. cit.

31 McKay, 1998, op. cit.

32 Moore O, Cassidy E, Carr A, *et al*. Unawareness of illness and its relationship with depression and self-deception in schizophrenia. *Eur Psychiatry*. 1999; **14**(5): 264–9.

33 Roe D, Kravetz S. Different ways of being aware of and acknowledging a psychiatric disability: a multifunctional narrative approach to insight into mental disorder. *J Nerv Ment Dis*. 2003; **191**(7): 417–24.

34 Davidson L, McGlashan TH. The varied outcomes of schizophrenia. *Can J Psychiatry*. 1997; **42**(1): 34–43.

35 Kapur S, Remington G. Atypical antipsychotics: new directions and new challenges in the treatment of schizophrenia. *Annu Rev Med*. 2001; **52**: 503–17.

36 Remington G, Kapur S, Zipursky RS. Pharmacotherapy of first-episode schizophrenia. *Br J Psychiatry*. 1998; **172**(33): 66–70.

37 Anthony WA. Recovery from mental illness: the guiding vision of the mental health service system in the 1990s. *Psychosocial Rehabilitation Journal*. 1993; **16**(4): 11–23.

38 Kirkpatrick H. A narrative framework for understanding experiences of people with severe mental illnesses. *Arch Psychiatr Nurs*. 2008; **22**: 61–8.

39 Ibid.

40 Roe D, Ben-Yishai A. Exploring the relationship between the person and the disorder among individuals hospitalized for psychosis. *Psychiatry*. 1999; **62**(4): 370–80.

41 Kirkpatrick, op. cit.

42 Roe, 1999, op. cit.

43 Roe, 2004, op. cit.

44 Rosenberg M. *Conceiving the self*. New York, NY: Basic Books; 1979.

45 Adams JR, Drake RE, Wolford GL. Shared decision-making preferences of people with severe mental illness. *Psychiatr Serv.* 2007; **58**(9): 1219–21.

46 Roe D, Goldblatt H, Baloush-Klienman V, *et al.* Why and how people with a serious mental illness decide to stop taking their medication: exploring the subjective process of making and activating a choice. *Psychiatr Rehabil J.* 2009; **33**(1): 366–74.

47 Roe D, Lachman M. The subjective experience of people with severe mental illness: a potentially crucial piece of the puzzle. *Isr J Psychiatry Relat Sci.* 2005; **42**(4): 223–30.

48 Roe, 2009, op. cit.

49 Sells JD, Stayner DA, Davidson L. Recovering the self in schizophrenia: an integrative review of qualitative studies. *Psychiatr Q.* 2004; **75**(1): 87–97.

50 McKay, 2002, op. cit.

51 McGorry, op. cit.

52 Ridgway P. Restoring psychiatric disability: learning from first person recovery narratives. *Psychiatr Rehabil J.* 2001; **24**(4): 335–43.

53 McCay EA, Beanlands H, Leszcz M, *et al.* A group intervention to promote healthy self-concepts and guide recovery in first episode schizophrenia: a pilot study. *Psychiatr Rehabil J.* 2006; **30**(2): 105–11.

54 McCay EA, Beanlands H, Zipursky R, *et al.* A randomized controlled trial of a group intervention to reduce engulfment and self-stigmatization in first episode schizophrenia. *Australian e-Journal for the Advancement of Mental Health.* 2007; **6**(3): 1–9.

CHAPTER 4

Understanding the Context
of the Individual

This (fourth) chapter of the book presents aspects of the context of people with SMI and their relation to PCC. As every person is influenced to some extent by his or her past, present and expected future circumstances or context, it is imperative to address such context as relevant in relation to PCC for persons with SMI. Context is also addressed in other chapters of the book, such as in Chapter 5, The Person/Patient-Provider/Clinician Relationship, where providers and their relationships and clinical communication with service users are addressed (and can be viewed as part of the health care context of the person with SMI); in Chapter 6, Management and Finding Common Ground, where the ethnic features of service users are addressed (and can be viewed as part of the biological and social context of the person with SMI); and in Chapter 7, Prevention and Health Promotion, where peer relationships and support are addressed (and can be viewed as part of the social context of the person with SMI).

Section 4.1, *Collaborating with Families of People with Serious Mental Illness*, argues that family collaboration plays an important role in maximizing the social support that service users with SMI receive from (and give to) their loved ones. The section presents common elements of effective family collaboration. Section 4.2, *Trans-Cultural Issues in Person-Centered Care for People with Serious Mental Illness*, examines the important role of culture in PCC, by examining the cultural and social context of the service user, the role that culture plays in the expression and experience of SMI, and approaches to incorporating cultural elements into the therapeutic relationship and providing care that is culturally relevant. This section draws heavily upon Canada's aboriginal population and its historical and cultural context to illustrate the role trans-cultural issues can play in PCC. Section 4.3, *Environmental Interventions in Relation to People with Serious Mental Illness*, argues for and illustrates the effects of the environment on persons with SMI, focusing on three environmental areas that are amenable to intervention: housing, public stigma and the financing of services. Interventions related to each of these areas are described and discussed in light of principles of PCC. Section 4.4, *Mental Health Systems and Policy in Relation to People with Serious Mental Illness*, argues that PCC should consider the person in the context of numerous systems, and illustrates how the mental health care organization is one such system that can have policies that either support or undermine PCC. The section also addresses policy and law in relation to PCC.

4.1 Collaborating with Families of People with Serious Mental Illness

Kim T. Mueser and Susan Gingerich

INTRODUCTION

Families play an important role in the treatment of people with SMI for several reasons. Because serious psychiatric disorders often develop early in adult life, and they can have devastating effects on the individual's ability to work, go to school or care for oneself, families often step in to provide the needed emotional and material supports.[1] This active caregiving role can be stressful and burdensome, especially considering that relatives often do not fully understand SMI and its treatment. Furthermore, families may have difficulty getting accurate information about their relative's illness and are sometimes confronted with mental health providers who have outdated beliefs about families causing SMI,[2] leading to mistreatment and poor collaboration.[3] High levels of stress in the family can both worsen the quality of family life and precipitate relapses and re-hospitalizations of the person with SMI.[4] A final reason for working with families is that relatives often know more about how the service user is functioning and about his or her needs than anyone else. Thus, families are in an ideal position to support the service user's involvement in treatment and pursuit of personal goals.

As described by Rudnick and Roe,[5] person-centered approaches should be contextualized; that is, the person's history and current circumstances must be considered. Families are a part of everyone's history, and for most people, also part of their present lives, and therefore should be recognized as important sources of support and hands-on assistance. In this section we provide guidelines for working with families of people with SMI as part of a person-centered approach. We describe the characteristics of family friendly agencies, explore a range of family intervention methods, and provide suggestions for how service providers can engage service users and their relatives in working collaboratively with the treatment team. Finally, additional resources for both family members and mental health providers are provided for further learning.

Goals of Family Work

Family work is guided by four major goals:

1. Establish a genuinely collaborative relationship between family members and the treatment team
Such a relationship involves recognizing that both the family and the mental health providers share a common concern for treating the service user's psychiatric disorder and helping him or her achieve personal goals, and that each party has unique and valuable contributions to make towards those goals.

Example

Jim was hospitalized for the treatment of an acute episode of his schizoaffective disorder. Jim's parents, Sarah and David, appreciated it when Jim's social worker contacted them soon after his symptoms had been stabilized and explained that Jim's treatment team wanted to collaborate with them in helping Jim stay out of the hospital and live as independently as possible. Sarah and David met with Jim's social worker along with Jim and were introduced to the other members of Jim's treatment team. As a family, they then had several meetings with the social worker, in which they expressed some concerns about Jim, including his belief that he was getting messages from the TV and radio and the fact that he slept most of the day and was up most of the night. The social worker validated their concerns and provided basic information about the nature of schizoaffective disorder and the principles of treatment. The social worker also expressed interest in Jim's talents and skills, and his past accomplishments at home and school. Sarah and David began to participate in treatment-planning meetings along with Jim and his treatment team. The team members listened attentively to Sarah and David and were very responsive when they supported Jim in stating that one of his goals was to complete high school and attend a trade school in which he could learn how to be a welder. By learning more about Jim's illness, and collaborating with him and his treatment team on helping him work towards his vocational goal, Sarah and David were able to become valued members of Jim's treatment team, to motivate and facilitate Jim's involvement in treatment, and to further stabilize Jim's symptoms and enable him to return to school.

2. Provide basic information to family members about the nature of SMI

Psychoeducation is used to provide information about symptoms, to dispel myths about mental illness, to explain the principles of treatment in order to reduce blame in the family, and to foster the ability of relatives to monitor the illness. It is particularly important to establish hope for recovery, wherein families see their loved one as being able to "live, work, and love in a community in which one makes a difference".[6] It can vary in length or format (*see* later subsection on "Family Intervention Methods").

Example

When Abraham reported auditory hallucinations, withdrew from social interactions and stopped engaging in activities he used to enjoy, his parents and sister were confused and concerned. After Abraham received a diagnosis of schizophrenia, he and his family were relieved to know that there was an illness that explained his symptoms, but at the same time they were discouraged because they knew little about mental illness and its treatment and endorsed many stigmatizing beliefs about people with mental illness. The whole family attended a brief psychoeducation program (six sessions), which addressed the following topics: basic facts about schizophrenia (including correcting common myths about the illness), staying on track with personal goals, the role of medications, participating in rehabilitation programs, reducing family stress and improving communication. Throughout the process, the service provider infused a tone of hope and optimism and provided several examples of people with schizophrenia who lead rewarding, fulfilling lives in the community. The psychoeducation helped the family communicate about the illness, develop coping strategies and support Abraham in his goal of going to college.

3. Teach family members how to monitor the course of the illness and develop a relapse prevention plan

Family work should take advantage of the high level of contact between services users and relatives by teaching relatives about the illness and helping them develop a plan to minimize the disruptive effects of hospitalizations by catching potential relapses early. Relatives often know the service user the best and are frequently in a position to see early warning signs of relapse far sooner than service providers, who may see the person only once a month or even less frequently.

Example

Ariel and her husband worked together to identify her personal early warning signs of relapse (feeling nervous and irritable, spending more time alone, and hearing a low murmur of voices) and developed a relapse prevention plan to respond to that included reducing stress in the household, practicing deep breathing, going on walks with her husband, and contacting her service provider to explore the possibility of temporarily increasing her medication dosage.

4. A final important goal of family work is to reduce stress on everyone in the family and to improve the quality of all family members' lives

This can lower the burnout of involved relatives, help all family members move forward in their lives, and reduce stress-related relapses and re-hospitalizations of the person with SMI.

Example

Maria's marriage to Juan, who had bipolar disorder, was fraught with stress due to the unpredictable nature and course of his illness. Of particular concern was that Juan's episodes of severe depression were often accompanied by suicide attempts, with Maria having to call for emergency help and hospitalization. As a result of these traumatic experiences, Maria felt in a constant state of stress and found it difficult to leave Juan alone for fear that he would make another suicide attempt in her absence. On Juan's part, he felt like he was always under surveillance, which contributed to more stress in their relationship. Maria and Juan participated in a family program that was effective at reducing the stress in the couple's lives in three ways. First, a relapse prevention plan was developed for Juan that prompted him to seek help, and if necessary inpatient hospitalization, when he first noticed that he was feeling depressed and having thoughts about hurting himself, in order to prevent the disruptive effects of suicide attempts. Second, with Juan's encouragement, Maria decided to pursue her goal of completing her bachelor's degree in accounting, which she had stopped when Juan developed bipolar disorder. Third, Juan also supported Maria in reconnecting with some old friends and in joining a health club, which increased Maria's well-being, her social support, and her physical condition. Maria's activities away from the house also decreased the stressful effects of feeling that she always had to be watchful of Juan, who in turn experienced less stress by not feeling that he was constantly being watched.

Characteristics of Family-Friendly Agencies

Family work is most effectively implemented in an agency that recognizes the normal concerns of relatives, appreciates the role relatives can play in helping a loved one on the road to recovery, and is welcoming to family members – a *family-friendly agency*. Routine exploration of family involvement should be conducted with all service users, using a broad definition of "family" that includes people who are not relatives but have a caring relationship with the person, other than mental health providers.

All family members should have access to support and basic information about their relative's illness in the context of a family-friendly agency.[7,8,9] Staff members need to be knowledgeable about SMI, its treatment, and the experience of family members, and demonstrate an empathic, respectful, non-judgmental attitude towards relatives. The agency waiting room needs to be comfortable, large enough to accommodate multiple family members (including children) waiting for appointments, and provide information brochures about psychiatric illnesses, their treatment, and resources for families.

A spectrum of family services should be available at the agency to meet the diverse needs of families (as described below), as well as a liaison person who can refer families to organizations for families, such as the NAMI in the U.S., the Schizophrenia Society and AMI-Quebec of Canada, Ypsilon in the Netherlands, and Otsma (the Israeli equivalent of NAMI). The agency should have flexible hours to respond to the needs of families, including the ability to provide evening appointments to accommodate working family members. Table 4.1 summarizes the characteristics of family-friendly agencies.

TABLE 4.1 Characteristics of Family Friendly Agencies

1. Staff members have a respectful, non-judgmental attitude about families and recognize the role families can play in supporting recovery
   - all staff members convey respect to families and help them navigate the agency and get the information and support they need
   - staff members receive training about the importance of involving families in supporting recovery, including current research that clearly shows that families do *not* cause mental illness
   - staff members receive training in engaging service users in family work
   - staff members receive training in engaging families, understanding their needs and concerns, and exploring with them ways of supporting their relative's recovery.
2. The agency is accommodating, welcoming and easy for families to navigate
   - a comfortable waiting area is provided for families
   - comfortable rooms of sufficient size are available for holding family meetings and multiple family groups
   - families receive clear directions about how to get to the agency, where to go within the agency, where to park and how to use public transportation to get to the agency
   - staff at the reception area (or equivalent) are trained to be helpful to families when they arrive at the agency
   - evening and weekend hours are available, as well as phone consultations and home visits
   - off-site locations are available for families who prefer to meet individually or in a multifamily group in the community, e.g. private rooms in libraries, churches, synagogues or offices of family organizations
   - staff provide accurate information about billing within the agency, e.g. knowledge of public and private insurance coverage for family meetings with and without the service user present.
3. The agency provides families with a full range of information about psychiatric illnesses and about available resources
   - brochures, handouts, flyers and information sheets are readily available, e.g. a magazine rack in the waiting room, and a staff member or volunteer is responsible for keeping the information orderly and up-to-date
   - the agency provides a lending library of books, magazines, videos and DVDs for families and service users
   - staff members are familiar with brochures and information sheets and have copies of their own to give out to service users and families
   - all staff are familiar with family services within the agency and know how to make referrals to these services, e.g. short-term family consultations, brief education, multi-family psychoeducation groups and individual family therapy
   - all staff are familiar with the resources provided outside the agency and how to make referrals to community resources, e.g. NAMI's Family-to-Family program and support groups

TABLE 4.1 Characteristics of Family Friendly Agencies (*continued*)

- the agency actively coordinates with family organizations on a regular basis, e.g. family organization speakers are present at staff meetings; agency staff members promote events sponsored by family organizations.

4. Staff members routinely explore family involvement with *all* service users
   - family involvement is assessed at intake with any new service user and documented
   - for service users not involved in family work, the service provider regularly re-evaluates the potential benefits of family work with the service user, e.g. every six months the service provider explores the service user's current family involvement and interest in involving family members in treatment
   - consent forms for permission to contact family are readily available to staff, who are trained to explain them to service users
   - family members have access to the treatment team and are informed about how to contact their team.

5. The agency addresses the varying needs of families with a spectrum of family services, providing at least the basic interventions within the agency, and making outside referrals as needed
   - appointment of a family coordinator (or similar position) who develops, coordinates, and oversees services provided to families within the agency
   - all service providers receive training in engaging families, including families in treatment planning, and providing brief family consultation or brief psychoeducation services
   - at least two service providers are trained to provide more intensive family programs, e.g. individual family therapy programs such as behavioral family therapy and multi-family psychoeducation groups) and offer these services to interested families
   - the agency holds regular events that reach out to families, e.g. open houses, summer picnics, winter holiday parties, guest speakers, graduation ceremonies from rehabilitation programs, resource fairs, open family education forums or events for a Mental Illness Awareness Week.

Family Intervention Methods

Families can play a vital role in the treatment and rehabilitation of people with an SMI. Because every family is different, and each family has its unique needs, a spectrum of family services is needed in order for agency staff to work collaboratively and productively with families.[10] We briefly describe a few family services that together comprise the full spectrum of a competent, family friendly agency. We do not describe services offered by family organizations, such as NAMI's educational programs (*see* www.nami.org/template.cfm?section=Education_Training_and_Peer_Support_Center), although families should be informed about such non-mental health provider services.

1. Regular involvement of family members in treatment planning and review

Having family members participate in treatment planning and review meetings provides a forum to discuss the concerns and goals of family members, correct misconceptions they may have about the disorder, obtain information about how the service user is functioning, and to help families play an active role in supporting the service user's progress towards goals and following up on treatment recommendations. Routine involvement of family members in treatment team meetings also serves to build a collaborative relationship with the family that can be maintained over the course of the service user's treatment.

Example

Eliza's parents, Rachel and Adam, were devastated when she developed her first episode of psychosis after going away to college at age 18. Eliza had to drop out of school and return home to get treatment for her disorder. Her parents' concerns were allayed when the director of a special program for people with first episode of psychosis, where Eliza was receiving her treatment, contacted them and expressed the importance of their involvement in Eliza's treatment; he arranged to meet with them to describe the program in more detail. During this meeting, Rachel and Adam were pleased to find out that in addition to learning about psychosis and its treatment, they would be included with Eliza in all treatment-planning and review meetings with other members of her treatment team. Participation in these meetings ensured that the treatment team understood and valued Rachel and Adam's perspectives and concerns about Eliza's needs. For example, Rachel and Adam's input in these meetings was critical to the treatment team addressing Eliza's alcohol and cannabis use, and her irregular adherence to her prescribed medications, which interfered with her goal of returning to school and obtaining her degree.

2. Brief family consultation or therapy

Families often have very specific needs that can be effectively addressed through a limited number of consultation sessions, e.g. one to five sessions, with a mental health provider.[11] Family consultation can involve just the relatives or include the service user as well, and it can take place at either the agency or another convenient location for the family. The approach begins with a connecting phase aimed at developing a working relationship between the service provider and family, which is followed by a discussion of the problems the family is facing, and prioritizing what the family would most like to accomplish through the consultation, e.g. the family wants to understand the service user's illness and find a safe place for him or her to live. Then, a plan is developed and implemented to address those needs. Depending on the family's specific goals, a range of therapeutic strategies can be used, such as empathic listening, providing information about mental illness and its treatment, practical assistance in solving problems, referral to resources in the community, and communicating and coordinating with other treatment providers.

Another approach similar to the family consultation method described above is the McMaster model of family therapy.[12] This model takes a family systems approach to providing short-term (five to 10 sessions) therapy for families of people with SMI, including the service user.[13] The program is divided into four stages, including assessment, contracting, treatment and closure. The treatment stage is primarily devoted to teaching the family strategies for resolving conflict related to the targeted goal(s), such as problem solving, compromise, and negotiation, with family members assuming responsibility for implementing the actual changes. A wide range of problems can be addressed in the program, such as the mother needing more help around the house or the service user stopping his or her medication, leading to symptom relapses.

Example

Teo and his family participated in a brief family consultation. Teo lived at home with his parents but wanted to get his own apartment. He contacted his mental health provider, who invited the whole family (Teo, his mother, father and older brother) to meet with her for consultation on this issue. Together they explored Teo's independent-living skills, his financial resources and his living preferences. They also identified community and family resources. At the end of four sessions, Teo and his family had developed a plan for Teo to learn more cooking and laundry skills from his mother, apply for a supported apartment program with his father's assistance, and start spending occasional weekends at his brother's apartment where he could practice grocery shopping and making meals for the two of them. A follow-up meeting was planned for three months later.

---

3. Brief Psychoeducation

This involves providing information about mental illness to families over a relatively brief period of time, such as four to 12 weeks. Sessions can be led by either mental health providers, trained family members, or both and conducted in a group format or with individual families. Brief psychoeducation usually includes the whole family and follows a set curriculum addressing topics such as basic facts about specific mental illnesses, medications, rehabilitation, reducing family stress and improving communication. Although brief psychoeducation tends to have a limited effect on preventing relapses, families often find it useful for addressing many of their questions, and it may serve to engage some families in more intensive interventions.[14,15]

Example

Ed's wife, Nancy, developed major depression in her mid-50s, which was associated with losing her job, a deterioration in her hygiene and appearance, and loss of interest and enjoyment of life, including in their three adult children. When Ed helped Nancy get into treatment at their local community mental health center, he and Nancy also met with a counselor for six sessions to learn about her depression and its treatment. Their three adult children attended two of the sessions. The whole family was relieved to learn that major depression is no one's fault, and that there are effective treatments for it. Ed was encouraged to learn that he could play a role in Nancy's treatment by helping her incorporate taking medications into her daily routine, scheduling regular enjoyable activities to do together, and helping her challenge her negative, self-defeating thinking. Nancy's children expressed their love and concern for her and suggested some outings they could take together on the weekends.

4. Multi-Family Psychoeducation Groups

These groups are for all interested family members, including the service user. The groups are led by service providers, and meet for 1–1.5 hours either once every two weeks or monthly for nine months or longer. A variety of strategies may be used in leading psychoeducation groups, including presenting information on different topics, eliciting the experiences and coping strategies of family members for dealing with problems, and using group-based problem solving to address common issues faced by families.[16] Psychoeducation in groups offers several advantages over individual-based approaches, including family members sharing their experiences with others and getting social validation, instilling hope in families by seeing how other families have learned to work together and help the service user achieve his or her goals, building social networks, and improved cost-efficiency.

Example

After meeting individually with one of the co-leaders and attending a one-day psychoeducational workshop with other families, the Davidson family (Miki and her mother, father, and sister) joined a multi-family group that met twice a month for 90 minutes. They got to know several other families and reported relief at "realizing we're not alone." They enjoyed the socializing at the beginning and end of each group, and found the group-based problem solving very helpful. After a few months of attending, they brought up their difficulties in coming up with an activity they could all enjoy together. Several group members had experienced this problem, too, and came up with possible solutions. After evaluating the pros and cons of each possible solution, the Davidson family decided to play a card game that they used to enjoy. They decided to start by playing for 45 minutes and planned the day and time, with Miki offering to make a snack to eat while they were playing. At the next meeting, they reported to the group that they had enjoyed playing cards and planned to do it once a week, with each person taking a turn selecting the card game to be played.

5. Individual Family Therapy

Individual family work is warranted in families who do not benefit from brief family consultation or psychoeducation, who cannot be engaged in multi-family groups, or who experience high levels of distress or dysfunction despite participation in multi-family groups. Family therapy for SMI is not based on outdated theories that the family is the cause of mental illness,[17] but rather focuses on reducing stress and conflict in the family, and improving their ability to manage the psychiatric disorder. Family sessions can be conducted at the agency or at home, and are usually provided for at least nine months. Some family therapy approaches are based on adapted family systems theory,[18] some are eclectic,[19] and some are cognitive-behavioral in orientation.[20,21] For example, behavioral family therapy (see the following vignette) is organized into five components, including: 1. Engagement of the family; 2. Individual and family assessment; 3. Psychoeducation; 4. Communication skills training; 5. Problem solving training; and 6. Termination.[22]

Example

After Janice's eighth hospitalization in 10 years following the onset of her schizoaffective disorder, her mother, Helen, was contacted by a psychologist and their local treatment center, who described to her a new family program designed to help service users stay out of the hospital and achieve their goals. Janice, Helen and Janice's brother, Edwin, who also lived at home with Janice and their mother, participated in a behavioral family therapy program over a 13-month period of time. Initially they met with their therapist at their home on a weekly basis, followed by meeting every other week, and then meeting monthly for several months towards the end. At the beginning of the program, the therapist met individually with each family member to assess his or her understanding of schizoaffective disorder, and to identify goals of treatment for each member. These meetings helped the family members connect with the therapist and feel that their concerns were understood and validated. Following these meetings, education was provided about schizoaffective disorder, its treatment, and the role of the family in helping individuals recover. The family was very interested in learning about schizoaffective disorder. The therapist explained that Janice was really the "expert" in the disorder, and her description of some of her symptoms was enlightening, as it was the first time they had ever discussed her symptoms together as a family. Next, training in communication skills was provided using techniques such as modeling and role-playing, followed by homework assignments to practice the skills in order to improve communication and reduce stress and tension in their daily home life. Following this, the family was taught a step-by-step method for solving problems effectively and with low stress, in order to help the members support each other and work towards their personal goals. In several problem-solving sessions, Janice's interest in working with animals was addressed, first by helping her find a volunteer job at a local animal shelter walking dogs, and then several months later obtaining a paying job working at that same animal shelter. Another problem-solving meeting addressed Helen's desire for more help around the house preparing meals and cleaning up, which led to specific chores for each family member to address this need. Over the 13 months that the family participated in behavioral family therapy, Janice had no relapses or re-hospitalizations and made significant progress towards her personal goals. At a two-year follow-up, Janice had still not been hospitalized, and all of the family members reported significantly reduced levels of tension and high levels of satisfaction with their family life.

6. Monthly Facilitated Open Forums

Having a standard monthly meeting that is an open forum for all service users and relatives can help families access critical information they might otherwise have difficulty obtaining. Open forums do not require a stable group membership or a commitment from participants. A forum can be hosted by any mental health provider. Doctors often draw especially large crowds because many family questions center on medications, and most service users and relatives have little opportunity to interact with psychiatrists. Different speakers can also be arranged at these monthly forums, although a consistent leader/facilitator can help build group cohesion.

Example

Josh regularly attended the monthly forum held by the mental health agency, often bringing a friend or relative with him. He liked the fact that there was a schedule with a range of topics such as managing stress, meeting new friends, positive communication skills, coping with anxiety, finding jobs, developing hobbies and learning about new medications. He and his family appreciated the regular leadership by a staff member from the mental health center and also enjoyed the guest speakers, who ranged from social workers to doctors, attorneys and hobby experts. Although the membership of the group varied over time, they got to know several other families. The group even scheduled special meetings at holiday times so that they could celebrate and share each other's special holiday dishes together.

7. Written Resources

Several books are available to mental health providers that describe effective methods for collaborating with families. Some books focus on family experiences and overall approaches to family work,[23,24,25,26,27,28,29] whereas others focus on how to implement specific family programs.[30,31,32,33,34,35,36,37,38] For example, one psychiatric hospital had a special section in their library dedicated to family related references. With input from service users and family members, the staff selected a "book of the month" for a regular discussion group that was co-led by a mental health provider and a librarian. A family checked out several books and attended the discussion group when the subject of the featured book particularly interested them.

Engaging Service Users in Working with Their Families

For most families, it is easier to engage the service user first, and to then separately engage the other family member(s) to discuss the family program. After confirming that the family can benefit from the program, the whole family can begin to participate. The initiation of family work usually begins with the service user, who must give permission for the service provider to contact his or her relatives. Engaging the service user is the key to a successful family program, and thus attention is needed to assure that all service providers have strong engagement skills. Before engagement is attempted, it is critical that family work is a strong recommendation of the service user's treatment team, rather than just an option worth exploring. This enables the service provider to explain to the service user (and relatives) that the family program is recommended by the team as part of the person's treatment.

The timing of engagement can also be critical. Although it is feasible to engage a service user in family work at any point in the illness, crises such as the first development of psychosis or a relapse requiring a hospitalization present a unique opportunity. Service users and relatives are less likely to claim that "everything is fine" immediately following a crisis and tend to be more open to family collaboration. This is especially true if the crisis has not yet been fully resolved, e.g. the service user is still in the hospital, and the service user and relatives are both eager for it to be over.

Service providers should not assume that most service users want their families involved in their treatment, and in fact should be aware that many service users are afraid of it due to misconceptions they may have about family therapy. Therefore, the first priority is to develop a good rapport with the service user, which includes showing interest in him or her, empathic listening, understanding his or her current perceptions of how things are going, and exploring possible changes he or she would like to make. Identifying possible goals the service user would like to achieve can be followed by a discussion of what the service user has done to achieve those goals, and the obstacles he or she has encountered. This discussion leads naturally into exploring the service user's relationships with family members, whether they have been helpful in achieving goals, and possible ways in which these relationships have been unhelpful or have interfered with goal attainment. In discussing the service user's family relationships, the service provider may learn that he or she has had multiple negative experiences with family members or has even experienced abuse. Although this is only the case for a small minority of service users, it is important for service providers to be sensitive to the possibility and to evaluate any potential harm that may result from initiating family work before making recommendations.

In discussing the potential benefits of involving family members with service users, the service provider should first explain that family work is recommended by their treatment team, and then provide a brief description of the program to summarize how it works. In describing the program, it is essential to distinguish it from traditional family therapy approaches by explaining that the emphasis is on providing information and teaching skills in a calm, mutually respectful manner, with the focus on the future rather than the past. Motivational interviewing strategies can be useful in helping service users evaluate the potential advantages and disadvantages of involving their relatives in their treatment.[39] This can be accomplished by reviewing one or two of the service user's most important goals, and then for each goal evaluating the pros and cons of working with their family in terms of achieving that goal. When high levels of stress and tension exist in the family, the service provider can explain that an important focus of the family program will be on reducing that conflict by teaching communication and problem-solving skills.

Several meetings with service users may be necessary to motivate them to participate in the program, and it may be useful to encourage them to talk with other members of their treatment team. Interested but ambivalent service users can be invited to participate in a limited number of family sessions, e.g. one to three, and to then decide whether they want to continue. Service users who express concern that the family program may impose yet another burden on their relatives can be assured that the focus of the program is not on just the service user, but rather on improving the lives of *everyone* in the family.

Some service users may experience additional challenges in deciding whether to participate in family work. For example, some individuals with SMI have been abandoned by their family for a variety of reasons, including the family being "burned out" from trying to deal with the individual's illness without sufficient knowledge or support and from the widespread stigma that is directed towards families as well as individuals with SMI. Service users who are estranged from their families are often apprehensive about re-establishing contact. The service provider can review with the service user the positive changes that have occurred since the estrangement, e.g. the individual may have made progress toward managing his or her illness more effectively, or may have taken steps towards personal goals, or may have reduced his or her substance use, and how this might affect the family's attitude towards him or her. The service provider can explore small steps that the service user might take to re-establish a connection, such as sending a short letter or making a brief phone call to family members that focuses on recent positive events and expresses interest in their well-being. The service provider can also offer to make the initial contact with estranged family members. Another example of a challenge experienced by service users during the engagement process is difficulty understanding the nature and benefits of family work due to cognitive impairments or intrusive symptoms. In such instances, the service provider is advised to break down the information about the family program into small chunks and to hold a series of short but frequent conversations about the subject rather than attempting to cover everything in one or two lengthy sessions.

Engaging Family Members

When the service user is motivated to participate in family work and has given permission to contact relatives, attention turns to engaging them. Engagement involves developing rapport with relatives, exploring their experience with the service user's mental illness, evaluating their needs and making initial plans to address these needs, both through family services provided by the agency and through community resources. Service providers must keep in mind the wide cultural diversity of service users and their families.[40,41] For example, in some cultures it is important to speak to the father first, whereas in others it is the mother who should be approached initially. Some cultures prefer more formal forms of address, whereas others feel more comfortable with informal interactions. Some families may benefit from a translator, starting with the very first contact, and many families benefit from translated written materials, including program descriptions and educational handouts. It is difficult to generalize cultural differences. However, service providers are encouraged to ask the service user for suggestions to guide their initial interactions with relatives and to use empathic listening in every contact with the family to decrease cultural misunderstandings.

The time and effort needed to engage relatives can be minimal, including as few as one or two phone calls or meetings, or it may require more contacts and meetings. Regardless of the time required to engage families, it is an essential part of the process of family collaboration. Engagement involves providing families with information to help them make informed decisions, developing positive expectations for future work with the treatment team, and exploring the benefits of participating in a family program.

After the service user has agreed to work with his or her family, the service provider should make the initial contact with the key relative as soon as possible. This contact can take place either by phone or in person at a mental health agency or hospital. When the initial contact is by phone, the service provider's main goal is to connect with the relative, describe the treatment team's recommendation for the program, briefly describe the program(s) and arrange to meet in person to describe the program(s) in more detail and to answer any questions that may arise.

One challenge sometimes encountered by mental health providers when engaging the relatives of service users with SMI is when another relative also has SMI. There are two common reasons this occurs. First, vulnerability to specific mental illnesses is partly determined by genetic factors,[42] and people with SMI are more likely to have relatives with similar disorders than people without SMI. Second, social selection factors related to SMI, such as living in poverty,[43] having a SUD,[44]

Example

The following in an example of the first conversation between a service provider and the mother of a service user:

Service provider:	Hello. May I speak with Mrs. Hanson please?
Mrs. Hanson:	This is Mrs. Hanson.
Service provider:	Hello, Mrs. Hanson. This is Lanita Bower. I'm calling from the New Beginnings Mental Health Center. I'm the social worker on your son Ross's treatment team. I believe he mentioned to you that I'd be calling?
Mrs. Hanson:	Yes, Ross mentioned it. I'm not sure what this is about, though. Is there some problem?
Service provider:	No, not at all. In fact, I am calling to talk to you about some new family services that we're offering here to the families of everyone we work with. These programs are designed to help family members understand more about mental illness and to work together to help the person stay well and achieve his goals. Your son's treatment team recommends participating in one of these programs. When I talked to Ross about it, he thought that having his family involved in such a program might be helpful and that you and perhaps his dad and his sister might also be interested to know more about what we're offering. Do you have a few minutes to talk right now? About 10 or 15 minutes?
Mrs. Hanson:	Yes, I guess so. But I have to catch an 11:30 bus for a lunch date.
Service provider:	I really appreciate your taking the time to talk to me. I'll be careful to finish the call by 11:00 so you can catch your bus. Would that be OK?
Mrs. Hanson:	Yes, that should be fine. So what's this all about?
Service provider:	Families are very helpful when someone has a mental illness, and we want to make sure that they get all the information and support they need. Each person and each family is unique though, so we have put together several different family programs. Would you like to hear a little about some of the programs we offer?
Mrs. Hanson:	Yes, I would. I must admit we had a bad experience at a family program at another agency about 10 years ago. All they did was blame us for things we did wrong.

Service provider:	I'm very sorry that happened. Some of the older family programs were critical like that, but not ours. We feel strongly that families are very helpful to the people we work with, and we want to support families in every way we can. We also want to reduce the stress that families are under. It might help to hear a few examples of what our programs are like. One program is "Family Consultation," which involves having just a few meetings where your family can get answers to their questions or get help with problems they may be having. Another program is "Individual Family Therapy." We use a model called Behavioral Family Therapy, which involves meeting as a family on a regular basis for several months to learn practical facts about mental illness, strategies for communicating effectively, and skills for solving problems together as a family – all skills that other families similar to yours have found helpful. Still another program is "Multi-Family Psychoeducation Groups," which involve meeting together with other families on an ongoing basis to get information, support and help in solving each other's problems. What do you think so far?
Mrs. Hanson:	Sounds interesting. We've had a hard time understanding Ross's problems. Sometimes we just don't know what to do or how to help him the best.
Service provider:	You are certainly not alone. A lot of families have told us that. Mental illness can be very confusing and it can be difficult to get good information or suggestions for what to do. What are the kinds of things you might like to learn more about in a family program?
Mrs. Hanson:	I don't really understand Ross's diagnosis, which the doctor says is "schizophrenia." And I don't get why Ross has lost interest in things he used to enjoy.
Service provider:	Those are very good questions, and I'd like you to know that those are exactly the kinds of topics which would be covered in the family programs I mentioned earlier. But I see by the clock that our time is almost up, and I know you need to get ready to catch your bus. I'd like to set up a time for us to talk further. I would be very interested in answering some of your questions in more detail and hearing more about your experiences as a family. I'd also like to figure out together whether one of the family programs at the agency may be helpful to you. Do you think other

	people in your family, like your husband and daughter, would be interested to join us for a meeting? We find that the more family members involved, the better.
Mrs. Hanson:	Well, they would probably both be interested, but they work.
Service provider:	I'm glad to say that we have evening hours here at the agency. For example, we're open on Tuesdays and Thursdays until 8 p.m. Or if it's more convenient for you, we could meet at your home or someplace else in the community. For example, the Oakmont Library has private rooms for meetings.
Mrs. Hanson:	I'd rather meet at the agency. I've given Ross a ride there before, and it's pretty close to where my husband and daughter work. They get off at 5 p.m. and could come straight from work.
Service provider:	Sounds good. How about next Thursday at 6 p.m.? Just to confirm some details, our address is 108 Oak Street. There's a public parking lot across the street that's well-lit. It's also near the Oakmont bus station.
Mrs. Hanson:	I think Thursday at 6 will work. I'll talk to my husband and daughter and let you know if they can come with me next Thursday.
Service provider:	That would be great. Again, my name is Lanita Bower, and my phone number is 111-222-3333. I'm in room 108, right next to the receptionist's desk. Also, please give me a call if you have any questions or concerns before then. I really look forward to meeting you and the rest of your family in person.

homelessness,[45] or the stigma of mental illness,[46] may result in service users having greater contact and developing closer relationships with other people with SMI.

When more than one family member has SMI, family collaboration can be effective at helping to manage the other relatives' mental illness as well, as described below.[47] This can be best achieved by striving to engage at least one additional person in the family (or a close friend) to participate in the family sessions. However, even in the absence of the participation of a family member who does not have SMI, e.g. working with a couple who both have SMI, family collaboration can be a helpful approach to teaching both individuals about their own and each other's psychiatric disorder(s), leading to improved monitoring of the illnesses, more informed decision-making and adherence to recommended treatments, closer coordination with the treatment team, and better outcomes. Family collaboration methods also need to accommodate to the special needs of families with multiple members with

SMI, such as presenting information more slowly and frequently checking for understanding, being attentive to additional needs for case management, and seeking opportunities to involve in treatment family members with SMI who are not currently receiving psychiatric services. Person-centered family collaboration with such families has great potential for teaching members how to share the responsibility of managing their SMIs together, and supporting one another in moving forward in their lives and achieving their personal and collective recovery goals.

Another strategy for engaging families in collaborative family work is for service providers to inform relatives about resources that can help them better understand the service user's mental illness, treatment options and the role of the family in creating a low-stress environment that is supportive of the service user's goals and recovery. Several books have been written for family members about mental illness,[48,49,50,51] schizophrenia,[52,53,54,55] and depression and bipolar disorder.[56,57,58,59,60,61] As families learn more about mental illness and their role in helping their service user relative, motivation to work collaboratively with service providers often increases. These books can also be useful resources for health providers to help them better understand the experiences of families and the important role relatives can play in helping the service user manage his or her mental illness and make progress in recovery.

More suggestions about engaging service users and family members, and strategies for addressing common concerns during the engagement process, are provided by Mueser and Glynn,[62] Murray-Swank, Dixon and Stewart,[63] and the Family Institute for Education, Practice and Research.[64]

CONCLUSION

Families are a critically important asset for many service users with SMI, based on their concern for their loved one, the high level of contact they often have, and the emotional and material support they provide. Families coping with SMI also often experience extraordinary amounts of stress, which can both worsen the quality of relatives' lives and precipitate symptom relapses in service users. However, mental health providers often overlook the important role of families in service users' lives, their needs and their potential as allies in the treatment of mental illnesses. Family collaboration is based on the recognition that families have much to offer as partners with mental health providers in the treatment of SMI, and that mutual respect, SDM and a focus on recovery are important ingredients to a successful relationship.

REFERENCES

1 Lefley HP. *Family Caregiving in Mental Illness*. Thousand Oaks, CA: Sage; 1996.
2 Fromm-Reichmann F. Notes on the development of treatment of schizophrenics by psychoanalytic psychotherapy. *Psychiatry*. 1948; **11**(3): 263–73.
3 Appleton WS. Mistreatment of patients' families by psychiatrists. *Am J Psychiatry*. 1974; **131**(6): 655–7.

4 Butzlaff RL, Hooley JM. Expressed emotion and psychiatric relapse. *Arch Gen Psychiatry.* 1998; **55**(6): 547–52.

5 Rudnick A, Roe D. *See* Section 1.1, *Foundations and Ethics of Person-Centered Approaches to Individuals with Serious Mental Illness.*

6 Deegan PE. Recovery: the lived experience of rehabilitation. *Psychosocial Rehabilitation Journal.* 1988; **11**: 11–19.

7 Cohen AN, Glynn SM, Murray-Swank AB, *et al.* The family forum: directions for the implementation of family psychoeducation for severe mental illness. *Psychiatr Serv.* 2008; **59**(1): 40–8.

8 Corrigan PW, Mueser KT, Bond GR, *et al. The Principles and Practice of Psychiatric Rehabilitation: an empirical approach.* New York, NY: Guilford Press; 2008.

9 Mueser KT, Glynn SM. *Behavioral Family Therapy for Psychiatric Disorders.* 2nd ed. Oakland, CA: New Harbinger; 1999.

10 Cohen, op. cit.

11 Family Institute for Education, Practice and Research. *Competency Training in Family Consultation.* Albany, NY: New York Office of Mental Health; 2007.

12 Ryan CE, Epstein NB, Keitner GI, *et al. Evaluating and Treating Families: the McMaster approach.* New York, NY: Routledge; 2005.

13 Miller IW, Keitner GI, Ryan CE, *et al.* Family treatment for bipolar disorder: family impairment by treatment interactions. *Journal of Clinical Psychiatry.* 2008; **69**: 732–40.

14 Glynn SM, Pugh R, Rose G. Benefits of attendance at a state hospital family education workshop. *Psychosocial Rehabilitation Journal.* 1993; **16**: 95–101.

15 Pickett-Schenk SA, Cook J, Steigman P, *et al.* Psychological well-being and relationship outcomes in a randomized study of family-led education. *Archives of General Psychiatry.* 2006; **63**: 1043–50.

16 McFarlane WR. *Multifamily Groups in the Treatment of Severe Psychiatric Disorders.* New York, NY: Guilford Press; 2002.

17 Fromm-Reichmann, op. cit.

18 Anderson CM, Reiss DJ, Hogarty GE. *Schizophrenia and the Family.* New York, NY: Guilford Press; 1986.

19 Kuipers L, Leff J, Lam D. *Family Work for Schizophrenia: a practical guide.* 2nd ed. London: Gaskell; 2002.

20 Mueser, op. cit.

21 Barrowclough C, Tarrier N. *Families of Schizophrenic Patients: cognitive behavioural intervention.* London: Chapman & Hall; 1992.

22 Mueser, op. cit.

23 Atkinson JM, Coia DA. *Families Coping with Schizophrenia.* Oxford: John Wiley & Sons; 1995.

24 Froggatt D, Fadden G, Johnson DL, *et al. Families as Partners in Mental Health Care: a guidebook for implementing family work.* Toronto: World Fellowship for Schizophrenia and Allied Disorders; 2007.

25 Hatfield AB, Lefley HP. *Surviving Mental Illness: stress, coping, and adaptation.* New York, NY: Guilford Press; 1993.

26 Karp DR. *The Burden of Sympathy: How Families Cope with Mental Illness.* New York, NY: Oxford University Press; 2001.

27 Lefley H. *Family Psychoeducation in Serious Mental Illness: models, outcomes, applications.* New York, NY: Oxford University Press; 2009.

28 Marsh DT. *Serious Mental Illness and the Family: the practitioner's guide.* Kaslow FW, editor. New York, NY: John Wiley & Sons; 1998.

29 Vine P. *Families in Pain: children, siblings, spouses, and parents of the mentally ill speak out.* New York, NY: Pantheon Books; 1982.

30 Mueser, op. cit.

31 Ryan, op. cit.

32 McFarlane, op. cit.

33 Anderson, op. cit.

34 Barrowclough, op. cit.

35 Anderson A. Comparative impact evaluation of two therapeutic programs for mentally ill chemical abusers. *International Journal of Psychosocial Rehabilitation.* 1999; **4**: 11–26.

36 Falloon IRH, Boyd JL, McGill CW. *Family Care of Schizophrenia: a problem-solving approach to the treatment of mental illness.* New York, NY: Guilford Press; 1984.

37 Miklowitz DJ. *Bipolar Disorder: a family-focused treatment approach.* 2nd ed. New York, NY: Guilford Press; 2008.

38 Sherman MD. *Support and Family Education: 14-session education program for people who care about someone with a mental illness.* Oklahoma City, OK: Oklahoma City Veterans Affairs Medical Center; 2000.

39 Miller WR, Rollnick S, editors. *Motivational Interviewing: preparing people for change.* Second ed. New York, NY: Guilford Press; 2002.

40 Lefley HP. Culture and mental illness: the family role. In: Hatfield AB, editor. *Families of the Mentally Ill.* New York, NY: Guilford Publications; 1987. pp. 30–59.

41 McGoldrick M, Giordano J, Pearce J, editors. *Ethnicity and Family Therapy.* 2nd ed, New York, NY: Guilford; 1996.

42 Jang KL. *Behavioral Genetics of Psychopathology.* Hillsdale, NJ: Lawrence Erlbaum; 2006.

43 Bruce ML, Takeuchi DT, Leaf PJ. Poverty and psychiatric status: longitudinal evidence from the New Haven Epidemiologic Catchment Area Study. *Archives of General Psychiatry.* 1991; **48**: 470–4.

44 Mueser KT, Noordsy DL, Drake RE, *et al. Integrated Treatment for Dual Disorders: a guide to effective practice.* New York, NY: Guilford Press; 2003.

45 Susser E, Struening EL, Conover S. Psychiatric problems in homeless men: lifetime psychosis, substance use, and current distress in new arrivals at New York City shelters. *Archives of General Psychiatry.* 1989; **46**: 845–50.

46 Corrigan PW, editor. *On the Stigma of Mental Illness: practical strategies for research and social change.* Washington, DC: American Psychological Association; 2005.

47 Mueser, op. cit.

48 Amador X, Johnson A-L. *I'm Not Sick, I Don't Need Help! Helping the Seriously Mentally Ill Accept Treatment: a practical guide for families and therapists.* Peconic, NY: Vida Press; 2000.

49 Morey B, Mueser KT. *The Family Intervention Guide to Mental Illness: recognizing symptoms and getting treatment.* Oakland, CA: New Harbinger Publications; 2007.

50 Sherman MD, Sherman DM. *I'm Not Alone: a teen's guide to living with a parent who has a mental illness.* Edina, MN: Sea of Hope Books/Beaver Pond Press; 2006.

51 Woolis R. *When Someone You Love Has a Mental Illness.* Revised ed. New York, NY: Jeremy P. Tarcher/Penguin Books; 2003.

52 Gur RE, Johnson AB. *If Your Adolescent Has Schizophrenia: an essential resource for parents.* New York: Oxford University Press; 2006.

53 Mueser KT, Gingerich S. *The Complete Family Guide to Schizophrenia: helping your loved one get the most out of life*. New York, NY: Guilford Press; 2006.

54 Levine J, Levine IS. *Schizophrenia for Dummies*. Hoboken, NJ: Wiley; 2009.

55 Torrey EF. *Surviving Schizophrenia: a manual for families, consumers and providers*. 5th ed. New York, NY: HarperTrade; 2006.

56 DePaulo Jr JR. *Understanding Depression: what we know and what you can do about it*. New York, NY: Wiley; 2002.

57 Evans DL, Andrews LW. *If Your Adolescent Has Depression or Bipolar Disorder: an essential resource for parents*. New York, NY: Oxford University Press; 2005.

58 Fast JA, Preston J. *Take Charge of Bipolar Disorder: a 4-step plan for you and your loved ones to manage the illness and create lasting stability*. Boston, MA: Warner Wellness; 2006.

59 Miklowitz DJ. *The Bipolar Disorder Survival Guide: what you and your family need to know*. New York, NY: Guilford Press; 2002.

60 Mondimore FM. *Adolescent Depression: a guide for parents*. Baltimore, MD: Johns Hopkins University Press; 2002.

61 Rosen LE, Amador XF. *When Someone You Love is Depressed: how to help your loved one without losing yourself*. New York, NY: Fireside; 1997.

62 Mueser, op. cit.

63 Murray-Swank AB, Dixon LB, Stewart B. Practical interview strategies for building an alliance with the families of patients who have severe mental illness. *Psychiatr Clin North Am*. 2007; **30**: 167–80.

64 Family Institute for Education, Practice and Research, op. cit.

4.2 Trans-Cultural Issues in Person-Centered Care for People with Serious Mental Illness

Nina Desjardins, Jennifer Gritke and Bill Hill

INTRODUCTION

PCC of people with SMI by definition respects the service user's values and choices, which are frequently informed by that individual's culture. Culture impacts how SMI is manifested, how it is experienced and how it responds to care. This section will examine the essential elements of a person-centered approach to trans-cultural care. This approach includes examination of the cultural and social context of the person presenting for care, the role that culture plays in the expression and experience of SMI, and approaches to incorporating cultural elements into the therapeutic relationship and providing care that is culturally relevant. Additionally, the provider's recognition and understanding of his or her own culture and its role in the therapeutic care relationship will also be examined. The culture of Canada's First Nations peoples will be used in depth to illustrate how the skill set and values of the person-centered approach are well suited to working with various populations, but we will also use examples from other countries. The first two authors wrote this section, except for the example near the end, which the third author wrote. As culture and family cannot be separated, we will assume their interdependence; we refer the reader to Section 4.1, *Collaborating with Families of People with Serious Mental Illness*, for a detailed discussion on families.

This section will focus on how to provide person-centered cross-cultural care; however, it is also important for the provider to be mindful of some instances when focusing on cross-cultural care may not be appropriate. One instance is that providers may mistakenly make assumptions about the service user's level of acculturation. While a provider may be attempting to be mindful of cultural difference, assuming that there is a significant cultural difference within the care relationship without first assessing the service user's self-identified level of acculturation goes against the principles of the person-centered approach. Even if the service user has recognized a high level of identification with his or her culture, it does not necessarily mean that a person-centered approach should focus on the service user's culture while providing care. A person-centered approach would allow the service user and provider to explore together the extent to which culture may or may not be important in the care relationship.

The provider should also be careful not to conflate cultural difference with structural violence; that is, they should be sure to reflect on whether they are assuming that a service user's cultural background has significantly influenced their life circumstances, or whether systematic and institutionalized social, political and economic forces have had a more important bearing on them.[1] A provider using a person-centered approach must become aware of the service user's perceptions of the relative importance of culture versus structural violence on their life and adjust the focus of their care accordingly.

Culture and Mental Illness

A group's culture can be defined as "the sum of learned knowledge and skills – including religion and language – that distinguishes one community from another and which, subject to the vagaries of innovation and change, passes on in a recognizable form from generation to generation."[2] Culture acts as a lens through which the external is interpreted, which in turn constructs experience through the shaping of cognition.[3] Cognitive processes vary across cultures. Cognitive bias leads to the anticipation of information, which in turn directs behavior and influences how outcomes of that behavior are interpreted. Thus, culture can create reality.[4] Recent developments in neurobiology demonstrate that brain structure can be changed by environment and learning,[5,6,7] indicating that brain structure is unlikely to be identical across cultures. Similarly, psychiatric diagnoses and symptoms cannot necessarily be assumed to be identical across cultures.[8,9] Mental illness, then, is at least partially a construct of culture in that it is behavior that has been collectively cognized, interpreted as abnormal, and then "validated" by the scientific method.

The Medical Culture

A provider's training may potentially limit his or her ability to practice effectively across cultures, particularly in the field of mental health. In fact, one can think of the field of biomedicine as constituting its own particular culture, in which providers often are fully immersed.[10] Those practicing a disease-centered approach to mental illness rely on objective, evidence-based sensory experience for knowledge, discounting what is not measurable. The scientific method sets limits on inquiry, and vital information can be passed over if culture is not considered, possibly devaluing or ignoring the service user's subjective experience. Providers may not be fully aware of the degree to which psychiatry is embedded in the medical culture that has developed out of Western biomedicine,[11] and more importantly, may not be aware of the influence the medical culture may have on PCC for people with SMI. It is essential for providers to acknowledge their role in the culture of Western biomedicine and attempt to examine and be self-reflective about how the history, values, beliefs and traditions of the culture of Western biomedicine affect the care that is provided to people with SMI. This may pertain to service users from a Euro-American cultural background that do not understand or believe in some or all of the facets of biomedical culture. It also pertains to people from non-mainstream or minority cultures that hold beliefs, values and traditions that may be at odds with Western biomedicine. For example, Tseng and Steltzer[12] note that the typical Western psychiatry practice of weekly one-hour sessions with service users is not necessarily universal, and that people who have come from other parts of the world may not be used to following a regimented care schedule. A provider who does not understand the discrepancy between appointment practices in different cultures may endanger the provider-service user care relationship if he or she is not aware of and sensitive to such cultural differences.

Person-Centered Cross-Cultural Care in Mental Health

Culture influences how an illness is experienced, expressed, i.e. "idioms of distress," diagnosed, and treated.[13] By influencing expectations and interpretations, culture can also influence clinical outcome. Cultural schemas determine whether or not symptoms are recognized as such, and what explanations are attributed to manifestations of SMI.[14] Given that the service user's subjective experience is central to PCC,[15] consideration of cultural factors on both sides of the service user/provider dyad is a critical aspect of assessing and treating people with SMI. Awareness of the cultural values and biases one brings into the care relationship is a vital part of this process.

While the DSM-IV-TR Cultural Formulation[16] (*see* Table 4.2) can be used as a framework for cross-cultural assessment and care, this approach is disease-centered and is biased towards Euro-American or Western culture. Because many non-Western models of healing are not disease-centered, a person-centered cross-cultural assessment must take this bias into account. People are shaped by their culture's history and worldview, and in many non-Western cultures exist within a social context that is more collectivistic than individualistic. The process of acculturation further shapes a person's experience and attitudes. Person-centered cross-cultural care should thus consider the elements listed in Table 4.3.

TABLE 4.2 DSM-IV TR Outline for Cultural Formulation

1. Cultural identity of the individual
2. Cultural explanations of the individual's illness
3. Cultural factors related to psychosocial environment and functioning
4. Cultural elements of the relationship between the individual and clinician
5. Overall cultural assessment for diagnosis and care

TABLE 4.3 Elements of Person-Centered Cross-Cultural Care

1. Cultural context – the history, worldview, values and traditions of the person's culture
2. Social context – the person's experience in relationship to others
3. Cultural identity – how the person defines himself or herself in relation to his or her culture
4. Level of acculturation
5. Cultural explanations for presenting issue
6. Cultural elements of the therapeutic relationship (including provider's self-assessment)
7. Culturally relevant care

The elements of person-centered cross-cultural care for people with SMI will be discussed in detail, with several cultural examples being used, in particular the culture of Canada's First Nations.

Cultural Context

When a provider is caring for someone with SMI who has a different cultural background, it is crucial that the provider be aware of the context, i.e. the history, worldviews, values and traditions of that culture. People from different cultural backgrounds may not subscribe to current mainstream and accepted understandings of psychiatric disorders, and may subscribe to alternative cultural explanations.[17] Historical and current experiences of discrimination, racism and cultural trauma may also have a significant impact on the service user's life experiences and beliefs.

In Canada, First Nations people have a distinct cultural context that may have an important bearing on a provider/service user care relationship for people with SMI. Although there is considerable diversity of values and traditions across the 614 First Nations communities that exist in Canada today, there are common features that are relevant to the care of people with SMI. The legal distinctions Status, Non-Status, Inuit and Metis refer to the distinctions between those who are legally considered wards of the Canadian state as legally defined by the Indian Act and those who are not. *Status* confers some benefits such as hunting and fishing rights, health care benefits, and some funding for post-secondary education. *Non-Status* refers to those who have lost or never had status. *Metis* people have origins in the intermarriage between Europeans (particularly French) and aboriginal people and have a unique cultural identity. The *Inuit* are a distinct people not legally defined by the Indian Act, but are included in the Canadian government's definition of "aboriginal." Aboriginal people in Canada account for 3.8% of Canada's population,[18] with the majority (60%) living off reserve in urban settings.[19] A sub-set of aboriginal people migrate between various cities and reserves, resulting in increased intertribal and interethnic marriage. This section will use the term *aboriginal* to describe ethnic identity, the term *First Nations* when referring to diversity, and *community* to refer to bands or tribal groups. Many aboriginal people choose to use their tribal affiliation when discussing ethnic heritage, e.g. Mohawk, Six Nations, or Cree. Canada's aboriginal people have decreased life expectancy, higher rates of preventable deaths, and infant mortality twice the national average.[20] Precise mental health statistics are unavailable for a number of reasons,[21] however, as a group aboriginal people have higher rates of suicide,[22] violence,[23] and incarceration.[24,25] It is also likely that they have higher rates of substance abuse.[26,27] A number of factors have contributed to these challenges, including lower socioeconomic status, acculturation stress and loss of identity. Aboriginal people also under-utilize the services available to them because of the perception that mainstream services are not responsive to their needs, congruent with their values or culturally safe.[28,29]

Historical Context

If the service user comes from a different cultural background than the care provider, it is beneficial to have an understanding of the historical context of that culture. The historical context can have a significant influence on the past and current experiences of the service user. A provider treating a service user who is a refugee or migrant from a country with great upheaval or war in the past would be well-served to have at least a basic understanding in the historical context of the service user's culture, as well as an interest in learning more as it may relate to the service user's care. Kinzie and Leung note that providers should know about the "high likelihood of massive trauma in some ethnic groups," citing the effects of war, ethnic cleansing and guerilla activities in refugees groups from places such as Indochina, Bosnia, Somalia and Central America.[30] Similarly, historically negative cross-cultural relations and a history of discrimination and marginalization of certain cultural groups within a larger society are issues that providers need to be aware of, as a particular historical context may color a provider and service user care relationship.

In Canada, colonialism has strained First Nations relations with mainstream culture. Although Canada is a multicultural society with a growing population of immigrant minorities, its aboriginal people have a unique history that requires special consideration. Ethnocentrism provided a rational for domination and assimilation of what were seen as socially, morally and intellectually inferior societies. Colonization of North America occurred from the 16th century onward, with a gradual depopulation of indigenous populations through disease and habitat destruction. The signing of treaties and the Indian Act of 1876 in Canada marked a turning point in First Nations history with the creation of the reserve system. Aboriginals on reserves received the benefits of food, shelter, health care and education. However, the Indian Act also banned religious ceremonies and removed Indians from their traditional way of life, which had been intimately connected to the land. Ultimately, many traditions went underground or were lost. Currently, poverty, poor water quality, lack of running water and substandard housing are common on reserves.[31] Many treaty rights are lost when individuals leave the reserve, and thus the system perpetuates the "ghettoization" of Canada's aboriginal people.

Another event which had a lasting and negative impact on Aboriginal culture was residential school education. Although the government of Canada issued an official apology in 2008 for the abuses that occurred in the residential school system, understanding of this history is not widespread across Canada's general populace. These church/government-run schools first opened in 1879 with the aim of assimilating aboriginal children by forcibly removing them from the influence of family and home. These schools took away their names, forbade their languages, and subjected the children to torture and abuse in the name of suppressing their culture.[32] The last school (Gordon Residential School in Saskatchewan) closed in 1996.[33] While some would say these schools were misguided but well-intentioned efforts to better the life of aboriginal people, others maintain they were calculated moves at cultural genocide and a crime against humanity.[34] The resulting trauma and loss of identity is considered an etiological factor in the multitude of mental health difficulties seen in this population today and are considered direct causes of lost parenting skills and disruption in social structure.[35,36] For many it is difficult to reconcile with the system that committed these crimes and thus the rift between First Nations and mainstream society remains vast.

These historical traumas have been found in other Aboriginal cultures as well. The Australian government also forcibly removed thousands of Aboriginal children from their parents, in an attempt to assimilate them into Australian society over a 150-year period, up to the 1980s.[37] This removal of aboriginal children resulted in "broken families, diminished physical and mental health, loss of language, culture and connection to traditional land, loss of parenting skills and enormous distress."[38] This historical trauma was first addressed nationally with the introduction of "National Sorry Day" in 1997, which was intended to commemorate and honor what is known as the "Stolen Generation."[39] On February 13, 2008, Prime Minister Kevin Rudd read an apology in Parliament directed to Australian aboriginals for the traumas caused by the Stolen Generation.

Worldview

Learning about the worldview of a service user from a cultural background that is unfamiliar or different from the care provider's is important. One's worldview encompasses perceptions, attitudes, beliefs and behaviors, and understanding that worldview may result in more effective and respectful PCC.

It is important to stress the diversity of cultural traditions across Canada's First Nations; however, there is some overlap in worldview. Cultures can generally be described as socio-centric or egocentric.[40,41] In socio-centric societies, the individual is oriented towards the collective and values interdependence and interconnectedness. Behavior is determined by social roles within the group. Cooperation, mutual support and helping behavior are highly valued. North American indigenous societies, for the most part, fall into this category. Egocentric societies, on the other hand, value self above the collective, and emphasis is on individual freedom and competition. Another useful general concept is whether a society is based on a dominance hierarchy or egalitarian. Hierarchies can be based on race, gender or class – for example, India's caste system. Mainstream North American society is egocentric and hierarchical, which is reflected in criticisms of the mainstream health care system, which is said to be hierarchical, i.e. doctor: nurse, doctor: service user. Within this context, aboriginal people report feeling "marginalized" and like outsiders.[42]

Values and Traditions

Understanding the traditions and values of another person's culture can be challenging. An understanding of the service user's culture can unfold as the therapeutic alliance evolves, but it may also be useful for the provider to undertake his or her own research.

With respect to First Nations people, approaching a traditional healer for specific teachings with respect to the local community and attending community events may be desirable and can aid credibility.[43,44] Some hospitals in Canada have elders or First Nations liaison personnel that can facilitate this process. Local aboriginal health access centers may also be sources of support. Table 4.4 summarizes some values that are said to be common in many First Nations communities.[45,46,47] A present-time orientation can be translated loosely as doing things when the time is right, and to do so one must be living in the present and in tune with creation. The ethic of non-interference refers to respecting the individual's autonomy by refraining from coercive or directive behavior. Elders are universally important as sources of knowledge and leadership. Note, however, that in some communities this structure has been compromised because of residential schools. Holism refers to the inseparability of mind, body, spirit, community and environment, which ties into the socio-centric belief that the "I" exists in relation to the larger "we" of family, community and Creation. This is the "meaning of family" referred to in Table 4.4. For this reason, the individual cannot be assessed without also assessing his or her relationships with his or her body, spirit, family, community and environment. This approach correlates to holism, non-interference, i.e. non-directiveness, and egalitarianism, all of which are espoused in the person-centered approach.[48]

Acculturation, Identity and Terminology

The cultural change that people experience when contact is made with another culture is called acculturation. There are a number of choices available to the individual when this occurs. The importance of determining the level of acculturation of an individual has been identified in a number of works.[49,50,51,52] For example, Garrett[53] identifies five basic levels of acculturation (*see* Table 4.5).

Castillo[54] points out that in a hierarchical society, personality development is affected by the role a person is assigned in the hierarchy and how he or she adapt to it. This is particularly important when an individual's race and culture have been stigmatized. He describes a number of choices available in this situation: submission, attempting to hide by copying the dominant group, overachieving, violent resistance or violence to self. For example, in the case of Canada's aboriginal people, some posit that the effect of cultural genocide has led to a construct of mainstream

---

TABLE 4.4 Values found commonly among First Nations

1. Present-time orientation
2. Harmony with nature
3. Ethic of non-interference
4. Deep respect for elders
5. Cooperative relationships with others
6. Modesty
7. Holism
8. Meaning of family

TABLE 4.5 Five Basic Levels of Acculturation

1. **Traditional** – generally speak and think in their native language; practice only traditional customs and beliefs
2. **Marginal** – may speak both the native language and the mainstream language; may not, however, fully accept the cultural heritage and practices of the tribal group or fully identify with mainstream cultural values and behaviors
3. **Bicultural** – generally accepted by dominant society; simultaneously able to know, accept and practice both mainstream values and the traditional values and beliefs of their cultural heritage
4. **Assimilated** – generally accepted by dominant society; embrace only mainstream culture and values
5. **"Pantraditional"** – may not have been raised with the traditions of their nation, but return to traditional ways, or choose to participate in pantraditional activities of their, or closely related, cultures

society as predatory, devaluing and racist. The relationship that a service user from a racial or cultural background that has been stigmatized has to a construct such as this will inevitably impact the therapeutic relationship. This relationship can be manifested in several ways. Submission to the aggressor may be manifested as a negative self-image, marginalization, or possibly as passivity and compliance. Resistance to the aggressor can be manifested as anger – through violence to others, violence to self, or more productively, through achievement, dominance or political involvement. Identification with the aggressor has been postulated to be the source of family violence and alcohol abuse.[55] A person-centered approach would seek to assist the service user in developing a congruent relationship with dominant society and with his or her cultural identity, with the individual defining what that relationship will be.

Cultural Explanations of Presenting Issue

In formulating our understanding of a service user's difficulties, it is important to understand the explanations his or her culture may be providing. Whether or not that explanation has validity in the lens of the provider's training is not important. Curing a disease is "likely to have poor outcome if the disease that is diagnosed is not simultaneously the illness that has brought the client in for treatment."[56] Healing occurs when the person's subjective experience of illness is treated.

Depression, Suicide and Substance Abuse

Although providers should have a basic knowledge and understanding of possible cultural influences on service user's experiences with depression, suicidal ideation and substance abuse, a provider attempting to use a PCC approach would be remiss if he or she focused on perceived cultural explanations without delving into the service user's subjective experience. In modern First Nations mental health dialogue, the effects of colonization, loss of identity, residential schools, rapid cultural change and historical abuse are among many explanations for the high rates of depression, alcoholism and suicide in this population. Attempting to fit an individual into any one of these frameworks runs contrary to the values of PCC. This is not to say that the individual is not suffering, but that it is how the service user conceptualizes that suffering is what matters. O'Nell's work with the Flathead people of Montana is an interesting study of cultural meaning of depression in one tribal group.[57] In that group, depression was an expression of solidarity rather than suffering.

Culture-Bound Syndromes

Culture-bound syndromes are "recurrent, locality-specific patterns of aberrant behavior and troubling experience that may or may not be linked to a particular DSM-IV diagnostic category."[58] Examples of culture-bound syndromes are widely available. *Koro* can be found in some Southeast Asian and African cultures and is posited to be an anxiety attack resulting from the belief that excessive shrinking of the penis into the abdomen will cause death.[59] *Amok*, as found in Malaysian culture, is viewed by some as an indiscriminate, mass homicidal act in reaction to stress or loss.[60] *Dhatu loss* in India is the belief that a loss of sperm or vaginal discharge reduces vitality, which may represent emotional distress or loss of empowerment.[61] There are three frequently described culture-bound syndromes in North American aboriginal cultures: *the windigo psychosis*, *ghost sickness* and *pibloktok*.[62] It may be tempting for providers to turn to culture-bound syndromes in assessing service users from different cultural background, however, some critiques of culture-bound syndromes exist. In his critique of the evidence regarding these disorders, Waldram[63] makes a strong case for these being "wayward psychiatric mythologizing" rather than stand-alone disorders. He goes on to point out that the disorders characterize aboriginals as primitive, anxious, hysteric and childlike. The concern here is that the existence of these diagnoses reflects the colonial bias that "other cultures had uniquely irrational ideas and incomprehensible behavior."[64] In persisting with the Western impulse to classify and categorize, we run the risk of ignoring the individual's underlying subjective experience. A person-centered approach to unusual symptoms or syndromes is to consider them to be culturally specific ways of expressing suffering, i.e. idioms of distress, rather than disease syndromes.

Psychosis

Studies attempting to discern any differences in rates of psychosis for various cultural and ethnic groups are fraught with methodological difficulties; however, some studies have noted higher rates of psychosis among certain cultural groups. One cultural group in particular, which has been the subject of multiple studies on schizophrenia, is the African-Caribbean community in the UK.[65] McKenzie, Fearon and Hutchinson found that various studies have reported rates of schizophrenia to be two to 14 times higher for African-Caribbeans than for whites in the UK.[66] Despite this finding, it is important to note that methodological biases and assumptions make the process of studying rates of psychosis among different cultural groups difficult, as does the process of untangling multiple layers of political, social, economic, geographic and cultural factors and meanings.

Besides an awareness of potentially higher rates of psychosis in various cultural groups, the cultural understanding and manifestations of psychosis by the culture must also be considered. For example, hearing voices may not be received as auditory hallucinations in some cultures, but instead may indicate that one is a conduit for spirits. For North American aboriginals, the literature is surprisingly scant. This may be because communities have become reticent to share knowledge because of past negative experiences with being diagnosed through the lens of Euro-American psychiatry. Belief in witchcraft, spirits and bad medicine are within cultural norms, and it is important to approach the matter without bias. However, sometimes these can be used as explanations for perceptual disturbances such as auditory hallucinations. Cultural explanations for psychosis also exist, and individuals with schizophrenia can be assigned specific roles within the social or religious structure of a community. Most of what has been written about psychosis in this context is epidemiological in nature and indicates that the incidence of schizophrenia in the North American aboriginal population is roughly equal to that of the general population.[67,68]

CULTURALLY RELEVANT CARE

Cultural Safety

Cultural safety is a relatively new concept that developed out of work with indigenous peoples' concerns with mainstream health care in New Zealand.[69] Cultural safety takes the concept of cultural competence a step further; it acknowledges the power differentials and colonial attitudes inherent in the Euro-American medical model, which is experienced as demeaning and devaluing by indigenous peoples. This concept echoes many of the concepts heretofore covered but has originated from within the indigenous community. Freeth[70] describes culturally safe care when she describes a "locus of evaluation" external to the provider where "the views, opinions and judgments" of the service user are more valid than the provider's. Kirmayer[71] also echoes this concept: "people who were once the object of ethnographic study have their own say in how their worlds are to be interpreted." The person-centered approach to cross-cultural care recognizes that the service user is the expert about his or her culture.

Lessons from Traditional Healing

Providing culturally relevant care also includes respecting alternative methods of healing that the service user may be accessing. Understanding the service user's view of health and healing can aid in strengthening the therapeutic alliance. The legitimacy of traditional forms of healing is recognized by all indigenous cultures, although practitioners of the biomedical model may dismiss these practices as primitive and superstitious.

Modern healing movements in First Nations communities – so-called pan-Amerindian healing[72,73] – are based on the traditional beliefs and values described in Table 4.4. Traditional methods of healing such as the sweat lodge,[74] healing circles and restorative justice[75,76] are gaining acceptance in the mainstream. Ceremonies provide structure and meaning to transitions that are central to the healing process, where old ways of being are abandoned and new identities are formed.[77,78] Currently the most universal symbol associated with the First Nations healing is that of the medicine wheel – a circle divided into four quadrants by a cross. It is used as a teaching model. One common teaching is that the self consists of mind, body, emotions and spirit, and that balance among these is paramount for good health. Healing our relationships – to ourselves, to each other, and to society – is one of the aims of traditional medicine. The goal is not to "cure" a disease, but to enable us to live well. From this point of view, the goal in care of SMI should not necessarily be the eradication of symptoms – it should be for individuals to live their lives according to goals they have set for themselves.

Other aspects of providing culturally relevant care are summarized below.[79,80,81]

➤ Show respect. Refrain from devaluing (or idealizing) the person's culture, but hold it in esteem. Acknowledge the difference in cultures and be open to discussing differences.

➤ Allow time for trust to develop rather than focusing on feelings or presenting problems; discuss other issues instead. It may take several sessions before the service user begins to discuss what brought him or her there. Allow him or her to tell his or her story, without interruption, in his or her own time.

➤ Be aware of non-verbal communication patterns. Respect the use of silence without "waiting it out."[82] Similarly, lack of eye contact may be a sign of respect. Do not read non-verbal communications as a lack of appreciation or lack of cooperation.

➤ Be patient.

➤ Meet with family and other important supports. Be open to allowing family to come into sessions. Allow as much time for this as necessary.

➤ Integrate care with the person's culture. If possible, learn about the service user's culture first hand from the service user, family and community supports. Attend non-medical events in the community. Integrate your care with supports within the cultural community, including traditional healers.

Example

A situation requiring a culturally competent person-centered approach to an aboriginal person with SMI:

A social worker at a regional psychiatric hospital in Canada was asked to come to a ward by a psychiatrist to assist in interpreting some behaviors and symptoms that were being exhibited by an aboriginal woman. The social worker was of aboriginal descent, and he had often incorporated facets of traditional cultural practices into his work with mental health service users. The psychiatrist was interested in a traditional perspective of this particular service user's condition.

The psychiatrist explained that the woman was not responding well to several different psychotropic medications. She had a long history of substance abuse and was diagnosed with schizophrenia. Prior to admission, she had been involved in a serious car accident while under the influence of drugs and alcohol. Upon admission, she was speaking to unseen persons and asking others if they could see and hear them. She was speaking of colors and directions, and was adamant that what she was saying and seeing existed. Her symptoms had remained the same no matter which medication or dosage was tried. She had been in hospital for over six weeks with little progress in her mental health condition, however, she had abstained from alcohol and illicit drug use. The doctor asked if the social worker would interview this individual in order to form an opinion on her condition. Were the service user's words delusional or cultural?

In preparation for the visit, the social worker wrapped and tied a portion of tobacco in a small 4"x4" red cloth. A tobacco tie is an offering of traditional medicine to honor the person with whom you are to speak. The offering is a protocol meant to show respect and to facilitate good communication, good energy and ancestral inclusion in the conversation. This offering of tobacco was meant to serve one of two purposes. If the service user was familiar with traditional cultural practices, she would understand that the social worker knew traditional protocols to speak about personal matters. If she was not a traditional person, the offering of tobacco would be explained with the aim of providing comfort through the sharing of teachings from one native person to another.

When the tobacco tie was offered, the service user took it, inverted it and moved it in the fashion of playing an accordion, and said, "Look, the White Eagle, you are a White Eagle, looking out for me coming in from the White Door. You are my speaker. Thanks to Creator for the Speaker. Oh, look, your beautiful White Buffalo Son. I like your fan. What a beautiful fan. Help me speak, can you? I have burning medicines on my tongue, can't speak or see sometimes. He keeps giving me burning medicines, medicines that burn my tongue and eyes. He's not trying to hurt me, but he can't hear me."

The colors mentioned by the service user can be related to a Medicine Wheel. A Medicine Wheel is a traditional native circular symbol separated into four colored quadrants of red, yellow, black and white. Each quadrant addresses aspects of an individual's physical, emotional, mental and spiritual health and relates to specific features of the cardinal directions. The service user's reference to the "White Door" can be related to clarity and the northern direction. Traditionally, the eagle is a messenger. The social worker seemed to be perceived as a messenger of clarity, someone who could interpret the words of the woman for her doctor.

It was learned that the service user had been taught by her Elders to be a seer and to speak in the vernacular of white doors, eagles and buffalos. This individual had been named in her own language. The name can be loosely translated as someone who "understands" in two worlds; she was one who stood with one foot in sprit world and one foot in this physical world.

The social worker related that, weeks earlier, his own son had been described by an Elder as having the quiet, gentle strength of a buffalo. As well, the social worker had just been gifted a beautiful fan made from a goose wing and the branch of a cedar tree, and it was indeed beautiful. This individual with an SMI said words that were seemingly incomprehensible to others, but they held meaning for her traditional interviewer.

The service user spoke with the social worker about the car accident. The service user spoke quite lucidly about the events that led up to the accident and subsequent admission. She would carry on a conversation and stay focused on the topic and then would speak again about colors and directions.

As the social worker continued to speak with the service user, he came to the conclusion that she was gifted, albeit she was experiencing positive symptoms of her schizophrenia as well.

Following the initial interview, the social worker and psychiatrist met with the service user together. The social worker explained that the service user's manner of expressing herself was indeed cultural, and, in his opinion, somewhat gifted. It was important to note that her manner of expressing ideas such as colors and animals needed to be taken into account when devising measurements of dosages to combat the other symptoms she was experiencing.

Over the three weeks following the initial meeting of the social worker and service user, subsequent visits took place. The woman's condition gradually stabilized, her medications were more effective and she required less of them as she was no longer being treated for what had originally been thought to be positive symptoms of her illness. These symptoms had become a matter of perspective. Many Elders in native communities would be considered gifted seers if they were to speak with such vision and accuracy.

The social worker concluded that although this individual had a serious mental illness, she was simply trying to express herself in her cultural language. The psychiatrist can be seen as an exceptional caregiver. He was proactive in trying different methods, medications and approaches, including cultural interpretation, to calm the woman's symptoms.

This example illustrates how two health care modalities were combined to bring positive results to the cross-cultural needs of a service user with SMI. We hope that such approaches will be more commonly used and further developed and studied in the future.

CONCLUSION

The values and practices required to provide person-centered cross-cultural care have been discussed. These include gaining a working knowledge of another culture and understanding the culture from the service user's point of view. This means they must be assessed in their context, not ours: their historical context, the context of their relationships and the context of their community. This approach also seeks to provide care that is culturally relevant and treats the service user's subjective experience, as opposed to his or her diagnosis. Parallels exist between the person-centered model of care, current thought in cross-cultural psychiatry and current thought in the field of First Nations mental health. Although historically Western psychiatry has been tainted by the bias of colonialism, a new paradigm is emerging that is both safe and relevant to people from non-Western cultural backgrounds. Duran[83] speaks of a post-colonial paradigm that will "accept knowledge from differing cosmologies as valid in their own right"; it is our opinion that the practice of a "post-colonial psychiatry" is possible. Such practice entails moving beyond the bio-medical model, respecting the service user's subjective experience and choices, and reflecting upon the impact one's own culture has upon the therapeutic dyad.

REFERENCES

1 Farmer P. *Infections and Inequalities: the modern plagues*. Berkeley, CA: University of California Press; 1999.
2 Lewis IM. *Social Anthropology in Perspective*. Cambridge, UK: Cambridge University Press; 1985.
3 D'Andrade RG. Cultural meaning systems. In: Shweder RA, Levine RA, editors. *Culture Theory: essays on mind, self, and emotion*. Cambridge, UK: Cambridge University Press; 1984. pp. 88–119.
4 Neisser U. *Cognition and Reality: principles and implications of cognitive psychology*. New York, NY: WH Freeman; 1976.
5 Kirmayer LJ, Minas H. The future of cultural psychiatry: an international perspective. *Can J Psychiatry*. 2000; **45**: 438–46.
6 Kirmayer LJ. Mind beyond the net: implications of cognitive neuroscience for cultural psychiatry. *Transcultural Psychiatry*. 2000; **37**(4): 467–94.
7 Kandel ER, Hawkins RD. The biological basis of learning and individuality. *Scientific American*. 1992; **262**(3): 78–86.
8 Kleinman A, Eisenberg L, Good B. Culture, illness, and care: clinical lessons from anthropologic and cross-cultural research. *Annals of Internal Medicine*. 1978; **88**: 251–8.
9 Kleinman A, Good B, editors. *Culture and Depression: studies in the anthropology and cross-cultural psychiatry of affect and disorder*. Berkeley, CA: University of California Press; 1985.

10 Tseng W, Seltzer J, editors. *Cultural Competence in Clinical Psychiatry*. Washington, DC: American Psychiatric Publishing, Inc.; 2004.

11 Ibid.

12 Ibid.

13 Kleinman A. *Patients and Healers in the Context of Culture: an exploration of the borderline between anthropology, medicine, and psychiatry*. Berkeley, CA: University of California Press; 1980.

14 Kleinman A. *The Illness Narratives: suffering, healing, and the human condition*. New York, NY: Basic Books; 1988.

15 Freeth R. *Humanising Psychiatry and Mental Health Care: the challenge of the person-centred approach*. Oxford, UK: Radcliffe Publishing; 2007.

16 American Psychiatric Association. *Diagnostic and Statistical Manual of Mental Disorders, 4th Edition, Text-Revised (DSM-IV-TR)*. Washington, DC: American Psychiatric Association; 2000.

17 Tseng, op. cit.

18 Statistics Canada. *2006 Census Data*. Ottawa, ON: Statistics Canada; 2007.

19 Statistics Canada. *1991 Aboriginal Peoples Survey*. Ottawa, ON: Statistics Canada; 1994.

20 Health Canada. *A Statistical Profile on the Health of First Nations in Canada*. Ottawa, ON: Health Canada; 2000.

21 Smilie J. A guide for health professionals working with aboriginal peoples: the socio-cultural context of aboriginal peoples in Canada. *Journal of the Society of Obstetricians and Gynaecologists of Canada*. 2000; **22**: 1070–81.

22 Advisory Group on Suicide Prevention. *Acting on What We Know: preventing youth suicide in First Nations*. Ottawa, ON: Health Canada; 2003.

23 Brzozowski J, Taylor-Butts A, Johnson S. Victimization and offending among the Aboriginal population in Canada. *Juristat: Canadian Centre for Justice Statistics*. 2006; **26**(3): catalogue no. 85-002-XIE.

24 Ross R. *Dancing with a Ghost: exploring Indian reality*. Markham, ON: Octopus Publishing Group; 1992.

25 Ross R. *Returning to the Teachings: exploring aboriginal justice*. Toronto, ON: Penguin Canada; 1996.

26 Health Canada. *A Statistical Profile on the Health of First Nations in Canada, 1999 to 2003*. Ottawa, ON: Health Canada; 2009.

27 Wardman D, Khan N, el-Guebaly N. Prescription medication use among an aboriginal population accessing addiction treatment. *Can J Psychiatry*. 2002; **47**(4): 355–60.

28 Renfrey GS. Cognitive-behavior therapy and the Native American client. *Behavior Therapy*. 1992; **23**: 321–40.

29 Johnson JL, Cameron MC. Barriers to providing effective mental health services to American Indians. *Ment Health Serv Res*. 2001; **3**(4): 215–23.

30 Kinzie JD, Leung PK. Culture and outpatient psychiatry. In: Tseng W, Streltzer J, editors. *Cultural Competence in Clinical Psychiatry*. Washington, DC: American Psychiatric Publishing, Inc.; 2004. pp. 37–51.

31 First Nations Regional Longitudinal Health Survey (RHS) 2002/03. *Results for Adults, Youth and Children Living in First Nations Communities* [online]. Ottawa, ON: Assembly of First Nations/First Nations Information Governance Committee; 2007. Available at: www.rhs-ers.ca/sites/default/files/ENpdf/RHS_2002/rhs2002-03-technical_report.pdf (accessed 26 May 2011)

32 *Highlights from the Report on the Royal Commission on Aboriginal Peoples: people to people, nation to nation* [online]. 1996. Available at: www.ainc-inac.gc.ca/ap/pubs/rpt/rpt-eng.asp (accessed 26 May 2011).

33 Assembly of First Nations. *History of Indian Residential Schools* [previously available online]. Cited from: www.afn.ca/residentialschools/history.html (accessed 18 Nov 2009).

34 Chrisjohn R, Young S. *The Circle Game: shadows and substance in the Indian Residential School experience in Canada.* Penticton, BC: Theytus Books; 1997.

35 Braveheart MYH. The historical trauma response among Natives and its relationship with substance abuse: a Lakota illustration. *J Psychoactive Drugs.* 2003; **35**(1): 7–13.

36 Kirmayer LJ, Brass GM, Tait CL. The mental health of Aboriginal peoples: transformations of identity and community. *Can J Psychiatry.* 2000; **45**: 607–16.

37 National Sorry Day Committee. *History of Sorry Day.* Available at: www.nsdc.org.au/home/index.php?option=com_content&view=section&layout=blog&id=7&Itemid=15 (accessed 3 May 2011).

38 Ibid.

39 Ibid.

40 Greenfield PM, Keller H, Fuligni A, *et al.* Cultural pathways through universal development. *Annual Review of Psychology.* 2003; **54**: 461–90.

41 Castillo RJ. *Culture and Mental Illness: a client-centered approach.* Pacific Grove, CA: Brooks/Cole Publishing Company; 1997.

42 Brown AJ, Fiske J, Thomas G. *First Nations Women's Encounters with Mainstream Health Care Services and Systems.* Vancouver, BC: British Columbia Centre of Excellence for Women's Health; 2001.

43 Renfrey, op. cit.

44 Kelly L, Brown JB. Listening to native patients. *Can Fam Physician.* 2002; **48**: 1645–52.

45 Renfrey, op. cit.

46 Brant CC. Native ethics and rules of behavior. *Can J Psychiatry.* 1990; **35**: 534–9.

47 Garrett MT, Herring RD. Honoring the power of relation: counseling Native adults. *Journal of Humanistic Counseling.* 2001; **20**(2): 139–60.

48 Freeth, op. cit.

49 Renfrey, op. cit.

50 Johnson, op. cit.

51 Garrett, op. cit.

52 Waldram JB. *Revenge of the Windigo: the construction of the mind and mental health of North American aboriginal peoples.* Toronto, ON: University of Toronto Press; 2004.

53 Garrett, op. cit.

54 Castillo, op. cit.

55 Duran E, Duran B. *Native American Postcolonial Psychology.* Albany, NY: State University of New York Press; 1995.

56 Castillo, op. cit.

57 O'Nell TD. *Disciplined Hearts: history, identity and depression in an American Indian community.* Berkeley, CA: University of California Press; 1996.

58 American Psychiatric Association, op. cit.

59 Ibid.

60 Ibid.

61 Trollope-Kumar K. *Speaking Through the Body: leukorrhea as a bodily idiom of communication in Garhwal, India* [Ph.D. thesis]. Hamilton, ON: McMaster University; 2001.

62 American Psychiatric Association, op. cit.

63 Ibid.

64 Kirmayer, Minas, 2000, op. cit.

65 McKenzie K, Fearon P, Hutchinson G. Migration, ethnicity and psychosis. In: Morgan C, McKenzie K, Fearon P, editors. *Society and Psychosis*. Cambridge, UK: Cambridge University Press; 2008. pp. 143–60.

66 Ibid.

67 Beals J, Novins DK, Whitesall NR, *et al*. Prevalence of mental disorders and utilization of mental health services in two American Indian reservation populations: mental health disparities in a national context. *Am J Psychiatry*. 2005; **162**: 1723–32.

68 Robert WR, Gottesman II, Albaugh B, Goldman D. Schizophrenia and psychotic symptoms in families of two American Indian tribes. *BMC Psychiatry*. 2007; **7**: 30.

69 Papps E, Ramsden I. Cultural safety in nursing: the New Zealand experience. *International Journal for Quality in Health Care*. 1996; **8**(5): 491–7.

70 Freeth, 2007, op. cit.

71 Kirmayer, Minas, 2000, op. cit.

72 Kirmayer, Brass, Tait, 2000, op. cit.

73 Garrett, op. cit.

74 Smith DP. The sweat lodge as psychotherapy: congruence between traditional and modern healing. In: Moodley R, West W, editors. *Integrating Traditional Healing Practices into Counseling and Psychotherapy*. Thousand Oaks, CA: Sage Publications Inc; 2005. pp. 196–209.

75 Ross R, 1992, op. cit.

76 Ross R, 1996, op. cit.

77 Castillo, op. cit.

78 Duran, op. cit.

79 Renfrey, op. cit.

80 Kelly, op. cit.

81 Garrett, op. cit.

82 Ibid.

83 Duran, op. cit.

4.3 Environmental Interventions in Relation to People with Serious Mental Illness

Philip T. Yanos and Stephanie A. Robilotta

INTRODUCTION

In spite of a long history of emphasis on biological determinism, there is growing research evidence that social factors can play an important role in shaping individual outcomes and recovery for people with SMI. Nevertheless, biomedical conceptualizations of SMI continue to pay relatively little attention to the influence of social structure on recovery, instead emphasizing genetic and biological explanations for outcome variation. This perspective is exemplified by DSM-IV-TR.[1] which states that "worse outcome" for schizophrenia is most likely explained by "poorer premorbid adjustment, lower educational achievement . . . structural brain abnormalities, more prominent negative signs and symptoms, more evidence of cognitive impairment." This emphasis on factors of presumed biological origin often explicitly excludes social factors as being relevant. This perspective was exemplified by a response to an article discussing the impact of poverty on conditions such as homelessness in this population,[2] where the author stated that it is misguided to emphasize economic disadvantage since it is the "clinical consequences" of mental illness that lead to any associated social disability.

Despite the traditional lack of emphasis described, evidence for the impact of environmental conditions on people with SMI has been mounting for some time now.[3,4] What is less clear, however, is how to translate insights regarding the impact of environmental conditions into appropriate, person-centered interventions for people with SMI. In this section, we review evidence for the impact of environmental conditions on people with SMI and discuss corresponding intervention work in three key areas: interventions addressing housing, public education interventions designed to reduce endorsement of stigmatizing views in order to reduce the incidence of stigmatizing experiences, and social policy interventions designed to improve access to treatment and remove enduring structural barriers to coping resources (such as medication). These areas were selected based on findings from prior reviews by the first author,[5,6] indicating that there is good evidence for the impact of these social factors on outcomes for people with SMI. The goal of the section is to highlight promising areas for intervention and bridge the gap between this work and the PCC perspective. Note that other sections in this book address environmental factors such as stigma, e.g. Section 3.1, *The Lived Experience: narratives through the lens of wellness*, and Section 3.2, *The Relationship Between the Person with a Serious Mental Illness and His or Her Disorder*; however, our section will discuss this topic in more detail as well as review appropriate interventions.

Housing of People with Serious Mental Illness

The impact of housing conditions on people with SMI was not historically considered to be important, since people with SMI traditionally resided in state hospitals and other institutional settings. Beginning with the accelerated advent of deinstitutionalization in the 1970s,[7] a variety of community-based housing options were developed, including board-and-care facilities, nursing homes, single-room-occupancy hotels, supportive community residences, and, most recently, supported independent housing. The oldest of these housing options, board-and-care facilities and nursing homes, typically provide little opportunity for independence or privacy, and have been derided as a form of "trans-institutionalization" that differs little from hospitalization;[8] nevertheless, they persist as a major form of housing in many locations.[9] The considerable variability in the types of housing available for people with SMI has brought to light the potential importance of housing conditions on outcomes such as quality of life, social functioning and community integration for this population.

Evidence for the impact of type of housing comes from a variety of sources. Early cross-sectional studies confirmed that greater independence in housing status, e.g. living independently versus in a custodial environment, was related to better life satisfaction.[10,11] Nelson *et al.*[12] similarly found that residents in group homes and supportive apartments displayed higher levels of personal empowerment and emotional well-being than the participants in board-and-care facilities. Although some studies have not identified a clear "gradient" in the relationship between all variations in independence in housing and life satisfaction, the findings that individuals living in the community report more life satisfaction than individuals residing in long-term inpatient settings has been consistently replicated (*see* reference 13).

Among persons with SMI living in the community, research has examined the impact of living in the least restrictive environment (supported independent housing) versus more restrictive congregate settings, e.g. community residences. The evidence supports that, compared to people living in transitional congregate settings, those who live in scatter-site independent housing use dramatically fewer public services such as hospitals, jails and shelters, and use more outpatient services.[14] They also have substantially better success in maintaining their housing rather than returning to homelessness or long-term institutionalization.[15] Independent scattered-site housing is associated with greater satisfaction with housing than residence in congregate housing.[16,17,18] With regard to community participation, findings are more mixed, but suggest an advantage for independent housing. Recent quasi-experimental work by Siegel *et al.*[19] comparing residents in supported independent housing and congregate settings in New York City indicated that supported housing residents reported greater satisfaction with housing and exhibited less use of crisis services over time compared to those housed in congregate settings. However, they did not show significant advantages in physical community integration and tended to increase in isolation. More recently, another study has suggested that independent living settings may provide a key advantage for some persons with

SMI. Mausbach *et al.*[20] found that middle-aged and older adults diagnosed with schizophrenia who lived in independent housing settings had significantly better community functioning overall than individuals living in custodial settings, and that this was not explained by demographic differences. The authors also examined whether "functional capacity," i.e. social skills, predicted community participation but found that capacity only improved functioning among persons living independently. This study suggests that independent housing may be necessary to provide the "opportunity" for improved community participation, and that restrictive environments may dampen such opportunities, an argument previously made by Yanos, Felton, Frye and Tsemberis.[21]

Cross-sectional evidence has also linked neighborhood characteristics of housing location to community integration.[22] This research found that individuals with mental illness residing in neighborhoods classified (based on census-level socioeconomic and political characteristics) as "liberal, nontraditional" had better community integration than individuals residing in both more conservative and poorer neighborhoods. Enduring stressors and community problems such as neighborhood poverty are hypothesized to strongly influence the likelihood of experiencing transitory stressors such as criminal victimization or domestic abuse. The rationale for this is that residence in impoverished areas with higher rates of crime places individuals of greater risk of being criminally victimized. There is evidence for this hypothesis from cross-sectional studies indicating that residence in poor urban areas is associated with higher rates of criminal victimization among people with mental illness.[23,24]

Housing: promising interventions

Housing options have been generally offered to persons with SMI in a haphazard way; there are therefore few models of clear "interventions" in which type of housing is targeted to the individual needs and preferences of mental health service users. An exception in this regard is the "Housing First" model developed by the program Pathways to Housing in New York City.[25] In contrast with a "continuum of care"[26] approach, in which housing and mental health/substance abuse treatment are emphasized and individuals are placed in housing programs suited to their level of functional ability as determined by providers, this approach assumes that service users prefer independence and will show better engagement in treatment after this need has been met. Though it has yet to be designated an "EBP," the Housing First model has garnered a considerable amount of empirical support and is currently considered to be an emerging best practice. Empirical support for Housing First comes primarily from a four-year, randomized study comparing Housing First to the Continuum of Care model in New York City. This study demonstrated dramatically higher rates of housing stability and lower rates of homelessness among Housing First participants.[27,28] There is also evidence that persons randomly assigned to Housing First demonstrated significantly better social community integration than individuals assigned to Continuum of Care 48 months after initial assignment.[29] Evaluations of Housing First by other research groups have shown favorable outcomes as well,[30] and a recent review of the literature concluded that Housing First, supplemented by off-site Assertive Community Treatment (ACT) teams, is the most effective means to reducing homelessness and re-hospitalization among persons with SMI.[31]

Example

The following is an illustration of how Housing First can be helpful to service users with SMI:

Joseph was an individual diagnosed with schizophrenia who had become homeless. He had become distanced from his family and was generally avoidant of contact with the mental health system, which he found to be too coercive; and he refused to take psychotropic medication. Prior to being offered Housing First services, Joseph was offered several opportunities to live in congregate facilities, which he refused because he did not feel that he could tolerate the restrictive environment they offered; instead he chose to remain homeless. Eventually Joseph was offered Housing First services, which he accepted, moving into his own apartment for the first time. Through gradual engagement with the ACT team over the course of several months, he agreed to begin taking medication and would meet with team members to discuss his goals and aspirations. As he took medication, his symptoms became less prominent, and he eventually identified the goal of becoming a yoga instructor, which he was encouraged to pursue by the ACT team. Together with one of the ACT team members, he identified community resources for pursuing this goal and developed a gradual plan for how to pursue it. Over the course of several years, and with occasional setbacks, Joseph took several classes and was eventually able to achieve his goal of becoming an instructor, which facilitated his contact with other community members and improved his sense of well-being.

This example illustrates how the more person-centered approach that the Housing First model offers can facilitate engagement and potentially recovery for mental health service users.

The Housing First model of intervention certainly has considerable appeal as a model of providing housing that is consistent with the principles of PCC. The potential promise of this was highlighted by a recent qualitative examination of the factors impacting the engagement of homeless persons with SMI and substance abuse concerns into services in New York City.[32] This study found that the opportunity to obtain independent housing is a major factor contributing to the engagement of persons in this population, while rules and restrictions linked to other housing approaches are associated with lack of engagement. Thus, Housing First may offer unique opportunity for persons with SMI who are "difficult to engage" to *be* engaged in treatment, and provide opportunities for recovery.

However, some important limitations of the Housing First model should be emphasized. One limitation is that it assumes that service users prefer independence. Though research supports that this is generally the case,[33] it is by no means universal. Therefore, there may be a disjoint between being offered housing in an independent setting and actual service user preference. Another possible limitation is that, due to restrictions of the housing market, the model is not always able to match service user preference in terms of the location of the housing,[34] and service users may therefore be dissatisfied with the neighborhood in which their apartment is located.[35] Thus, a modification of the Housing First model might allow services users the opportunity to consider a trade-off between location and restrictiveness and allow service users the choice of living either in a congregate setting or independent apartment. Such a modification would provide maximum flexibility to service users with SMI and would be most consistent with PCC principles.

Social Stigma

There has recently been increased recognition of the impact of stigma on people with SMI. Broad population surveys indicate that many among the general public hold stigmatizing views about persons with schizophrenia and other forms of SMI.[36,37] Stigmatizing views include increased expectations of dangerousness as well as the view that people with SMI are incompetent and cannot maintain employment.[38,39,40] Associated with these views, the public also reports a tendency to avoid those with SMI, especially schizophrenia.[41] There is also strong evidence that stigma predominates in the media, which can have a strong influence on individual attitudes.[42] A recent analysis of all U.S. newspaper media stories referring to mental illness during a six-week period in 2002[43] found that the largest proportion of stories emphasized dangerousness and violence, while only a small minority emphasized recovery. Stories emphasizing dangerousness were also most prominently featured and were typically found on the front pages of newspapers. The negative effect that the practices of the media can have on the intensity of stigmatizing attitudes in the general public has been supported by experimental research, which found that exposure to an section emphasizing violence was related to harsher subsequent attitudes toward people with mental illness.[44]

Although the research described above has documented the prevalence of stigmatizing views in the community and the media in particular, research has not yet linked the prevalence of such attitudes to individual-level outcomes related to recovery such as life satisfaction, hopefulness and social functioning. However, cross-sectional studies have linked the experience of individual stigmatizing interactions to worse outcomes, such as decreased self-efficacy and poorer life satisfaction.[45,46,47] It is therefore plausible that community-level stigma impacts recovery-relevant outcomes among mental health service users by increasing the likelihood of their experiencing stigmatizing interactions, although a direct link has yet to be demonstrated.

Example

The following is an illustration of how social stigma can affect service users with SMI:

Stephen is an individual diagnosed with bipolar disorder from a middle-class background who has completed college and has had several previous work experiences. After recently experiencing a manic episode, he is hesitant to look for work again because he is afraid that his employers will sense that there is something "wrong" with him when they note the gaps in his resume. He also has a strong interest in spirituality but avoids attending services in his religious community because he has had previous experiences indicating that he will be "evaluated" for his social status when he attends services. He believes that these interactions will be humiliating because they will make it apparent that he has not achieved anything in his life, and that others in the community will suspect his mental illness. He also has several friends from high school and college that he would like to speak with, but he avoids doing so because the last time they saw him was when he was manic, and some of his friends had commented that he was "psycho" at the time. When he thinks about his life, Stephen is very self-denigrating as a result of his mental illness and experiences depressed mood as a result.

Awareness and concern about stigma had a clear impact on Stephen's functioning and well-being.

Social Stigma: interventions

A number of different interventions to combat social stigma have been enacted in a variety of locations. As well summarized by Corrigan and Penn,[48] and more recently by Corrigan and O'Shaughnessy,[49] these interventions tend to fall into three categories: protest, public education and contact-related interventions. Below, we briefly discuss these types of interventions and research supporting their effectiveness.

Protest interventions attempt to combat stigmatizing depictions in the media by way of letter-writing campaigns, demonstrations and other forms of protest. Although there are specific examples whereby a protest turned out to be effective (for example, the protest of the television show *Wonderland* led to its cancellation), Corrigan and O'Shaughnessy[50] have convincingly argued for the limitations of such approaches. Drawing on social psychology research regarding "rebound effects," they have shown that members of the public react to efforts to control what they can see or read. As a result, there is little evidence to support that such interventions are effective at changing public attitudes toward people with SMI.

Public education interventions generally attempt to change stigmatizing views by presenting positive images of people with mental illness through public service announcements, television commercials, magazine advertisements and posters. More intensive educational interventions involving informational videos and lectures may also be used with targeted groups such as high school or college students. Corrigan *et al.*[51] summarized findings regarding educational interventions and found them to be generally positive but also to have relatively small and short-term effects.

The final category of interventions involves **contact**. Contact interventions aim to bring people into direct contact with persons with SMI (and particularly persons who will provide an example that counters stereotypes) as a way of decreasing stigma. Corrigan *et al.*[52] emphasized that contact is most effective when the contact person "moderately disconfirms stereotypes" so that they are not seen as "exceptions." Reviewing studies involving contact, Corrigan *et al.*[53] concluded that contact-oriented interventions produce greater and more lasting changes in stereotypical attitudes than educational interventions, and that contact is therefore the best strategy for changing stigma.

A limitation of direct contact interventions, however, is that such interventions cannot be easily disseminated on a population-level, and are therefore most likely to be useful when targeted to specific groups that are likely to come into contact with people with SMI, e.g. police officers, primary care staff, etc. There appears to be a need to combine contact interventions with educational approaches. An interesting integrated approach to combining public education and elements of contact is the "Like Minds, Like Mine" effort conducted in New Zealand.[54] This ongoing initiative combines mass media advertising combating stigma with one-minute documentaries of well-known New Zealanders and "ordinary persons" who have experienced mental illness. Through a series of themed television and radio campaigns, e.g. "Know me before you judge me," the initiative targets specific stigmatizing views (such as that people with SMI are incompetent or cannot work) by introducing persons from a variety of cultural backgrounds and describing their work and family lives before explaining that they have a mental illness. By profiling either celebrities or other persons that the general population can presumably relate to, the campaign introduces an element of "contact" on a mass scale. Surveys tracking attitudes about mental illness before and after early campaigns for the "Like Minds" initiative found that New Zealanders significantly increased in their endorsement of non-stigmatizing attitudes, such as "people who've had a mental illness can still lead a normal life." The findings of this initiative suggest that elements of contact can be integrated into public education in order make them more effective and allow widespread application.

While there is no obvious link between interventions to combat stigma and the principles of PCC, mass scale interventions to combat stigma may potentially have two-fold impact on the lives of people with SMI that would be consistent with this approach. First, individuals experiencing symptoms of mental illness should be more likely to seek treatment and should feel less constrained by concerns over the stigmatizing views of others if community stigma is reduced. They may seek help earlier and be less likely to be brought into services through involuntary means because their symptoms may not have progressed to such a point. Thus, individuals can be more free to choose treatment under circumstances of decreased stigma. Second, decreased community stigma should also impact persons who regularly interact with people with SMI, including family members and providers, and it may be more likely for such individuals to respect the choices and individual preferences of such persons.

An additional concern regarding stigma interventions that concerns PCC involves sensitivity to cultural differences in the ways that mental illness is construed. Although the "Like Minds" campaign in New Zealand incorporated an emphasis on addressing the views of Maori and other ethnicities,[55] there has been scant discussion of this issue in the stigma-intervention literature more generally. Ideally, a person-centered approach to combating stigma would incorporate different cultural constructions of mental illness into its intervention approaches.

Treatment Resource Availability

The development of effective antipsychotic and other medications for the treatment of schizophrenia and other serious mental disorders has spurred excitement for the potential of such approaches to further recovery from SMI. However, a major barrier to the use of such treatments is social constraints that can affect the ability of individuals to access such services. For example, health insurance is frequently necessary in order for persons to be able to afford medications that can facilitate recovery. In addition, treatment programs need to be available in order for persons to be able to access them. From this perspective, treatment resources, such as the availability of mental health services and the existence of social programs to fund them, may exert an important influence on the use of coping strategies such as help-seeking and medication adherence.

Supporting the importance of funding is cross-sectional evidence demonstrating a positive association between having adequate health insurance coverage and/or medication benefits and the use of services such as antipsychotic medication and outpatient services.[56,57,58,59] Particularly compelling evidence for this relationship also comes from a time-series study showing that changes in local mental health policy can have a direct negative impact on psychotropic medication use.[60] Specifically, Soumerai et al.[61] found that the imposition of a monthly payment cap for the purchase of medication among Medicaid beneficiaries in New Hampshire led to a marked decrease in the use of psychotropic medications among people with schizophrenia; after political action led to withdrawal of the payment cap, medication use rapidly returned to prior levels.

Other studies have demonstrated that the availability of psychosocial services to people with SMI can have an impact on relevant outcomes. For example, in some geographic locations only inpatient mental health services are available and community-based services such as ACT or SE programs are not available. An interesting "natural experiment" assessed the impact of changes in mental health policy in Israel in 2000 on people with schizophrenia.[62] The policy changes involved the investment of funds in rehabilitation services that were not previously available, including vocational rehabilitation, housing, case management and peer support services. The study compared the likelihood of rehospitalization for people with schizophrenia originally hospitalized in 1990–1991 versus 2000–2001 (this study used Israel's comprehensive national data set and therefore reflects "population-level" data rather than a sample). The study found that 63% of the first group (those before the policy change) versus 41% for the second group were rehospitalized within three years. There were also important differences in length of hospitalization. These findings support the view that the change in policy which provided better access to treatment helped improve the lives of a national cohort of people with mental illness.

Treatment Resources: promising interventions

Given that barriers affecting the availability of medication and other treatment resources (such as EBPs) can significantly affect both the use of such resources and subsequent outcomes related to recovery, it is therefore essential that interventions be developed to maximize the availability of such resources. However, a major stumbling block in countries such as the U.S. is the absence of a "single-payer" model for financing mental health care.[63] Thus, many individuals who lack insurance may remain unable to afford necessary medications. Furthermore, in other locations, insured persons may not receive other evidence-based services, such as SE, because these services are not reimbursed by insurance providers.

Addressing this problem by means of intervention clearly requires coordination on a number of levels. One intervention model that was applied toward this end with a particularly in-need population was the Access to Community Care and Effective Services and Support (ACCESS) model, which provided coordinated mental health, housing, substance abuse and social services to homeless persons with SMI and which was studied in a large demonstration project (*see* reference 64 for an overview) Although it was found that the systems integration program led to improved housing stability for persons with SMI, it was also found that other service user outcomes were not improved by the systems integration project. As a result, Goldman *et al.*[65] concluded that systems integration does not "promote better client outcomes above and beyond what can be achieved with good clinical services, such as ACT." Thus, systems integration as an intervention in itself seems to have limitations in how it can impact recovery-related outcomes.

Perhaps a more promising line of intervention, therefore, relates to "systems transformation" efforts that begin with the philosophical principles of PCC, making adjustments to the service system in response to this overarching principle. Tondora *et al.*[66] reviewed promising efforts to transform local systems of care following from the principles of "person-centered planning." Their perspective, the key elements of structural organization relate more to the philosophical principles underpinning service delivery, e.g. choice, respect and self-determination, rather than the "nuts and bolts" of treatment systems. While their review identified several promising elements that service systems can follow, it remains to be seen if the implementation of such principles will have a meaningful impact on outcomes related to recovery.

CONCLUSION

In this section, we have reviewed evidence for the impact of environmental conditions on people with SMI and discussed corresponding intervention work in the areas of housing, social stigma and access to treatment. We conclude that environmental conditions indeed have a significant impact on the lives of people with SMI, and that structural interventions are needed in these areas. We have identified a few promising interventions in these areas that are relatively consistent with the principles of PCC, including: the Housing First model in the area of housing, combined public information and contact interventions for stigma reduction, and person-centered planning for systems reorganization. Combining such interventions with the promising individual-level person-centered interventions discussed throughout this volume can make a more comprehensive contribution to facilitate the recovery of people with SMI.

REFERENCES

1 American Psychiatric Association. *Diagnostic and Statistical Manual of Mental Disorders, 4th Edition (DSM-IV)*. Washington, DC: American Psychiatric Association; 1994.

2 Nelson SH. 'Role of social disadvantage in crime, joblessness, and homelessness among persons with serious mental illness' [comment]. *Psychiatric Services*. 2002; **53**: 573.

3 Yanos PT, Moos RH. Determinants of functioning and well-being among persons with schizophrenia: An integrated model. *Clinical Psychology Review*. 2007; **27**: 58–77.

4 Yanos PT, Knight EL, Roe D. Recognizing a role for structure and agency: integrating sociological perspectives into the study of recovery from severe mental illness. In: McLeod J, Pescosolido B, Avison W. *Mental Health, Social Mirror*. New York, NY: Springer; 2007. pp. 407–33.

5 Yanos, Moos, 2007, op. cit.

6 Yanos, Knight, Roe, 2007, op. cit.

7 Mechanic D. *Mental Health and Social Policy: the emergence of managed care*. 4th ed. New York, NY: Allyn & Bacon; 1998.

8 Ibid.

9 Yanos PT. Beyond "Landscapes of despair": the need for new research on the urban environment, sprawl, and the community integration of persons with severe mental illness. *Health Place*. 2007; **13**: 672–76.

10 Lehman AF, Slaughter JG, Myers CP. Quality of life in alternative residential settings. *Psychiatr Q*. 1991; **62**(1): 35–49.

11 Lehman AF, Kernan E, DeForge BR, *et al*. Effects of homelessness on quality of life of persons with serious mental illness. *Psychiatr Serv.* 1995; **46**(9): 922–6.

12 Nelson G, Hall BG, Bowers WR. Predictors of the adaptation of people with psychiatric disabilities in group homes, supportive apartments, and board-and-care homes. *Psychiatric Rehabilitation Journal.* 1999; **22**(4): 381–9.

13 Brunt D, Hansson L. The quality of life of persons with serious mental illness across housing settings. *Nord J Psychiatry.* 2004; **58**(4): 293–8.

14 Culhane DP, Metraux S, Hadley T. Public service reductions associated with placement of homeless persons with severe mental illness in supportive housing. *Housing Policy Debate.* 2002; **13**: 107–63.

15 Gulcur L, Stefancic A, Shinn M, *et al*. Housing, hospitalization and cost outcomes for homeless individuals with psychiatric disabilities participating in continuum of care and housing first programmes. *J Community Appl Soc Psychol.* 2003; **13**: 171–86.

16 Newman SJ. Housing attributes and serious mental illness: implications for research and practice. *Psychiatr Serv.* 2001; **52**(10): 1309–17.

17 Wolf J, Burnam A, Koegel P, *et al*. Changes in subjective quality of life among homeless adults who obtain housing: a prospective examination. *Soc Psychiatry Psychiatr Epidemiol.* 2001; **36**(8): 391–8.

18 Schutt RK, Goldfinger SM, Penk WE. Satisfaction with residence and with life: when homeless mentally ill persons are housed. *Eval Program Plann.* 1997; **20**: 185–94.

19 Siegel C, Samuels J, Tang DI, *et al*. Tenant outcomes in supported housing and community residences in New York City. *Psychiatr Serv.* 2006; **57**(7): 982–91.

20 Mausbach BT, Depp CA, Cardenas V, *et al*. Relationship between functional capacity and community responsibility in patients with schizophrenia: differences between independent and assisted living settings. *Community Ment Health J.* 2008; **44**(5): 385–91.

21 Yanos PT, Felton B, Tsemberis S, *et al*. Exploring the role of housing type, neighborhood characteristics, and lifestyle factors in the community integration of formerly homeless persons diagnosed with mental illness. *J Ment Health.* 2007; **16**: 703–17.

22 Segal SP, Baumohl J, Moyles EW. Neighborhood types and community reaction to the mentally ill: a paradox of intensity. *J Health Soc Behav.* 1980; **21**(4): 345–59.

23 Hiday VA, Swartz MS, Swanson JW, *et al*. Criminal victimization of persons with serious mental illness. *Psychiatr Serv.* 1999; **50**(1): 62–8.

24 Lam JA, Rosenheck RA. The effect of victimization on clinical outcomes of homeless persons with serious mental illness. *Psychiatr Serv.* 1998; **49**(5): 678–83.

25 Tsemberis S, Asmussen S. From streets to homes: the pathways to housing consumer preference supported housing model. *Alcohol Treat Q.* 1999; **17**: 113–31.

26 Arons BS, Weiss SR. Role of the public sector. In: Schreter RK, Sharfstein SS, Schreter CA, editors. *Managing Care, Not Dollars: the continuum of mental health services.* Washington, DC: American Psychiatric Press; 1997.

27 Gulcur, op. cit.

28 Tsemberis S, Gulcur L, Nakae M. Housing first, consumer choice, and harm reduction for homeless individuals with a dual diagnosis. *Am J Public Health.* 2004; **94**(4): 651–6.

29 Gulcur L, Tsemberis S, Stefancic A, Greenwood RM. Community integration of adults with psychiatric disabilities and histories of homelessness. *Community Ment Health J.* 2007; **43**(3): 211–28.

30 Mares AS, Kasprow WJ, Rosenheck RA. Outcomes of supported housing for homeless veterans with psychiatric and substance abuse problems. *Ment Health Serv Res.* 2004; **6**(4): 199–211.

31 Nelson G, Aubry T, Lafrance A. A review of the literature on the effectiveness of housing and support, assertive community treatment, and intensive case management interventions for persons with mental illness who have been homeless. *Am J Orthopsychiatry.* 2007; **77**(3): 350–61.

32 Padgett DK, Henwood B, Abrams C, *et al.* Engagement and retention in services among formerly homeless adults with co-occurring mental illness and substance abuse: voices from the margins. *Psychiatr Rehabil J.* 2008; **31**(3): 226–33.

33 Minsky S, Reisser GG, Duffy M. The eye of the beholder: housing preferences of inpatients and their treatment teams. *Psychiatr Serv.* 1995; **46**(2): 173–6.

34 Yanos PT, Felton B, Tsemberis S, *et al.* Exploring the role of housing type, neighborhood characteristics, and lifestyle factors in the community integration of formerly homeless persons diagnosed with mental illness. *Journal of Mental Health.* 2007; **16**(6): 703–17.

35 Yanos PT, Felton B, Tsemberis, 2007, op. cit.

36 Martin JK, Pescosolido BA, Tuch SA. Of fear and loathing: the role of disturbing behavior, labels, and causal attributions in shaping public attitudes toward people with mental illness. *J Health Soc Behav.* 2000; **41**: 208–23.

37 Swindle R, Heller K, Pescosolido B, Kikuzawa S. Responses to nervous breakdowns in America over a 40-year period: mental health policy implications. *Am Psychol.* 2000; **55**: 740–9.

38 Link BG, Phelan JC, Bresnahan M, *et al.* Public conceptions of mental illness: labels, causes, dangerousness, and social distance. *Am J of Public Health.* 1999; **89**(9): 1328–33.

39 Pescosolido BA, Monahan J, Link BG. The public's view of the competence, dangerousness, and need for legal coercion of persons with mental health problems. *Am J Public Health.* 1999; **89**(9): 1339–45.

40 Phelan JC, Link BG, Stueve A, *et al.* Public conceptions of mental illness in 1950 and 1996: what is mental illness and is it to be feared? *J Health Soc Behav.* 2000; **41**: 188–207.

41 Martin, op. cit.

42 Corrigan PW, Markowitz FE, Watson AC. Structural levels of mental illness stigma and discrimination. *Schizophr Bull.* 2004; **30**(3): 481–91.

43 Corrigan PW, Ralph RO. Introduction: recovery as service user vision and research paradigm. In: Ralph RO, Corrigan PW, editors. *Recovery in Mental Illness: broadening our understanding of wellness.* Washington, DC: American Psychological Association; 2005. pp. 3–17.

44 Thornton JA, Wahl OF. Impact of a newspaper article on attitudes toward mental illness. *J Community Psychol.* 1996; **24**: 17–25.

45 Yanos PT, Rosenfield S, Horwitz A. Negative and supportive social interactions and quality of life among persons diagnosed with serious mental illness. *Community Ment Health J.* 2001; **37**: 405–19.

46 Dickerson FB, Sommerville J, Origoni AE, *et al.* Experiences of stigma among outpatients with schizophrenia. *Schizophr Bull.* 2002; **28**(1): 143–55.

47 Wright ER, Gronfein WP, Owens TJ. Deinstitutionalization, social rejection, and the self-esteem of former mental patients. *J Health Soc Behav.* 2000; **41**(1): 68–90.

48 Corrigan PW, Penn DL. Lessons for social psychology on discrediting psychiatric stigma. *Am Psychol.* 1999; **54**(9): 765–76.

49 Corrigan PW, O'Shaughnessy JR. Changing mental illness stigma as it exists in the real world. *Aust Psychol.* 2007; **42**: 90–7.

50 Ibid.

51 Corrigan PW, Mueser KT, Bond GR, *et al. Principles and practice of psychiatric rehabilitation: an empirical approach.* New York, NY: Guilford Press; 2008.

52 Ibid.

53 Ibid.

54 Vaughan G, Hansen C. "Like minds, like mine": a New Zealand project to counter the stigma and discrimination associated with mental illness. *Australas Psychiatry.* 2004; **12**(2): 113–17.

55 Ibid.

56 Rabinowitz J, Bromet EJ, Lavelle J, *et al.* Relationship between type of insurance and care during the early course of psychosis. *Am J Psychiatry.* 1998; **155**(10): 1392–7.

57 Rabinowitz J, Bromet EJ, Lavelle J, *et al.* Changes in insurance coverage and extent of care during the two years after first hospitalization for a psychotic disorder. *Psychiatr Serv.* 2001; **52**(1): 87–91.

58 McAlpine DD, Mechanic D. Utilization of specialty mental health care among persons with serious mental illness: the roles of demographics, need, insurance, and risk. *Health Serv Res.* 2000; **35**(1 Pt. 2): 277–92.

59 Yanos PT, Crystal S, Kumar R, *et al.* Characteristics and service use patterns of non-elderly Medicare beneficiaries diagnosed with schizophrenia: findings from the MBCS. *Psychiatr Serv.* 2001; **52**(12): 1644–50.

60 Soumerai SB, McLaughlin TJ, Ross-Degnan D, *et al.* Effects of limiting Medicaid drug-reimbursement benefits on the use of psychotropic agents and acute mental health services by patients with schizophrenia. *N Engl J Med.* 1994; **331**(10): 650–5.

61 Ibid.

62 Ibid.

63 Lehman AF. Quality of care in mental health: the case of schizophrenia. *Health Aff (Millwood).* 1999; **18**(5): 52–65.

64 Goldman HH, Morrissey JP, Rosenheck RA, *et al.* Lessons from the evaluation of the ACCESS program. *Psychiatr Serv.* 2002; **53**(8): 967–9.

65 Ibid.

66 Tondora J, Pocklington S, Gorgers AG, *et al. Implementation of Person-Centered Care and Planning: how philosophy can inform practice.* Chicago, IL: Department of Psychiatry, University of Illinois; 2008. Available at: www.psych.uic.edu/uicnrtc/cmhs/pcp.paper.implementation.doc (accessed 4 Mar 2011).

4.4 Mental Health Systems and Policy in Relation to People with Serious Mental Illness

Cheryl Forchuk

INTRODUCTION

A person-centered approach has become a standard feature of quality health care.[1,2] While the term itself retains some ambiguity as to its precise meaning,[3,4,5] there is a growing body of literature and evidence supporting person-centered practice,[6,7,8,9] especially as it relates to the care of persistent and/or severe illness.[10,11] While mental health issues are widespread in the population (an estimated one in four individuals), SMI is concentrated in an estimated one in 17.[12] The concept of PCC infers that there are other factors that exist which are outside the service user or "center." Although the focus of this approach is on the service user, the service user and the care provided to the service user exist within a constellation of other systems. These systems and their accompanying directives exert influence over health care practices, including service user care, while at the same time health care practices and beliefs exert an influence over these broader systems and policies.[13,14] A mental health care organization can have policies that support or undermine PCC practices. The relationships between agencies and service providers can influence service user centeredness. Broader policies also directly affect the care of service users as well as the practitioner's ability to engage in PCC. A wide range of contextual factors must therefore be considered to ensure that a comprehensive person-centered approach is undertaken.

Organization

A person-centered model of care may be implemented by an individual service provider, a team, an organization, or by an entire health care system.[15] Most practitioners providing services to people with SMIs do so on behalf of an organization. If organizations are to be person-centered, the person-centered perspective must be used to examine the organization's policies and practices. Although almost all policies and practices can potentially influence the nature of service user care, there are some which are particularly important to the ability of practitioners to maintain a person-centered focus of care. Some organizational structures are considered more conducive to a person-centered model than others.[16,17,18] Regardless of a health practitioner's personal attributes, there are certain key organizational elements that can be considered general prerequisites to PCC.[19] The need to implement person-centered mental health care remains great. PCC incorporates cultural sensitivity and addresses issues of access and acceptability of health care services.[20]

Organizational and administrative policies may give rise to an environmental context that influences the delivery of service user care.[21,22] Successful implementation of person-centered practice therefore necessitates an administrative style and culture supportive of such a model of care.[23,24] An organization's philosophy or mission statement tends to filter downwards to influence direct service user care practices and therefore it must reflect the values, beliefs and needs of the population being served.[25,26] Involving service users, their families,[27] and providers[28] in the development and/or revision of mission statements, agency policies and standards of care can help to ensure that agency mandates remain service user focused. Open communication and support from senior and middle-level management is essential and facilitates the establishment of rapport between organizational leadership and direct care providers. This in turn fosters meaningful collaboration and the establishment of a positive milieu in which information can be easily exchanged, challenged and cultivated.[29,30] Furthermore, organizational models that support provider participation in administrative roles and tasks create an atmosphere whereby service user centered issues can be raised and addressed in an efficient, timely manner.[31] Similarly, when service users and their families have a say in program planning, organizational policies and decision-making, such as through patient and family councils, barriers and concerns pertaining to service user centered practices can be identified and promptly resolved.[32]

Service users with SMIs often receive services over a lengthy period of time and may receive services from several agencies. Diagnoses of individuals with a SMI include dimensions of duration of illness and disability. Duration and disability of SMI create difficulties in carrying out tasks of everyday living.[33] Continuity of care and supporting relationships are therefore important considerations for agencies providing services to this service user population. At each stage a service user's relationship with relevant health care organizations will be briefly examined from a person-centered perspective and key questions for consideration will be set out.

To illustrate the systems issues, the examples of Mary and John will be used. Mary is currently 36 years old and was diagnosed with schizophrenia when she was 24. She is married with a six-year-old daughter and works in a consumer-run restaurant. John is 24 and has a history of depression and alcohol dependence. He has also struggled with homelessness since his teens.

Learning about the Agency

A service user's awareness of various health care services may depend on a variety of factors, including socioeconomic status, language and literacy.[34,35] Organizations should consider how a service user comes to learn about a particular health care service or agency. For instance, is information only available through other service providers or can the service user access this service or agency independently? In recent years, there has been an increasing tendency to use technology to reach potential service users. However, many service users with SMI are dealing with poverty issues that limit their ability to access information in this way. In one study of discharge practices,[36] about a quarter of the service users surveyed did not even have a telephone, let alone a computer. To overcome this barrier, a variety of approaches are likely needed including the utilization of pamphlets and brochures that would be made available in a variety of settings. If potential service users cannot directly learn about an agency, it sets the stage for the use of a less person-centered approach. For example, Mary has a lot of access to community resources since these are freely available at the consumer-run restaurant in which she works. Both Mary and her husband frequently search the Internet and find interesting sections and programs which Mary discusses with her service providers. On the other hand, John is quite isolated. He would benefit from employment programs, housing supports and addiction counseling. However, he feels overwhelmed by his problems and is not sure where to start. Since the age of onset was early, it interrupted his education, which makes understanding many brochures or information pamphlets quite difficult.

Referral to the Agency

It is often surprising how many agencies with "PCC" language in their vision and mission statements do not allow for self-referrals. Sometimes reimbursement practices require another practitioner to serve as a gatekeeper. For example, in Ontario, Canada, service users seeing specialized medical practitioners are generally not eligible for reimbursement unless the referral has come through the service user's primary care practitioner (family doctor or nurse practitioner). Community mental health agencies do not require a referral for reimbursement, yet referral practices operate as if this was in fact the case. Since individuals with an SMI may not always have a primary care provider, this existing practice creates a barrier for service users seeking to access required, specialized community services. Collaboration between primary care providers and community services will enhance primary care delivery of health care services to individuals with an SMI.[37] This matter is discussed in this book in detail in Section 5.3, *Shared/Collaborative Care for People with Serious Mental Illness.*

Assessment and Intake Processes

During the assessment and intake process, the question arises as to how much emphasis should be placed on the service user's story versus the referral agency material. Given these competing interests, the question arises as to what constitutes an effective assessment/intake form. One example of an assessment/intake form is the service user patterns form developed at the former Hamilton Psychiatric Hospital in Hamilton, Ontario. The form requires information about the service user to be written in his or her words. Bernardo and Forchuk[38] found that there was a significant difference in the language used by referring agencies compared to the language used by service users, a difference which indicated very different perceptions of the issues. For example, referring providers often spoke of "suddenly" worsening symptoms leading to a hospital admission. On the other hand, in the same situation, service users spoke of continued, unrelenting symptoms that they eventually could no longer cope with. If the initial assessment leading to intake is not based on the service user's perceptions of the problems at hand, it becomes very difficult to provide person-centered care. In keeping with a person-centered focus, it is important to take into account a service user's perspective as well as service user identified issues and goals during the assessment and intake process.[39,40,41] For example, Mary may have concerns that her personal strengths including employment and a supportive family are not adequately accounted for in the assessment process.

Assignment of Service Users

How is it determined which staff members will work with which service users? Does this matching process consider service user identified needs in relation to staff expertise? If so, how is this accomplished and how consistently are service users assigned to the same staff members? For example, if a service user is readmitted to the same hospital three months or a year after his or her last discharge, will he or she be assigned the same attending psychiatrist, nurses, social worker and other team members? In the context of nursing assignments, is there a primary nursing assignment in place or do nursing assignments change regularly? Organizational structures that enable caregiver continuity are fundamental to the person-centered process. Continuity of care from a consistent service provider, such as in the primary nursing context, facilitates the development of a trusting and meaningful therapeutic relationship between service users and their care providers.[42,43] Primary nursing is defined as an organizational model of care whereby continuity of care between nurse and service user is emphasized. Continuity of care includes direct caregiving, coordination, education and advocacy by the nurse from admission to discharge into the community.[44] A key issue related to continuity of assignment is that of the ratio of part-time to full-time staff.[45] It has been recommended that in order to maintain consistency and stability within multidisciplinary teams, 70% of nursing staff should have permanent, full-time status.[46,47] What happens if a problematic relationship develops between a service user and care provider? How easy would it be to switch providers in such instances, and what would be the potential negative consequences for the service user? Individual caseloads, service user acuity and environmental conditions must also be considered when service users are assigned to care providers, as all of these factors influence the amount of time and energy a clinician has available to invest in the therapeutic process.[48] For example, in deciding who should work with John it would be important to consider his complex needs regarding addiction and depression, his socioeconomic challenges and the developmental issues related to his age.

Terminating Relationships

In examining person-centered policies, an important consideration is how to end therapeutic relationships. For example, some agencies have rigid policies about conditions for continuing relationships, such as service users must be medication concordant or must be making therapeutic progress. Such policies are generally more agency-centered or provider-centered than person-centered. People with long-term mental illnesses often need a longer time to establish a therapeutic relationship and a longer time to therapeutically separate at the end of the relationship. This means that service users often need to continue seeing a service provider beyond the active working phase of their relationship. If they are being transferred to another agency or program, they may be assisted by a transitional process involving both new and old staff members until the new staff member has formed a working relationship with the service user.[49] Discharge planning must always start at the time of admission. However, even this may be inadequate due to a lack of staff time and the shortened length of the average service user stay.[50] The discharge process could be quite simpler for a person like Mary, who has a number of personal supports, compared to someone like John, who will have a number of ongoing needs and far fewer personal resources.

Models of Care Delivery

Embracing a person-centered model of care is possible only when all the members of a health care system or team contribute to the implementation process.[51] Organizations embracing this model must identify and eliminate barriers and must allow sharing of power, since large differences in the power of team members do not facilitate sharing power with the service user.[52] Bauman *et al.*[53] described three important elements of PCC as being communication, partnerships and a focus beyond a specific condition to a much broader focus on health promotion and healthy lifestyles. These three elements should be imbedded in any model of PCC.

Team Functioning and Interdisciplinary Teams

One must consider the various members of an interdisciplinary team and how their training and perspectives may influence their approach to PCC. Through open communication and a shared approach, the team can work toward creating a complementary and holistic experience for the service user.[54]

Overall, organizations that value and support interdisciplinary collaboration tend to yield better outcomes for their service users than those which do not.[55] The organizational climate within hospitals has been an underestimated determinant of poor service user outcomes and staff recruitment/retention failure.[56] Fostering positive working relationships among disciplines is therefore very beneficial, as it helps to create a positive work environment. Organizations that hold the well-being of their employees in high regard have lower rates of burnout and increased levels of job satisfaction and staff retention. Employees that feel valued are more emotionally available to invest energy and skill in their work, which in turn fosters the trust service users have with care providers and strengthens the overall quality of the therapeutic relationship.[57]

In keeping with the principles of PCC, documentation should remain service user focused, interdisciplinary, and goal oriented.[58] Charting should be respectful of service user values and beliefs. Negative language or the use of labels, such as "dysfunctional" or "compliant" versus "non-compliant," should be avoided. Such terms are merely problem focused and serve to minimize service user strengths, thus they are detrimental to the therapeutic process.[59,60] For example, a person like John may have faced many labels, e.g. "addict," that could influence how staff may perceive him.

Coordination and Collaboration

Reorganizing the health care system to maximize partnerships between service users and service providers is a priority in the context of managing chronic disease.[61] Collaboration with family members, consistent with service user wishes, is an important part of working with the service user. Since service user centered care focuses on the individual, if families are involved, the focus remains on the individual within the context of their family. For someone like Mary, this may be obvious. However, it is also important to explore issues of collaboration and support with John.

Educational Opportunities

Access to a variety of educational opportunities serves to enhance knowledge acquisition and skill development. In such a setting, care providers of all disciplines have an opportunity to explore the principles underlying PCC. Care providers have an opportunity to examine service user care practices and to challenge and build upon their existing knowledge base. Reflective practice is encouraged and is meant to assist care providers in clarifying personal values, beliefs and biases and how they relate to the service user's experience. They can then apply insights derived from reflective processes to their educational needs and objectives.[62] Through such practices, care providers are able to gain greater experience in employing therapeutic intervention to ensure positive health benefits for their service users. In addition, health care agencies need to consider current practices on an ongoing basis to ensure that treatment approaches are up to date and effective. Thus, health care agencies must ensure that policies are in place that promote research and the use of EBP. Dissemination strategies that provide care providers with sufficient time and an atmosphere of flexibility provide care providers with opportunities to explore the relevant literature, to engage in research and to engage in dialogue with other care providers, other agencies and other organizations. Such dissemination strategies help to ensure that care practices are up to date, evidence-based, and are relevant to the service user population.[63]

Evaluation

Evaluation strategies that assess the effectiveness of current care practices from the perspective of both service users and care providers are essential to ensure that current approaches to care for service users are meaningful and effective.[64] Monitoring care practices and incorporating consistent means of evaluation helps to identify strengths and weaknesses in a given model of care. Methods which elicit service user perspectives, for example through service user satisfaction surveys, can provide information regarding whether interactions are perceived as being positive or negative and can also determine if the service user's health care goals were being met.[65] Staff performance appraisals help to identify any concerns or issues that need to be addressed.[66]

Broader Systems and Determinants of Health

PCC occurs within a larger context and is influenced by established political, social and economic systems.[67] Broad determinants of health such as age, gender, culture, early child development, education, working conditions, access to social supports and socioeconomic status have a profound effect on the health status of individuals and entire communities.[68,69] For example, John may have become homeless due to changes in the availability of public housing, which dramatically diminished at the same time he first struggled with his depression. Living on the street then exposed him to a different social system and a group that heavily used alcohol as well as other substances to cope. Community development initiatives help to strengthen and empower communities to influence changes that are relevant to their health concerns.[70] Systems to consider include those directly related to the health care system, such as mental health legislation and advance directives as well as those related to broad determinants of health such as housing, income and employment. Coalitions comprised of providers and/or laypersons are one such means of influencing change.[71] Awareness of broad determinants would also include assessment of these issues on an individual level and their inclusion in the plan of care. Many of these issues are addressed in detail elsewhere in this book, such as in Section 4.1, *Collaborating with Families of People with Serious Mental Illness*, and in Section 4.2, *Trans-Cultural Issues in Person-Centered Care for People with Serious Mental Illness*.

CONCLUSION

PCC does not exist in a vacuum. Understanding the broader systems and policies that support or undermine PCC is essential for successful implementation of this health care approach. To implement PCC care that promotes community integration, there needs to be an awareness of the broader legislative and policy context existing in the hospitals and in the community.

REFERENCES

1 Anthony MK, Hudson-Barr D. A patient centred model of care for hospital discharge. *Clin Nurs Res*. 2004; **13**(2): 117–36.
2 Mead N, Bower P. Patient-centredness: a conceptual framework and review of the empirical literature. *Soc Sci Med*. 2000; **51**: 1087–110.
3 Anthony, op. cit.

4 Mead, op. cit.

5 Bensing J. Bridging the gap: the separate worlds of evidence-based medicine and patient-centred medicine. *Patient Educ Couns.* 2000; **39**: 17–25.

6 Anthony, op. cit.

7 Mead, op. cit.

8 O'Donnell M, Parker G, Proberts M, *et al.* A study of client-focused case management and consumer advocacy: the community and consumer service project. *Aust NZ J Psychiatry.* 1999; **33**: 684–93.

9 Registered Nurses' Association of Ontario. *Client Centred Care.* Toronto, Canada: Registered Nurses' Association of Ontario; 2006a (Rev. Suppl.).

10 Bauman AE, Fardy HJ, Harris PG. Getting it right: why bother with patient-centred care? *Med J Australia.* 2003; **179**: 253–6.

11 Von Korff M, Glasgow RE, Sharpe M. Abc of psychological medicine: organizing care for chronic illness. *BMJ.* 2002; **325**(7355): 92–4.

12 Kessler RC, Chiu WT, Demler O, *et al.* Prevalence, severity and comorbidity of twelve-month DSM-IV disorders in the National Comorbidity Survey Replication (NCS-R). *Arc Gen Psych.* 2005; **62**(6): 617–27.

13 Registered Nurses' Association of Ontario, 2006a, op. cit.

14 Restall G, Ripat J, Stern M. A framework of strategies for client-centred practice. *Can J Occup Ther.* 2003; **70**(2):103–12.

15 Registered Nurses' Association of Ontario, 2006a, op. cit.

16 Ibid.

17 Bauman, op. cit.

18 Restall, op. cit.

19 Registered Nurses' Association of Ontario, 2006a, op. cit.

20 Drake RE, Wilkniss SM, Frounfelker RL, *et al.* The thresholds-dartmouth partnership and research on shared decision making. *Psychiatric Services.* 2009; **60**(2): 142–5.

21 Registered Nurses' Association of Ontario, 2006a, op. cit.

22 Registered Nurses' Association of Ontario. *Establishing Therapeutic Relationships.* Toronto, Canada: Registered Nurses Association of Ontario; 2006b (Rev. Suppl.).

23 Registered Nurses Association of Ontario, 2006a, op. cit.

24 24. Registered Nurses Association of Ontario, 2006b, op. cit.

25 Restall, op. cit.

26 Anthony, op. cit.

27 Restall, op. cit.

28 Reid Ponte P, Conlin G, Conway JB, *et al.* Making patient-centred care come alive: achieving full integration of the patient's perspective. *J Nurs Admin.* 2003; **33**(2): 82–90.

29 Registered Nurses' Association of Ontario, 2006a, op. cit.

30 Registered Nurses'Association of Ontario, 2006b, op. cit.

31 Restall, op. cit.

32 Reid, op. cit.

33 Trainor J, Church K. A framework for support. In: Trainor J, Pomeroy E, Pape B, editors. *Building a Framework for Support: a community development approach to mental health policy.* Toronto, ON: Canadian Mental health Association; 1999. pp. 37–58.

34 Rafael, D. *Strengthening the social determinants of health: the Toronto Charter for a healthy Canada* [online]. 2003. Available at: http://depts.washington.edu/ccph/pdf_files/Toronto%20Charter%20Final.pdf (accessed 26 May 2011).

35 Vollman AR, Anderson ET, McFarlane J. *Canadian Community as Partner.* Philadelphia, PA: Lippincott, Williams & Wilkins; 2004.

36 Forchuk C, Martin ML, Chan L, *et al.* Therapeutic relationships: from hospital to community. *J Psychiatr Ment Hlt.* 2005; **12**(5): 556–64.

37 Parikh SV, Lin E, Lesage AD. Mental health treatment in Ontario: selected comparisons between the primary care and specialty sectors. *Can J Psychiatry.* 1997; **42**: 929–34.

38 Bernardo A, Forchuk C. Factors associated with readmission to a psychiatric facility. *Psychiatr Serv.* 2001; **52**(8): 1100–6.

39 Anthony, op. cit.

40 Bensing, op. cit.

41 Registered Nurses' Association of Ontario, 2006a, op. cit.

42 Ibid.

43 Registered Nurses' Association of Ontario, 2006b, op. cit.

44 Registered Nurses' Association of Ontario, 2006a, op. cit.

45 Registered Nurses' Association of Ontario, 2006b, op. cit.

46 Ibid.

47 Blythe J, Baumann A, Zeytinoglue I, *et al.* Full-time or part-time work in nursing: preferences, tradeoffs and choices. *Healthc Q.* 2005; **8**(3): 69–77.

48 Registered Nurses' Association of Ontario, 2006b, op. cit.

49 Forchuk, op. cit.

50 Anthony, op. cit.

51 Registered Nurses' Association of Ontario, 2006a, op. cit.

52 Ibid.

53 Bauman, op. cit.

54 Registered Nurses' Association of Ontario, 2006b, op. cit.

55 Registered Nurses' Association of Ontario, 2006a, op. cit.

56 Registered Nurses' Association of Ontario. *Ensuring the care will be there: report on nursing recruitment and retention in Ontario.* Toronto, Canada: Registered Nurses' Association of Ontario; 2000.

57 Bell J. The dysfunction of dysfunctional. *J Fam Nurs.* 1995; **1**(3): 235–7.

58 Registered Nurses' Association of Ontario, 2006a, op. cit.

59 Registered Nurses' Association of Ontario, 2006a, op. cit.

60 Bell, op. cit.

61 Bauman, op. cit.

62 Registered Nurses' Association of Ontario, 2006a, op. cit.

63 Registered Nurses' Association of Ontario, 2006b, op. cit.

64 Registered Nurses' Association of Ontario, 2006a, op. cit.

65 Ibid.

66 Ibid.

67 Restall, op. cit.

68 Rafael, op. cit.

69 Vollman, op. cit.

70 Ibid.

71 Restall, op. cit.

CHAPTER 5

The Person/Patient-Provider/ Clinician Relationship

This (fifth) chapter of the book presents various aspects of the relationships between persons with SMI and providers of mental and other health care, both for persons with SMI in general as well as for special populations with SMI. These relationships are crucial for PCC of persons with SMI, perhaps even more than for PCC in general, as a large component of the interventions of mental health care consists of these relationships. Other chapters of this book also address such relationships, e.g. Chapter 6, Management and Finding Common Ground, which addresses interventions such as medications, psychotherapy and rehabilitation, that are delivered to persons with SMI by providers whose relationships with the persons with SMI are crucial for successful and satisfactory service delivery; and Chapter 7, Prevention and Health Promotion, which addresses physical (medical) care for persons with SMI, where the relationships of the physical care providers with the persons with SMI are also important for successful and satisfactory service delivery.

Section 5.1, *Therapeutic Relationships with People with Serious Mental Illness*, argues that PCC is not possible without establishing and maintaining therapeutic relationships, and that this is particularly important in mental health settings since persons with SMI may have difficulty establishing trusting relationships. The section argues that consideration of both the service provider and the service user is essential for understanding therapeutic relationships. Section 5.2, *Clinical Communication with Persons who have Serious Mental Illness*, argues that clinical communication has amassed a large body of research, but is just recently being examined in relation to people with SMI. The section argues that given the considerable impact that communication can have on health outcomes, and the centrality of good communication to PCC, there should be a focus on clinical communication with people who have SMI. Section 5.3, *Shared/Collaborative Care for People with Serious Mental Illness*, claims that there are limited data and experience in relation to collaborative or shared (mental and primary) health care for people with SMI and describes a number of programs that focus on collaboration in mental health care delivery for persons with SMI. The section includes clinical application of the person-centered concept through examples and real-life experiences in delivering services through collaborative care.

Section 5.4.1, *Person-Centered Approaches for Adolescents with Serious Mental Illness*, reviews multiple considerations that contribute to the need for a pragmatic approach to successful PCC in relation to adolescents with SMI. These considerations include, among others, the phase of adolescent development. Section 5.4.2, *Dual Diagnosis: an individualized approach*, claims that dual diagnosis (the Canadian term for the common co-occurrence of psychiatric disorders in cognitively disabled individuals) is common in the population of the cognitively disabled, and that diagnosis of mental illness, including SMI, is a challenge in these individuals. The section emphasizes the importance of understanding the individual with dual diagnosis and his or her unique vulnerabilities, so that care can be individualized, resulting in effective PCC for this population. Section 5.4.3, *Serious Mental Illness: person-centered approaches in forensic psychiatry*, focuses on the application of person-centered approaches for individuals with SMI who have come in conflict with the law and, as a result, are often cared for in a forensic mental health care setting. The section argues and illustrates that it is possible to combine the demands of the justice system with PCC for this population. Section 5.4.4, *Treatment of Co-Occurring Substance Use Disorders using Shared Decision-Making and Electronic Decision-Support Systems*, claims that SUDs are common for people with SMI, and that many of the adverse outcomes related to SMI, such as relapse, homelessness and incarceration, are strongly associated with SUDs. The section briefly considers the "chronic" disease management model and offers guidelines for current mental health services in relation to people with such co-occurring disorders, including use of electronic systems.

5.1 Therapeutic Relationships with People with Serious Mental Illness

Cheryl Forchuk and Robin Coatsworth-Puspoky

INTRODUCTION

It could be argued that the underlying foundations of PCC as outlined by Rudnick and Roe in Section 1.1, *Foundations and Ethics of Person-Centered Approaches to Individuals with Serious Mental Illness,* also underlie the therapeutic relationship. These foundations include: person focused, person driven, person sensitive, and person contextualized. These foundations are necessary for the development of therapeutic relationships. The purpose and focus of such relationships is to meet the goals and needs of service users/persons while taking into account their uniqueness as individuals.

One difference between the concepts of *therapeutic relationships* and *PCC* is that therapeutic relationships explicitly consider at least two "persons": the service user and the service provider (the generic term *service provider* is used here to represent the helping person that may be from one of many disciplines). The focus of the therapeutic relationship remains fixed on the service user and not the service provider. Whether or not the relationship is service user driven would depend on the particular theoretical orientation of the service provider, but most theories of therapeutic relationships would endorse this view. However, the service provider also plays a major role in the development of a therapeutic or non-therapeutic relationship. Since it is assumed that the service provider also plays a significant role, strategies are used to enhance the service provider's level of self-awareness and self-reflection to ensure that the service user's goals and needs are being met by the relationship rather than the goals and needs of the service provider. Another related difference between the concepts of *therapeutic relationship* and *PCC* is that therapeutic relationships involve a focus on interpersonal processes. These processes include communication and the developing phases of the relationships.

This section will briefly review different theoretical and disciplinary perspectives of the therapeutic relationship, describe the development of therapeutic or non-therapeutic relationships, review factors related to the development of therapeutic relationships, discuss boundaries, and highlight specific issues related to therapeutic relationships and SMI.

Theories Related to Therapeutic Relationships

One of the challenges in discussing therapeutic relationships in relation to PCC is that there are many different disciplinary and theoretical perspectives of the therapeutic relationship. Some of these theories are more closely aligned with PCC than others. A small sample of these theories is listed below in Table 5.1 and illustrates

TABLE 5.1 Some Different Theoretical Perspectives on the Therapeutic Relationship

Name of Theorist	Discipline	Theory/Model	Examples of Major Concepts	Development Factors (Service User; Provider; Interpersonal)
Freud (1856–1939)	• Psychiatry	• Psychoanalysis theory	• Unconscious process (free association; dream analysis; resistance; transference; interpretation)	• Individual care approach used for enhancement of personal maturity and personal growth[1]
Sullivan (1892–1949)	• Psychiatry	• Interpersonal psychotherapy	• Participant observer • Parataxic distortion • Consensual validation	• Constant collaboration between service provider and service user • Assumption: service user will reenact relationship patterns with service provider[2]
Peplau (1909–1999)	• Nursing	• Nursing theory – interpersonal relations	• Interpersonal processes that occur between the service provider – service user • Phases of the relationship (orientation; working – identification and exploitation; resolution)	• Service user builds competencies (interpersonal, community living, problem solving) • Service provider has greater self-understanding through interaction • Interpersonal concepts: communication; pattern integration, and service user – service provider relationship[3,4]

Rogers (1902–1987)	• Psychology	• Humanistic theory	• Client-centered therapy
			  – Genuineness
			  – Unconditional positive regard
			  – Empathy
				• Therapeutic interventions include: removing environmental elements that are hindering growth and development, and to promote congruence of service user[5,6,7]

Perls (1893–1970)	• Psychology	• Gestalt theory	• Focuses on the present and reality	• Service user rebuilds thinking, feeling and acting into a connected whole[8,9]
Maslow (1921–1970)	• Psychology	• Hierarchy of needs theory	• Human behavior as a response to needs • How individuals are motivated	• As needs are met, service user moves towards self-actualization and development of full potential[10]

Orlando (1926—)	• Nursing	• Communication and validation	• To investigate and meet service user's immediate needs for help • Relationship built by sharing and validating perceptions, thoughts and feelings	• Service provider self-reflects on perception, thoughts and feelings; seeks to understand through processes such as validation; makes a deliberate, disciplined, professional response[11]
Klein (1882–1960)	• Psychology	• Object relations theory	• Exploring the role of a service user's mental representations of themselves and others and how these representations influence the relationships of the service user	• Service user discusses mental representations of themselves and others with service provider • Service provider notes how service user projects previous object relationships onto current relationships • Service providers try to change maladaptive mental representations by establishing a therapeutic relationship with service user[12]
Kohut (1913–1981)	• Psychology	• Self-psychology	• Emphasizes the important role of childhood development and experiences • Highlights the important role played by empathic relationships	• Service provider endeavors to become an idealized parent figure through transference in order to provide service user with a healthier sense of self and by getting service user to reflect on past relations[13]
Miller and Rollnick (current)	• Psychology	• Motivational interviewing	• Focuses on a service user's intrinsic motivation • The approach utilizes both person-centered and semi-direction • Emphasizes the importance of self-sufficiency	• Attempts to increase the service user's awareness of the potential consequences and risks resulting from his behavior • The service provider then helps the service user envision a better future and encourages the service user to motivate himself to achieve this future[14]

some of the diversity in perspectives. This table also identifies some of the facilitators of the therapeutic relationship from each theoretical perspective. The examples included originate from the disciplines of nursing, psychiatry and psychology, but all health care affiliated professions have placed some emphasis on therapeutic relationships, and many professions often borrow from the literature of other professions for theory, research and practice on this concept.

Similarities of Approaches

Regardless of the theoretical approach, there are some similarities which are common to all theories related to therapeutic relationships. For instance, the importance of the formation of a therapeutic relationship serves as a foundation for all of the relevant theoretical approaches. However, the nature and emphasis placed on the service user's role, the service provider's role and the interpersonal process role and technique varies between different approaches to therapeutic relationships. Regardless of theory, each theoretical approach provides an opportunity for service users to explore and express their thoughts and feelings to a service provider. Each approach will offer an explanation for service users' situations, which will allow service users to view their circumstances in a new light. Within the safety of the relationship, service users are afforded an opportunity to test out new behaviors. Despite their differences, the various theoretical approaches emphasize that change is possible, and thus all serve to provide service users with the hope of a better future.

Development of Relationships

Relationships can be seen as processes, and as with most processes, they have a beginning, middle and end. Peplau has described the beginning, middle and end phases of the therapeutic relationship as the orientation phase, the working phase and the resolution phase.[15,16]

The orientation phase can begin even before the first meeting between the service user and service provider. It starts when a person is assigned to a service provider and each person begins to have preconceptions about each other. For the service user, the preconceptions may be based on previous helpful (or unhelpful) relationships. The preconceptions maybe derived from assumptions based on other individuals coming from a similar discipline, gender, ethnic group, age group or countless other possibilities. Preconceptions can even be based on such features as eye color or hair length. Similarly, for the service provider, preconceptions can be based on a multitude of factors including gender, age, diagnosis, referral source, psychiatric history, past hospitalization pattern, housing status, income or resemblance to a person from the service provider's past. During the orientation phase, both service user and service provider attempt to move past their preconceptions by learning to view the other person as a "real" person. Establishing trust, a key task of this phase, is accomplished by testing consistent parameters of the relationship. These relationship parameters include the focus of the relationship, how often and how long each appointment will be, the nature of each person's role or roles, and the duration of the relationship. The time to establish trust can vary considerably from person to person and ranges from minutes to months. In a previous study on the orientation phase with people who had a long-term mental illness, it typically took months.[17] The development of trust is shaped by resources and the service providers' caring and/or uncaring behaviors.[18,19,20,21,22,23,24,25] In many cases, persons with SMI have problems trusting people. In the case of some illnesses – such as schizophrenia – paranoia or lack of trust is a prevalent symptom. In addition, in many instances mental illness first arises during adolescence or early adulthood, when individuals are developing their competencies in relationship building.

According to Stanhope, Marcus and Soloman,[26] the degree of trust existing between a service user and service provider is affected by the level of coercion perceived by the service user in terms of the services provided. The high rates of lifetime exposure to trauma in service users may not only increase service users' vulnerability in relationships, but may contribute to further trauma.[27] Service users' perceptions of the service provider not being available were associated with symptoms of PTSD and depression.[28] The degree of trust existing between a service user and service provider is further affected by the level of coercion perceived by the service user in terms of the services provided.[29] In general, this study found that the greater the feelings of perceived coercion and helplessness experienced by service users, the less likely they are to trust service providers. When case managers were perceived as coercive by service users, the service contact was evaluated as negative by the users and may result in long-term negative outcomes for service users.[30] In light of these realities, it is not surprising that it may take many meetings and a great deal of effort for a relationship of trust to develop between a service user and service provider.

The working phase commences when the service user identifies issues to be worked on in context of the relationship. This is the phase where treatment and/ or rehabilitation plans can be developed mutually and initiated. Very often the initial problems identified by the service user may be more superficial in nature than issues that they identify later on in the process. The process of identifying and resolving issues is similar to working through the layers of an onion; with each layer that is worked through, another deeper layer is revealed until the core is reached. How deeply each dyad works can depend on many things including the length of the relationship, the specific role of the helping person, the immediacy of concerns and the pain associated with dealing with the deeper layers. The helping person supports the service user in setting the pace and determining the depth and content of the working phase.

The resolution phase is the period commencing when the last problem is worked through until the time the relationship is terminated. It is a period for reflecting on what has been accomplished and for planning proactively for future sources of support in the absence of the service provider. For a person with a SMI this period may involve learning personal signs of relapse and identifying resources of help in the community. Developing a network of supportive relationships and a movement towards community integration are common in this phase.

Of course, not all relationships between service users and service providers are therapeutic. Non-therapeutic relationships can also develop throughout these phases. For example, in a qualitative study of the therapeutic relationship between service providers and service users with long-term mental illnesses,[31] most of the relationships progressed through the orientation, working and resolution phases as described above. Service users even used the words "phase," "level" or "stage" to describe the progression of the relationship. However, some dyads developed non-therapeutically. Although they started in the orientation phase, there was little consistency, and a relationship of trust did not develop. Service providers reported constantly changing therapeutic approaches since the relationship was not developing.[32] Similarly, service users would frequently change their approach and become aware that things were not working well. This situation has been labeled the "grappling and struggling" phase. Eventually things would become so uncomfortable during this phase that the dyad would collude to avoid each other. This phase was called "mutual withdrawal". Service providers would "run out of time" and be unable to see these service users. The service user would be off the ward or engaged in other activities during planned sessions. If they did meet, service providers would describe a strategy of keeping the meetings brief and service users would describe a strategy of keeping the conversations superficial. Needless to say, no therapeutic work would be accomplished in a relationship where the partners are avoiding each other. Similar phases were also identified by Coatsworth-Puspoky and others.[33] If a relationship has reached this phase, the simplest solution may be a therapeutic transfer.[34] In looking at one service provider with two different service users and one service user with two service providers over time, it was discovered that there was no statistical relationship between a service user or service provider having difficulty with the first and second person.[35] This supports the idea that each relationship is unique and that we should see problems as reflecting problem relationships rather than problem service users.

Factors Affecting Therapy

Service user factors, service provider factors and the environment influence the uniqueness of each service user-service provider relationship,[36,37,38] whereas the effectiveness of any type of care is influenced by service user variables and care variables. The influence of service user and service provider factors, care variables and environment will be discussed.

Service User Factors

Common service user variables capable of affecting care include the degree of openness to care and the degree of self-relatedness which refers to the ability to experience and understand internal states, thoughts and feelings.[39] Active service user participation was also identified as a factor influencing the relationship.[40] The length and number of previous hospitalizations experienced by a service user and service users' perceptions of the difference in power between themselves and the service provider influences service users' perceptions of trust, anxiety and preconceptions.[41,42,43] For example, Harry Jones has a long history of readmissions, which will make it more likely to take more time to establish a trusting relationship with his assigned nurse, Susan Smith. On the other hand, the relationship could be supported if there were similar positive relationships in the past and in particular if Susan reminded him of a particularly positive relationship.

Service Provider Factors

The service provider-service user relationship is not only influenced by preconceptions and initial impressions of the service user, but is also influenced by the preconceptions and initial impressions of the service provider.[44,45,46] Service providers' preconceptions are influenced by the number of years in mental health professions.[47,48,49] The attitude and personality of the service provider also influences the relationship.[50,51] In a qualitative study with service users (n=21), attitude includes the six subcategories of "being professional, conveying hope, working alongside, knowing and respecting the person, human quality, and connection."[52] Similar themes are reported by other researchers.[53,54,55,56] For example, service providers being committed to understanding the service user,[57,58,59] using their skills of listening, responding respectfully, problem-solving and exploring appropriately,[60,61,62,63] and providing an atmosphere of trust, warmth and genuineness[64,65,66,67,68] resulted in service users' feeling safe and secure within the relationship.[69,70] As well, how power was used by service providers within the relationship and how service users perceived the use of power also influenced the relationship.[71,72,73] Using the earlier example of Harry Jones and Susan Smith, Susan's view of Harry will be very influential in determining the nature of the evolving relationship. For example, she could label him negatively due to his frequent readmissions or his similarity to service users that were not successful in the past. Conversely, careful attention to power issues, such as giving control over topics and the timing of meetings, as well as conveying hope, could help the relationship move in a more positive direction.

Therapy Variables

Common therapy variables capable of such influence include the quality of the therapeutic relationship, which pertains to the level of empathy, genuineness and unconditional acceptance shown by the service provider, the fit between the problem and the type of treatment, and the fit between the service user and type of treatment.[74] The therapeutic relationship is influenced not only by service provider and service user factors, but also the environmental context where the relationship occurs. For example, consistency, listening and ensuring regular and private interactions were essential in the development of the therapeutic relationship.[75,76,77,78,79,80] As well, accessibility or availability of service providers to develop relationships with service users was created by ensuring that staffing levels were adequate for the area.[81,82,83] Increased paperwork and the biomedical model were factors cited as having an adverse effect on the therapeutic relationships.[84] In addition to increased paperwork, Hostick and McClelland[85] identified service provider factors (being moved between units, being uninvolved in decisions), system factors, management factors (priorities, styles and demands; uninterested, uncaring managers), additional external pressures and escalating workloads as adversely affecting the service provider relationship.[86] The researchers suggested that of all of the factors, the influence of management and managers may be the most detrimental.

The therapeutic service provider relationship is a template for the development of other interpersonal relationships.[87,88] For example, Frank and Gunderson[89] found that positive service user experiences with service provider relationships result in an increased ability to form and receive greater satisfaction from and have fewer disturbances within relationships with other people and other care providers.[90,91,92] In addition, the therapeutic alliance increases service user's compliance with treatment (therapy and medications) and decreases not only the frequency, but the duration of re-hospitalization.[93,94]

Boundary Issues in Relation to Different Standards of Practice

Boundaries are imaginary lines that delineate the relationship between the service provider and service user as professional and therapeutic and differentiate it from social relationships.[95,96,97,98] Professional boundaries address roles; time; place and space; money; gifts, services and related matters; clothing; language; self-disclosure; and physical contact.[99,100]

Regulated service providers, e.g., physicians, nurses, occupational therapists, psychologists and social workers, follow standards, guides or policies that define their role in establishing and maintaining professional boundaries with service users.[101,102,103,104,105] Boundaries in the service provider-service user relationship are established at the beginning of the relationship. Service providers are supportive of and work collaboratively with the service user to develop goals, make decisions, understand the meaning of behaviors, share information and develop the best solution for the service user. Establishing and maintaining boundaries is the responsibility of the service provider. "Boundaries define the helping pathway – for both service users and providers – and as such are integral to professional effectiveness."[106] When clear boundaries are established by service providers, service users receive care that is in their best interest, thereby preventing abuse and inequality of power within the relationship.[107,108,109,110]

Misuse of power by service providers results in service user abuse and violation or crossing of service user boundaries.[111,112,113,114,115,116] Boundary crossing or misuse of power occurs when service providers use the power in the relationship to meet their personal needs as opposed to the needs of service users.[117] Standards, guides and policies of the Colleges[118,119,120,121] and health care literature have identified warning signs that a boundary violation or crossing may occur. Examples of warning signs include sharing personal information and personal home contact information with the service user, dressing differently or keeping secrets. However, it should be noted that the sharing of personal information is considered to be appropriate in some circumstances; for instance, if personal information is used for the purposes of teaching the service user about effective coping methods utilized by the service provider when he or she was in a similar situation.[122] Service providers are responsible for contemplating the warning signs within their own practice and practice setting to ensure that service users' boundaries are not being violated.[123,124] When boundaries are crossed it may be intentional or unintentional, but it is considered abuse.[125] Abusive behaviors include verbal and emotional abuse, physical abuse, neglect, sexual abuse and financial abuse.[126]

Specific Issues: relationships and serious mental illness

Specific issues that may limit communication or participation within the therapeutic service provider-service user relationship include the service user's illness. This may include depression, cognitive impairments, or paranoia. Forchuk and others[127] identified paranoia and delusions, anxiety and anger as factors that service users were guarded about, as they feared service providers may use them against them. Symptoms of depression, cognitive impairment or paranoia may share many features such as a lack of trust, decreased interaction as a result of social interaction, or difficulties with concentration or communication.[128] For example, persons experiencing depression may have less interaction with others and less satisfaction with their relationships.[129] As well, trust in relationships becomes compromised when service providers encourage service users to confront their delusion or attempt to re-orientate those service users who are experiencing delusions.[130]

The age of onset of mental health challenges may limit social skill development, thereby impacting service users' abilities to communicate with service providers and other persons. Age may affect how service providers interact with service users and how service users interact with service providers. For example, with children and adolescents, Fontaine[131] suggests the use of open-ended questions and allowing ample time for service users to respond. Listening is when service providers will gather the majority of their information.[132] She cautions service providers to be aware that children or adolescents may not have been able to communicate their feelings or may not have the cognitive abilities to express their feelings.[133] This may also result in difficulties developing interpersonal competencies and peer and romantic relationships. Similarly, older adults with cognitive impairments may experience difficulties expressing their feelings verbally to service providers and significant others, thereby impacting relationships.[134] The development of therapeutic relationships between older service users and service providers may be impeded by visual and hearing deficits.[135,136] Impaired hearing in older adults results in decreased physical, mental and social functioning.[137] Visual and hearing deficits can be enhanced by ensuring service users' eyeglasses and hearing aids are functional and being worn, by minimizing background noises,[138] and by providing additional time for older service users to interpret and respond to messages in a conversation.[139,140]

CONCLUSION

Therapeutic relationships are foundational to PCC. Relationships develop through a process where service users can learn to trust the helping person and identify issues that need addressing. However, it is important to recognize that there are many different theoretical and professional perspectives existing on the nature of therapeutic relationships, which may influence perceptions about the role of the service user, the role of the helper/provider and the relative weight given to each technique or interpersonal process.

REFERENCES

1 Freud S. *A General Introduction to Psychoanalysis*. New York, NY: Washington Square Press; 1935.
2 Sullivan HS. *The Interpersonal Theory of Psychiatry*. New York, NY: WW Norton; 1953.
3 Peplau H. Interpersonal relations: a theoretical framework for application in nursing practice. *Nurs Sci Q*. 1992; **5**(1): 13–18.
4 Forchuk C, Hildegard E. *Peplau: interpersonal nursing theory*. Newbury Park, CA: Sage Publications; 1993.
5 Rogers CR. A theory of therapy, personality and interpersonal relationships, as developed in the cli1ent-centered framework. In: Koch S, editor. *Psychology: a study of a science*. Vol. 3. New York, NY: McGraw-Hill; 1959.
6 Rogers CR. *A Way of Being*. Boston, MA): Houghton Mifflin; 1980.
7 Rogers CR. *Counseling and Psychotherapy*. Boston, MA: Houghton Mifflin; 1942.
8 Perls FS. Four lectures. In: Fagan J, Sheperd IL, editors. *Gestalt Therapy Now*. Palo Alto, CA: Science and Behavior Books; 1970.
9 Perls FS. *In and Out of the Garbage Pail*. Lafayette, CA: Real People Press; 1969.
10 Maslow A. A theory of human motivation. In: Carr L, editor. *Motivation and Personality*. New York, NY): Harper & Row Publishers, Inc.; 1954.
11 Orlando IJ. *The Dynamic Nurse-Patient Relationship: function, process and principles*. New York, NY: GP Putnam; 1961.
12 Klein M. *The Writings of Melanie Klein*. London: Hogarth Press; 1975.
13 Kohut H. *The Restoration of Self*. New York, NY: International Universities Press; 1971.
14 Miller WR, Rollnick S. *Motivational Interviewing: preparing people to change*. New York, NY: Guilford Press; 2002.
15 Peplau H. Interpersonal relations in nursing. New York, NY: Putnam Sons; 1952.
16 Peplau H. Peplau's theory of interpersonal relations. *Nurs Sci Q*. 1997; **10**(4): 162–7.
17 Forchuk C. The orientation phase of the nurse-client relationship: how long does it take? *Perspect Psychiatr Care*. 1992; **28**(4): 7–10.
18 Coatsworth-Puspoky R, Forchuk C, Ward-Griffin C. Nurse client processes in mental health: recipient's experiences. *J Psychiatr Ment Health Nurs*. 2006; **13**: 349–55.
19 Forchuk C, Westwell J, Martin ML, *et al*. Factors influencing movement of chronic psychiatric patients from the orientation to the working phase of the nurse-client relationship on an inpatient unit. *Perspect Psychiatr Care*. 1998; **34**(1): 36–44.
20 Forchuk C, Westwell J, Martin ML, *et al*. The developing nurse-client relationship: nurses' perspectives. *J Am Psychiatr Nurses Assoc*. 2000; **6**(1): 3–19.
21 Forchuk C, Reynolds W. Client's reflections on relationships with nurses: comparisons from Canada and Scotland. *J Psychiatr Ment Health Nurs*. 2001; **8**(1): 45–51.

22 Horberg U, Brunt D, Axelsson A. Clients' perceptions of client-nurse relationships in local authority psychiatric services: a qualitative study. *Int J Ment Health Nurs.* 2004; **13**(1): 9–17.

23 Hostick T, McClelland F. "Partnership": a co-operative inquiry between community mental health nurses and their clients. *J Psychiatr Ment Health Nurs.* 2002; **9**(1): 111–17.

24 Koivisto K, Janhonen S, Vaisanen L. Patients' experiences of being helped in an inpatient setting. *J Psychiatr Ment Health Nurs.* 2004; **11**(3): 268–75.

25 Shatell MM, Starr SS, Thomas SP. "Take my hand, help me out": mental health service recipients' experience of the therapeutic relationship. *Int J Ment Health Nurs.* 2007; **16**: 274–84.

26 Stanhope V, Marcus S, Soloman P. The impact of coercion on services from the perspective of mental health care consumers with co-occurring disorders. *Psychiatr Serv.* 2009; **60**(2): 183–8.

27 Mueser KT, Trumbetta SL, Rosenberg SD, *et al.* Trauma and posttraumatic stress disorder in severe mental illness. *J Consult Clin Psychol.* 1998; **66**(3): 493–9.

28 Beattie N, Shannon C, Kavanagh M, *et al.* Predictors of PTSD symptoms in response to psychosis and psychiatric admission. *J Nerv Ment Dis.* 2009; **197**(1): 56–60.

29 Stanhope, Marcus, Soloman, 2009, op. cit.

30 Ibid.

31 Forchuk, Westwell, Martin, *et al.*, 2009, op. cit.

32 Ibid.

33 Coatsworth-Puspoky, Forchuk, Ward-Griffin, 2006, op. cit.

34 Forchuk, Westwell, Martin, *et al.*, 1998, op. cit.

35 Forchuk C. Uniqueness within the nurse-client relationship. *Arch Psychiatr Nurs.* 1995; **9**(1): 34–9.

36 Peplau, 1952, op. cit.

37 Forchuk, 1992, op. cit.

38 Forchuk, 1995, op. cit.

39 Passer M, Smith E, Atkinson M, *et al.* Psychology frontiers and applications. Toronto: McGraw-Hill Ryerson Ltd; 2003.

40 Forchuk, Westwell, Martin, *et al.*, 2000, op. cit.

41 Forchuk, 1992, op. cit.

42 Frank AF, Gunderson JG. The role of the therapeutic alliance in the treatment of schizophrenia: relationship to course and outcome. *Arch Gen Psychiatry.*1990; **47**(3): 228–36.

43 Coatsworth-Puspoky, Forchuk, Ward-Griffin, 2006, op. cit.

44 Forchuk, Westwell, Martin, *et al.*, 2000, op. cit.

45 Forchuk C. The orientation phase of the nurse-client relationship: testing Peplau's theory. *J Adv Nurs.* 1994; **20**(3): 532–7.

46 Lund VE, Frank DL. Helping the medicine go down: nurses' and patients' perceptions about medication compliance. *J Psychosoc Nurs Ment Health Serv.* 1991; **29**(7): 6–9.

47 Coatsworth-Puspoky, Forchuk, Ward-Griffin, 2006, op. cit.

48 Forchuk, 1994, op. cit.

49 Lund, Frank, 1991, op. cit.

50 Coatsworth-Puspoky, Forchuk, Ward-Griffin, 2006, op. cit.

51 Rydon S. The attitudes, knowledge and skills needed in mental health nurses: the perspective of users of mental health services. *Int J Ment Health Nurs.* 2005; **14**(2): 78–87.

52 Ibid.

53 Shatell, Starr, Thomas, 2007, op. cit.

54 Forchuk, Reynolds, 2001, op. cit.
55 Horberg, Brunt, Axelsson, 2002, op. cit.
56 Shatell, Starr, Thomas, 2007, op. cit.
57 Horberg, Brunt, Axelsson, 2002, op. cit.
58 Shatell, Starr, Thomas, 2007, op. cit.
59 Reynolds W. The influence of clients' perceptions of the helping relationship in the development of an empathy scale. *J Psychiatr Ment Health Nurs.* 1994; **1**(1): 23–30.
60 Forchuk, Reynolds, 2001, op. cit.
61 Horberg, Brunt, Axelsson, 2002, op. cit.
62 Koivisto, Janhonen, Vaisanen, 2004, op. cit.
63 Reynolds, 1994, op. cit.
64 Forchuk, Westwell, Martin, 1998, *et al.*, op. cit.
65 Forchuk, Reynolds, 2001, op. cit.
66 Horberg, Brunt, Axelsson, 2002, op. cit.
67 Shatell, Starr, Thomas, 2007, op. cit.
68 Stanhope, Marcus, Soloman, 2009, op. cit.
69 Horberg, Brunt, Axelsson, 2002, op. cit.
70 Koivisto, Janhonen, Vaisanen, 2004, op. cit.
71 Coatsworth-Puspoky, Forchuk, Ward-Griffin, 2006, op. cit.
72 Shatell, Starr, Thomas, 2007, op. cit.
73 Rydon, 2005, op. cit.
74 Beutler L, Machado PP, Neufeldt SA. Therapist variables. In: Bergin AE, Garfield SL, editors. *Handbook of Psychotherapy and Behavior Change.* 4th ed. New York, NY: Wiley; 1994.
75 Forchuk, Westwell, Martin, 1998, *et al.*, op. cit.
76 Forchuk, Westwell, Martin, *et al.*, 2000, op. cit.
77 Forchuk, Reynolds, 2001, op. cit.
78 Koivisto, Janhonen, Vaisanen, 2004, op. cit.
79 Shatell, Starr, Thomas, 2007, op. cit.
80 Gartland GJ. Teaching the therapeutic relationship. *Physiother Can.* 1984; **36**(1): 24–8.
81 Horberg, Brunt, Axelsson, 2002, op. cit.
82 Coatsworth-Puspoky, Forchuk, Ward-Griffin, 2006, op. cit.
83 Forchuk, Reynolds, 2001, op. cit.
84 Rydon, 2005, op. cit.
85 Hostick, McClelland, 2002, op. cit.
86 Ibid.
87 Frank, Gunderson, 1990, op. cit.
88 Forchuck, 1994, op. cit.
89 Frank, Gunderson, 1990, op. cit.
90 Forchuk, 1992, op. cit.
91 Horberg, Brunt, Axelsson, 2002, op. cit.
92 Forchuk, 1994, op. cit.
93 Frank, Gunderson, 1990, op. cit.
94 Olfson M, Mechanic D, Hansell S, *et al.* Predicting medication noncompliance after hospital discharge among patients with schizophrenia. *Psychiatr Serv.* 2000; **51**(2): 216–22.
95 College of Nurses of Ontario. *Practice Standard: therapeutic nurse-client relationship.* 2006. Available at: www.coto.org/pdf/sexual_abuse_prevention.pdf (accessed 5 May 2011).

96 College of Physicians and Surgeons of Ontario. *Policy Statement #4-08: maintaining appropriate boundaries and preventing sexual abuse.* 2008. Available at: www.cpso.on.ca/policies/policies/default.aspx?ID=1604 (accessed 5 May 2011).

97 Ontario College of Social Workers and Social Service Workers. *Code of Ehics and Standards of Practice Handbook.* 2nd ed [online]. 2008. Available at: www.ocswssw.org/docs/codeofethicsstandardsofpractice.pdf (accessed 26 May 2011).

98 Peternelj-Taylor C. Professional boundaries: a matter of therapeutic integrity. *Journal of Psychosocial Nursing.* 2002; **40**(4): 23–9.

99 College of Nurses of Ontario, op. cit.

100 College of Occupational Therapists of Ontario (COTO). Sexual abuse prevention guidebook. 1996. Available at: www.coto.org/pdf/sexual_abuse_prevention.pdf (accessed 5 May 2011).

101 College of Nurses of Ontario, op. cit.

102 College of Physicians and Surgeons of Ontario, op. cit.

103 Ontario College of Social Workers and Social Service Workers, op. cit.

104 COTO, op. cit.

105 The College of Psychologists of Ontario. *Standards of Professional Conduct.* 2005. Available at: www.cpo.on.ca/resources-and-publications/search.aspx?s=Standards%20of%20Professional%20Conduct (accessed 5 May 2011).

106 Everett B, Gallop R. The link between childhood trauma and mental illness. Thousand Oaks, CA: Sage; 2001.

107 College of Nurses of Ontario, op. cit.

108 College of Physicians and Surgeons of Ontario, op. cit.

109 Ontario College of Social Workers and Social Service Workers, op. cit.

110 COTO, op. cit.

111 Schafer P, Peternelj-Taylor C. Therapeutic relationships and boundary maintenance: the perspective of forensic patients enrolled in a treatment program for violent offenders. *Issues Ment Health Nurs.* 2003; **24**(6–7): 605–25.

112 College of Nurses of Ontario, op. cit.

113 College of Physicians and Surgeons of Ontario, op. cit.

114 Ontario College of Social Workers and Social Service Workers, op. cit.

115 Peternelj-Taylor, 2002, op. cit.

116 COTO, op. cit.

117 College of Nurses of Ontario, op. cit.

118 Ibid.

119 College of Physicians and Surgeons of Ontario, op. cit.

120 COTO, op. cit.

121 The College of Psychologists of Ontario, op. cit.

122 College of Nurses of Ontario, op. cit.

123 Ibid.

124 COTO, op. cit.

125 College of Nurses of Ontario, op. cit.

126 Ibid.

127 Forchuk, Westwell, Martin, *et al.*, 2000, op. cit.

128 Fontaine KL. *Mental Health Nursing.* 5th ed. Upper Saddle River, NJ: Pearson Education, Inc.; 2003.

129 Ibid.

130 Forchuk, Westwell, Martin, *et al.*, 2000, op. cit.

131 Fontaine, 2003, op. cit.

132 Ibid.

133 Ibid.

134 Piercy KW. When it is more than a job: close relationships between home health aides and older clients. *J Aging Health.* 2000; **12**(3): 362–87.

135 Fontaine, 2003, op. cit.

136 Larsen PD, Hazen SE, Martin JL. Assessment and management of sensory loss in elderly patients. *AORN J.* 1997; **65**(2): 432–7.

137 Strawbridge WJ, Wallhagen MI, Shema SJ, *et al.* Negative consequence of hearing impairment in old age: a longitudinal analysis. *Gerontologist.* 2000; **40**(3): 320–6.

138 Larsen, Hazen, Martin, 1997, op. cit.

139 Fontaine, 2003, op. cit.

140 Larsen, Hazen, Martin, 1997, op. cit.

5.2 Clinical Communication with Persons Who Have Serious Mental Illness

Orit Karnieli-Miller and Michelle P. Salyers

INTRODUCTION: THE IMPORTANCE OF COMMUNICATION IN PERSON-CENTERED CARE

This section addresses communication in PCC and refers the reader to other sections in this book, such as Section 5.1, *Therapeutic Relationships with People with Serious Mental Illness*, for discussion of related PCC matters. During the last two decades there has been increased public awareness of the important role of health care communication as a central clinical function. Clinical communication is critical in collecting information, enhancing service users' understanding of the situation and their treatment plan, increasing service user satisfaction, concordance to treatment recommendations, health outcomes,[1,2] and promotion of effective relationships.[3] Clinical communication skills include various interpersonal skills, such as verbalizing thoughts and feelings, speaking and understanding the same language, being attentive and responsive to non-verbal cues, explaining information (educating), checking for understanding and addressing emotions elicited.

All of these interpersonal communication features are impacted when a person is suffering from an SMI. For example, service users that are diagnosed with a personality disorder may engage inappropriately, including being hostile, seductive and/or distant;[4] similarly, psychoses can include delusional beliefs and odd behaviors. These behaviors may, in turn, lead to feelings of frustration, anger and discomfort by the health care provider and lead to a communication clash. Providers need to maintain flexibility and develop specific management strategies to enhance communication and tailor it to the service users' specific needs.[5]

Another important health care feature that impacts communication greatly is the increasing need for service users to become active collaborators in managing their care. This is an inherent part of the idea of recovery, or living successfully with SMI and other persistent health challenges.[6] In the broader health field, the principles of collaborative management of chronic illness involve the service user and health care provider working together to clearly identify problem areas, set goals, learn self-management skills and participate in active follow-up.[7] PCC and its communication includes attuned and empathic listening to service user experiences, perceptions and concerns; using simple, non-technical language at a level service users can understand;[8] respecting culture and beliefs; and providing the amount of information about the disease and care that the person desires. Systematic reviews have shown that this type of PCC translates into higher levels of trust and satisfaction, reduced emotional burden, and improved biomedical markers such as blood pressure and blood sugar control.[9] Relationships in which service users are activated to take greater control in their care are important predictors of concordance to treatment and improved physical health outcomes.[10,11] This way of thinking leads to the need for developing clinical communication strategies that are tailored to both service users and providers and are also relevant to the developments in the 21st century (such as Internet use, patient rights laws, etc.). One of the key communication strategies, SDM, is a collaborative, person-centered approach to care, emphasizing how service providers and users can best work together. This communicational strategy will be extensively discussed next.

Example

The following is an illustration of a service user's perspective concerning PCC communication with her psychiatrist, its influence on her satisfaction, and her level of involvement in SDM about her care:

Hadar, a 27-year-old female living with bipolar disorder, describes her relationship with her psychiatrist during an interview about service users' relationships with psychiatrists and preferences for decision-making. She states that her relationship with her psychiatrist is "a great one" and that he is the "best psychiatrist I had." When asked to elaborate, she says:

"He is nice, he talks to me at my level (eye-to-eye), and he does not patronize me. If he is deliberating about the best treatment for me, he tells me the reasons he is thinking of it. He explains himself. For example, I gained a lot of weight in my lithium treatment; I told him I want to stop with it. He explained that it will influence many other things: 'you might go into mania; you might suffer from depression. Your situation is good now; I do not want to change.' . . . . He explained what could happen to me and asked me if I am willing to take that risk. I said no. I do not want to be hospitalized again. . . . He listens to me when I come and tell him [if something works for me or not].

I want to know why I take the specific medication; in the past, psychiatrists just gave them to me without explaining why.

I like his personal person-to-person connection . . . he explains things to me. He tells jokes, smiles, gives compliments, tells me if something changes, tells me good stuff . . . it is pleasant to go there. He more or less tells me what the problem is and decides what the course of action will be.

. . . I like it that I can decide when to come. If I want to come, I can."

As shown in this excerpt, Hadar is describing an open communication style where information is shared. Pros and cons of each option are discussed, and the service user's concerns and expectations are heard and taken into consideration. In PCC the service user decides who will make the final decision about treatment; in this case it was the psychiatrist (hence this is not typical SDM). However, as Hadar prefers, this decision is based on a two-way discussion, including the psychiatrist hearing her, explaining and considering different choices and consequences. When the type of involvement and participation expected by the service user is met, there is higher likelihood for greater satisfaction with the relationship and care. Hadar's last sentence reflects autonomy to decide when to visit. This illustrates that PCC communication and SDM is not limited to treatments like medications, but also to the management of the relationship, the content and the manner.

This example also illustrates SDM in an Israeli context, where service providers still carry much traditional authority; hence service users tend to defer to care providers for their decisions. This raises the issue of cultural aspects of PCC, which are addressed in this book in Section 4.2, *Trans-Cultural Issues in Person-Centered Care for People with Serious Mental Illness.*

Shared Decision-Making as an Approach to Person-Centered Communication

A hallmark of person-centered communication is SDM, an interactive process where both the service user and the provider collaborate to decide on a care plan that best fits the service user's health care needs and life values. The basic idea underlying SDM is that service user preferences, values and needs are idiosyncratic and significant in making decisions regarding the best care for the individual.[12] SDM is based on a dialogue between the provider and the service user concerning different care options, adverse effects, risks and benefits and how these relate to the service user's life plan, values and preferences. The service user is the one who needs to live with the consequences of these decisions, and therefore his/her involvement is crucial.

Example

The following is an illustration of a service provider-service user interaction that demonstrates how SDM is applied in an actual clinical encounter:

This is an excerpt from an audio-taped medication check-up visit showing how a service provider and service user work together to make a treatment decision. After a long discussion of the current symptoms and how they are interfering with the service user's life, the service provider asks:

[Provider]:	Are these symptoms something that you want to continue to deal with on your own?
[Service user]:	No.
[Provider]:	Is there a medication change that you believe would be helpful to you? I have an idea, but I don't know if medication is the way you want to go.

[Service user]: Okay, what's the idea?

[Provider]: The idea is to add [drug 1]; take two at night and one in the morning. And the reason why I say [drug 1] is that it sounds a little bit like you're having some mood swings during the day and that maybe morning medicine might help. And there's also been new research that shows that [drug 1] helps to quiet voices, which we never really knew before because we've always considered [drug 1] to be only a mood stabilizer. So to me that's the easy one because you're on a very low dose of the [drug 1] and increasing it might help with that. There's another option, which would be to increase the [drug 2]. But that could potentially interfere with sleep.

The provider has opened up two options. She provides the rationale for the options, including recent research. In response, the service user talks about his sleep patterns, so the provider offers a third option and reminds him that the choice is his:

[Provider]: The other option is we could have you take three [drug 1] at night instead of two. You're on the extended release, and possibly taking three at night could help you sleep and theoretically it lasts through the next day. So there are lots of options, and you are in charge of deciding which one works best for you including doing nothing with the medicine and continuing to use your skills. That is entirely up to you.

They talk more about the dosage, side effects, and what would change, and the service user makes a decision.

[Service user]: Okay. All right, I would try that.

[Provider]: You would rather increase the [drug 2] than the [drug 1]?

[Service user]: Yeah, yeah.

[Provider]: Okay, now what I need you to watch out for is to watch out for sleep disturbance, which means maybe your sleep is going to break up even more. So watch for that because that can happen with the higher dose. And if that happens I need you to call me. Watch for increased agitation. I don't expect that to happen, but if it does again I want you to drop the dose back to where it was and give me a call.

They talk more about other aspects of the service user's life. At the end of the session, the provider checks in with the service user about his preference and his understanding of the decision they made.

[Provider]:   How are you feeling about increasing the [drug 2]?
[Service user]:   Sounds good, yeah.
[Provider]:   Okay, so how are you going to do the [drug 2]?
[Service user]:   Go from 30 to 45 . . .
[Provider]:   Which is how many?
[Service user]:   Go from one pill to one and a half.
[Provider]:   Okay.
[Service user]:   And then, if I have sleep problems or feel more anxiety, I will call you.
[Provider]:   Right. You got it.

Active participation in decision-making has been broadly advocated for health care service users, including those with SMI.[13,14] In addition, there are several reasons to believe that SDM fits well in the mental health field. First, in most mental illnesses, there is more than one treatment option available; involving the service user in the decision-making process provides the opportunity to choose the preferred option. Second, treatment options are often accompanied by side effects, some of which can be very unpleasant.[15] Third, mental health treatment for SMI requires a long-term approach, which can only be achieved through understanding the importance and implication of concordance and non-concordance to the treatment plan, real commitment to it and acceptance of the plan by the service user.[16] This commitment can occur only with true participation and mutual understanding in the decision-making process – that includes addressing the service users concerns, fears, uncertainties,[17] life plans and goals. Fourth, the process of SDM allows broadening the conversation to include service users' "personal medicines" (coping strategies that may or may not include conventional health care treatments) that can help in achieving real recovery goals.[18]

Although the ideas underlying SDM (including promoting accurate scientific information and having an active service user) are key to evidence-based medicine research on SDM, SMI is in its initial stages and lags considerably behind work in general medicine.[19,20] Initial studies have found that service users with moderate and severe depression are interested in receiving information and sharing the decision about their health.[21] Similarly, studies of service users with schizophrenia and general SMI expressed interest and preference to being involved in different decisions about their care, especially those involving psychiatric medication.[22,23] Furthermore, studies have shown that service users with SMI can participate actively in their own care and can achieve judicious care decisions.[24,25,26]

Challenges in Applying Shared Decision-Making in Psychiatry

SDM is a complicated process in both physical and mental health. However, some scholars believe that the SDM process may be more difficult with psychiatric service users because of unique challenges for this population.[27] One challenge is overcoming potentially impaired insight and lack of awareness of the illness.[28,29] For example, this may be particularly prominent in specific disorders, e.g. advanced stages of dementia, or specific stages of illness, e.g. acute psychosis. If a person does not acknowledge the existence of an illness, it is much more difficult to work with him or her on identifying and implementing care options. In these kinds of situations, Seale *et al.*[30] found that psychiatrists justified their own use of a more directive, authoritative, and/or coercive style. Various coercive persuasion manners have also been found in the general medicine field.[31] Of course, coercive persuasion methods can have a negative influence on the therapeutic alliance and relationship. Negotiation skills, for both service users and providers, in addition to the use of motivational interviewing skills (described below) can provide a helpful set of tools for talking with people about their health care goals and difficulties without resorting to coercion.

A second major related challenge is whether people with SMI have the capacity to engage in decisions regarding their care. Some health care providers doubt service users' capability to understand and rationally evaluate the information they receive.[32] Similarly, a diminished ability to concentrate or indecisiveness associated with depression may lead the health care providers to take a greater role.[33] Although some cognitive impairments may accompany SMI (such as deficits in attention and memory), the majority of people with SMIs are legally competent and able to make their own decisions.[34] In addition, tools such as advance directives (described below), can assist the person to be involved in decision-making in anticipation of times in which capacity may be impaired. Thus, although SDM may not be possible for some people with SMI at some times due to their lack of capacity to decide at those times, it is a worthwhile and realistic aspiration that increased capacity and SDM can be aimed at and achieved over time for many of these individuals.

A third key challenge of SDM in people with SMI is that sometimes symptoms themselves may interfere with communication and establishing rapport. For example, in situations of severe mistrust or paranoia in service users,[35] it may be difficult to provide information and form a partnership to evaluate care options together. Other positive symptoms present in psychosis such as pressured speech or flight of ideas may make it difficult to follow the person's train of thought. For people with severe negative symptoms of schizophrenia or depression, e.g. poverty of speech or anhedonia, active conversation also can be impaired. Similarly, reading non-verbal and facial expressions in people with severe negative symptoms can be difficult for novice health care providers and may interfere with their ability to relate and connect with the service users.

A fourth challenge lies in the beliefs and expectations of the health care providers. Despite advances in recovery outcomes for people with SMI, many practitioners maintain negative attitudes toward rehabilitation, mutual support and recovery, which can hinder the provision of PCC.[36,37] Treatment planning often fails to reflect recovery goals, i.e. what service users see as important in their own lives, and frequently does not include recipients of services in the planning process.[38] Practitioners often believe that service users need to be protected from stress and need to live in group homes and other protected settings,[39] even though there is convincing evidence to the contrary.[40] Similarly, many practitioners assume that service users are "not motivated" or not ready for competitive work,[41] leading to placement in sheltered workshops or day treatment programs. Medications are often prescribed without explanation, making it difficult if not impossible to understand their purpose.[42] These negative attitudes affect the quality and quantity of communication and level of trust.

Finally, SDM is not suited for everyone. Not all service users (with SMI or not) want an active role in their care.[43] Providers should be aware of a person's ability and willingness to participate in sharing the decision, based on their personal, social and economic resources. If there is resistance or conflict in the service user-provider relationship, it often indicates a move away from being person-centered, in cases where the goal and/or proposed solution do not match the service user's view.

Overcoming Challenges: skills and tools

Overcoming these challenges to SDM is not an easy task, and it requires practice change on the part of health care providers as well as empowering service users. The idea underlying SDM is partnership, and in partnership both roles must change in order to create a new balance in power and responsibilities.[44] Two primary strategies have been used to shift people away from the passive end of the spectrum towards a more active, collaborative approach: one is improving communication between service users and practitioners and the other is providing service users with decision aids.[45] Although we explore both types of strategies independently, the ideal scenario would involve a multifaceted approach aimed at both providers and service users.

Interventions focused on improving service provider-service user communication acknowledge the various communication skills needed to share a decision. These skills include listening and understanding service users' attitudes, values, beliefs and life plans; being able to assess service users' knowledge, preferred level of involvement, and type of information needed; providing the service user with an adequate amount of information about the illness and care options; explaining benefits, risks and adverse effects in an evidence-based and balanced manner; encouraging service users to express their beliefs and concerns; and negotiating and reaching an agreement regarding the decision, based on all factors involved.

One well-known model of communication skills in the general health field that enhances person-centered communication is the Four Habits Model.[46] This approach is based on sets of skills that are organized around four parts of a health care encounter: investing in the beginning, eliciting service users' perspectives, demonstrating empathy, and investing in the end. These habits and behaviors affect the success or failure of the whole encounter.[47] This model has been applied in several places and has proved to be effective in enhancing communication skills.[48,49] Adopting this model to work with SMI service users has the potential to enhance user satisfaction and involvement in care. The Four Habits approach facilitates positive relationships by communicating that topics "beyond" mental illness are important, allowing service users to tell their story, concerns and needs in their own words and pace, without interruption, and working toward establishing the meeting's agenda based on the service users' needs and concerns (habit one). The second habit involves comprehending the service user's perspective and understanding of the problem and its effects on him, including his lifestyle, work, family and daily activities. In the field of mental health, this would include understanding service users' personal medicine and preferences.[50] The third habit focuses on empathy – acknowledging the role of emotions in health decisions and behaviors and encouraging and reflecting emotions displayed by service users. The fourth habit aims to enhance service users' understanding of the rationale behind the treatment decision. To achieve this, health care providers are encouraged to communicate the information in lay terms, to frequently check for understanding and explore difficulties/disagreements with the treatment plan. Adapting the Four Habits Model can enhance health care providers' and service users' communication.

Another area of provider communication skills that is receiving growing attention is motivational interviewing,[51] a person-centered approach that builds on the service user's internal motivation to change. Motivational interviewing grew out of the addictions field, but has been applied in a variety of health care settings to help people with behavior change.[52] Basic principles of motivational interviewing include: expressing empathy, identifying discrepancies between personal goals and behaviors that need to be changed, avoiding argumentation, rolling with resistance and supporting self-efficacy. For people with SMI, motivational interviewing could be useful in a number of different ways including helping people take medications more regularly and increasing their ability to work effectively in SE programs.[53,54]

Because motivational interviewing is driven by what the service user values, this tool can also be used to explore and understand with service users how much involvement they would like to have and what steps are needed to reach their goals. Motivational interviewing could increase the level of rapport, which may be particularly helpful for service users experiencing certain symptoms as described above. This approach can also be particularly helpful when working with people who lack awareness or insight into their illness. By avoiding argumentation, identifying what the person wants to achieve, and exploring descriptively what gets in the way, i.e. discrepancies between values and behaviors, the health care provider and service user can identify steps to take without labeling. In this way, a person need not agree that he or she has a diagnosis of schizophrenia to work towards addressing life goals. In addition, motivational interviewing can provide a structure for providing information by eliciting the person's interest and willingness to hear information and afterwards by following up with questions on understanding and acceptance of the information (ask, provide, ask). In this way, the provider can give information, suggestions or opinions in a way that is acceptable to the person.

Aside from training health care providers, other interventions focus on empowering service users. One important approach is to provide them with better information about the care and the purpose of specific decisions.[55] Recently, tools have been developed aimed at improving communication in mental health by enhancing service user involvement in their care. These tools include decisional aids, leaflets and other materials focusing on educating service users and family members, as well as providers. For example, Priebe and colleagues[56] developed a computer-mediated communication tool to enhance service user-health care provider communication, and in a controlled study found significant positive effects on all three outcomes, i.e. quality of life, unmet needs for care and treatment satisfaction. Van Os and colleagues[57] created a 20-item, two-way communication checklist, filled by service users prior to their appointment. They found this tool efficient in improving communication and leading to changes in the care plan.

In addition to providing basic information, service users might need help overcoming their own hesitations to share thoughts, concerns or opinions.[58] Service users can be coached to ask more questions and be more assertive in providing their worldview and needs in the discussion with the provider. Deegan[59] refers to developing a "power statement" that helps service users talk about their recovery goals as well as fears, concerns, and personal medicines with providers. One innovative approach for SMI combines computerized education and exploration of values, preferences, and concerns along with peer counseling.[60] Focus groups from the pilot study indicated that both providers and service users liked the program and believed it helped the service user be more active and included in their care; a randomized trial of the program is underway. In the medical field, even brief interventions can have a significant impact on health outcomes.[61]

Another set of tools for service users involves written plans about care decisions that may be developed between service users, providers and other supporters. These may take a variety of forms including WRAP in which a service user outlines what they are like when they are well, what things help them stay well, e.g. daily walks, talking with a friend, how they know when they are getting sick, and what to do when that happens, including a specific crisis intervention plan.[62] WRAP plans are often developed with the assistance of other service users. Similarly, relapse prevention plans are formal documents created by service users and providers together that identify early warning signs and triggers that may lead to relapse and ways to cope in those instances.[63] A related set of tools are psychiatric advance directives, which are legal documents that describe desired care options if the person is not capable of making those decisions at the time, e.g. during an acute psychotic episode.[64] The beauty of these planning tools is that the service user's wishes for care are identified when the person is in a position to make decisions. However, the plans are not always followed by health care providers, particularly regarding hospitalizations.[65]

Future Directions

A wealth of information has been collected in the field of health care communication. However, there are few studies focusing specifically on SMI,[66] and those that do have relatively small samples.[67] Some promising approaches for communication skills are now being developed, and rigorous studies will be needed to help determine their efficacy. Health care communication approaches may need to be tailored for working with service users with specific symptoms, for example, engaging service users with severe negative symptoms or paranoia.[68] Further research is needed on the roles of the service user and the provider during interaction to identify what types of behaviors improve the quality of the communication. In this chapter we focused exclusively on communication skills between providers and service users. However, there is great need to further develop skills for SDM in interdisciplinary teams, communicating between colleagues, and involving family members and significant others in decisions about care. In this way, we will be able to identify and codify best practices of communication, by learning from the perspectives of all participants.

A critical factor for best communication practices will be to develop ways of implementing and sustaining changes over time. The inadequacy of training alone to effect actual practice change is well-established. Fixen and colleagues[69] have addressed some of the problems of implementing EBPs and maintaining changes after some intervention or training, but more work is needed to know what is effective in bringing about practice change. In addition, significant changes will need to involve system-level interventions. For example, advance directives can be useful tools, but may be meaningless if service user desires are not actually upheld in times of crisis. We need to understand the context of decision-making and how to create a system that will support real service user involvement in care.

CONCLUSION

In practice, there is no "quick fix" for communication that can be suited to all service users and providers, due to the differences in people's needs, capabilities, resources, worldviews and health care situations. However, SDM is a process that takes these factors into account and represents a way of truly collaborating with service users consistent with PCC. We believe SDM can and should be exercised for both minor and major issues when working with people with SMI. In fact, if SDM is adopted in day-to-day interactions it will naturally apply in higher-risk decisions and increase the likelihood of applying these decisions even during times when the service user may not be fully capable of expressing his or her wishes.[70] There is a growing number of tools to overcome challenges in applying SDM in psychiatric care aimed at providers (such as motivational interviewing and communication training) and aimed at service users (such as advance directives and computerized decision-making tools). More work will be needed in identifying most effective methods of implementing and sustaining person-centered communication.

REFERENCES

1 Rao JK, Anderson LA, Inui TS, *et al.* Communication interventions make a difference in conversations between physicians and patients: a systematic review of the evidence. *Med Care.* 2007; **45**(4): 340–9.

2 Street RL, Krupat E, Bell RA, *et al.* Beliefs about control in the physician-patient relationship: effect on communication in medical encounters. *J Gen Intern Med.* 2003; **18**(8): 609–16.

3 Karnieli-Miller O. *The Experiencing of Breaking and Receiving Bad News on Chronic Illness During Adolescence: an insiders' perspective of adolescents, parents and physicians* [dissertation]. Haifa, Israel: University of Haifa; 2006.

4 Ward RK. Assessment and management of personality disorders. *American Family Physician.* 2004; **70**: 1505–12.

5 Ibid.

6 Holman H, Lorig K. Patients as partners in managing chronic disease: partnership is a prerequisite for effective and efficient health care. *BMJ.* 2000; **320**(7234): 526–7.

7 Von Korff M, Gruman J, Schaefer J, *et al.* Collaborative management of chronic illness. *Ann Intern Med.* 1997; **127**(12): 1097–102.

8 Seale C, Chaplin R, Lelliott P, *et al.* Sharing decisions in consultations involving antipsychotic medication: a qualitative study of psychiatrists' experiences. *Soc Sci Med.* 2006; **62**(11): 2861–73.

9 Stewart M, Brown JB, Donner A, *et al.* The impact of patient-centered care on patient outcomes. *J Fam. Prac.* 2000; **49**(9): 796–804.

10 Ong LML, De Haes CJM, Hoos AM, *et al.* Doctor-patient communication: a review of the literature. *Soc Sci Med.* 1995; **40**(7): 903–18.

11 Michie S, Miles J, Weinman J. Patient-centredness in chronic illness: what is it and does it matter? *Patient Educ Couns.* 2003; **51**(3): 197–206.

12 Stewart, op. cit.

13 Lehman AF, Lieberman JA, Dixon LB, *et al.* Practice guideline for the treatment of patients with schizophrenia. 2nd ed. *Am J Psychiatry.* 2004; **161**(Suppl. 2): 1–56.

14 Hamann J, Cohen R, Leucht S, *et al.* Do patients with schizophrenia wish to be involved in decisions about their medical treatment? *Am J Psychiatry.* 2005; **162**(12): 2382–4.

15 Hamann, op. cit.

16 Naber D. Subjective effects of antipsychotic treatment. *Acta Psychiatr Scand.* 2005; **111**(2): 81–3.

17 Deegan PE. The lived experience of using psychiatric medication in the recovery process and a shared decision-making program to support it. *Psychiatr Rehabil J.* 2007; **31**(1): 62–9.

18 Ibid.

19 Montori VM, Guyatt GH. What is evidence-based medicine and why should it be practiced? *Respir Care.* 2001; **46**(11): 1201–14.

20 Adams JR, Drake RE. Shared decision-making and evidence-based practice. *Community Ment Health J.* 2006; **42**(1): 87–105.

21 Loh A, Leonhart R, Wills CE, *et al.* The impact of patient participation on adherence and clinical outcome in primary care of depression. *Patient Educ Couns.* 2007; **65**(1): 69–78.

22 Hamann, op. cit.

23 Adams JR, Drake RE, Wolford GL. Shared decision-making preferences of people with severe mental illness. *Psychiatr Serv.* 2007; **58**(9): 1219–21.

24 Salyers MP, Matthias MS, Spann C, *et al.* The role of patient activation in psychiatric visits. *Psychiatr Serv.* 2009; **60**(11): 1535–9.

25 Becker DR, Drake RE, editors. *Improving Employment Outcomes for People with Severe Psychiatric Disabilities.* Washington, DC: American Psychiatric Publishing; 2001.

26 Bunn MH, O'Connor AM, Tansey MS, *et al.* Characteristics of clients with schizophrenia who express certainty or uncertainty about continuing treatment with depot neuroleptic medication. *Arch Psychiatr Nurs.* 1997; **11**(5): 238–48.

27 Bhugra D. Decision making by patients: who gains? *Int J Soc Psychiatry.* 2008; **54**(1): 5–6.

28 Amador XF, Gorman JM. Psychopathologic domains and insight in schizophrenia. *Psychiatr Clin North Am.* 1998; **21**(1): 27–42.

29 Hamann J, Leucht S, Kissling W. Shared decision making in psychiatry. *Acta Psychiatr Scand.* 2003; **107**(6): 403–9.

30 Seale, op. cit.

31 Karnieli-Miller O, Eisikovits Z. Physician as partner or salesman? Shared decision-making in real-time encounters. *Soc Sci Med.* 2009; **69**(1): 1–8. Epub 2009 May 20.

32 Hamann J, Langer B, Winkler V, *et al.* Shared decision making for in-patients with schizophrenia. *Acta Psychiatr Scand.* 2006; **114**(4): 265–73.

33 Loh, op. cit.

34 Grisso T, Appelbaum PS. The MacArthur treatment competence study. III. Abilities of patients to consent to psychiatric and medical treatments. *Law Hum Behav.* 1995; **19**(2): 149–74.

35 Levine RH. A researcher's concern with ethics in human research. *J Calif Alliance Ment Ill.* 1994; **5**(1): 6–8.

36 Corrigan PW, McCracken SG, Edwards M, *et al.* Staff training to improve implementation and impact of behavioral rehabilitation programs. *Psychiatr Serv.* 1997; **48**(10): 1336–8.

37 Chinman MJ, Kloos B, O'Connel M, *et al.* Service providers' views of psychiatric mutual support groups. *Community Psychology.* 2002; **30**: 1–18.

38 Chinman M, Allende M, Bailey P, *et al.* Therapeutic agents of assertive community treatment. *Psychiatr Q.* 1999 Summer; **70**(2): 137–62.

39 Carling PJ. *Return to Community: building support systems for people with psychiatric disabilities.* New York, NY: Guilford Press; 1995.

40 Won YI, Solomon PL. Community integration of persons with psychiatric disabilities in supportive independent housing: a conceptual model and methodological considerations. *Ment Health Serv Res.* 2002; **4**(1): 13–28.

41 Braitman A, Counts P, Davenport R, *et al.* Comparison of barriers to employment for unemployed and employed clients in a case management program: an exploratory study. *Psychiatric Rehabilitation Journal.* 1995; **19**(1): 3–8.

42 Mann SB. Talking through medication issues: one family's experience. *Schizophr Bull.* 1999; **25**(2): 407–9.

43 Thompson AG. The meaning of patient involvement and participation in health care consultations: a taxonomy. *Soc Sci Med.* 2007; **64**(6): 1297–310. Epub 2006 Dec 13.

44 Towle A, Godolphin W. Framework for teaching and learning informed shared decision making. *BMJ.* 1999; **319**(7212): 766–71.

45 Adams, Drake, 2006, op. cit.

46 Frankel RM, Stein T. Getting the most out of the clinical encounter: the Four Habits Model. *The Permanente Journal.* 1999; **3**(3): 79–88.

47 Ibid.

48 Stein T, Frankel RM, Krupat E. Enhancing clinician communication skills in a large health care organization: a longitudinal case study. *Patient Educ Couns.* 2005; **58**(1): 4–12.

49 Runkle C, Wu E, Wang EC, *et al.* Clinician confidence about conversations at the end of life is strengthened using the Four Habits approach. *J Psychosoc Oncol.* 2008; **26**(3): 81–95.

50 Deegan, 2007, op. cit.

51 Miller WR, Rollnick S. *Motivational Interviewing: preparing people to change addictive behavior.* New York, NY: Guilford Press; 1991.

52 Britt E, Hudson SM, Blampied NM. Motivational interviewing in health settings: a review. *Patient Educ Couns.* 2004; **53**(2): 147–55.

53 Rusch N, Corrigan PW. Motivational interviewing to improve insight and treatment adherence in schizophrenia. *Psychiatr Rehabil J.* 2002 Summer; **26**(1): 23–32.

54 Larson JE, Barr LK, Kuwabara SA, *et al.* Process and outcome analysis of a supported employment program for people with psychiatric disabilities. *American Journal of Psychiatric Rehabilitation.* 2007; **10**(4): 339–53.

55 Bhugra, op. cit.

56 Priebe S, McCabe R, Bullenkamp J, *et al.* Structured patient-clinician communication and 1-year outcome in community mental healthcare: cluster randomised controlled trial. *Br J Psychiatry.* 2007; **191**: 420–6.

57 Van Os J, Altamura AC, Bobes J, *et al.* Evaluation of the two-way communication checklist as a clinical intervention: results of a multinational, randomised controlled trial. *Br J Psychiatry.* 2004; **184**: 79–83.

58 Greenfield S, Kaplan S, Ware JE. Expanding patient involvement in care: effects on patient outcomes. *Ann Intern Med.* 1985; **102**(4): 520–8.

59 Deegan, 2007, op. cit.

60 Deegan PE, Rapp C, Holter M, *et al.* Best practices: a program to support shared decision making in an outpatient psychiatric medication clinic. *Psychiatr Serv.* 2008; **59**(6): 603–5.

61 Greenfield, op. cit.

62 Copeland ME. *Wellness Recovery Action Plan.* Brattleboro, VT: Peach Press; 1997.

63 Walling DP, Marsh DT, Frese FJ. *Relapse Prevention in Serious Mental Illness: the role of organized psychology in treatment of the seriously mentally ill.* San Francisco, CA: Jossey-Bass; 2000. pp. 49–60.

64 Appelbaum PS. Advance directives for psychiatric treatment. *Hosp Community Psychiatry.* 1991; **42**(10): 983–4.

65 Srebnik DS, Russo J. Consistency of psychiatric crisis care with advance directive instructions. *Psychiatr Serv.* 2007; **58**(9): 1157–63.

66 Hassan I, McCabe R, Priebe S. Professional-patient communication in the treatment of mental illness: a review. *Commun Med.* 2007; **4**(2): 141–52.

67 Adams, Drake, Wolford, 2007, op. cit.

68 Ward, op. cit.

69 Fixsen DL, Naoom SF, Blase KA, et al. *Implementation Research: a synthesis of the literature.* Tampa, FL: University of South Florida, Louis de la Parte Florida Mental Health Institute, The National Implementation Research Network (FMHI Publication #231); 2005.

70 Towle, op. cit.

5.3 Shared/Collaborative Care for People with Serious Mental Illness

Jatinder Takhar, David Haslam, Lisa McAuley and Jane Langford

INTRODUCTION

Historically, models of collaboration have been based on certain fundamental principles such as common purpose, open communication, paradigm and location of service, business management and relationships. While relationships remain central to the concept of the model, sharing of care among the different disciplines is the core element that promotes optimum treatments to improve service user care and satisfaction with the service.

This section will introduce readers to the shared care concept, with some background and description of different models of shared care that exist nationally, internationally and locally for people with SMI. The authors will use examples of successful implementation of these renowned models within the context of service user centeredness. The authors will further describe the process of care/referral, roles of each player within the context of this model, services within these models, examples of service users within the model, evaluation, strengths, challenges and the future. Although the discussion will focus largely on relevant experience in Ontario, experience from other jurisdictions will be noted too. Also note that this section assumes much of what is discussed in other sections of this book, such as Section 5.2, *Clinical Communication with Persons Who Have Serious Mental Illness*, hence the reader is referred to that and other sections in this book for pertinent background knowledge.

Background

Dating back to the 1970s, there has been recognition of the need for a closer working relationship within collaborative care models between psychiatrists and primary care physicians in the management of service users with psychiatric disorders. The reasons for this are varied and numerous; but central among them is the issue of health service resources, including their costs and the number of psychiatrists available to provide them. Another reason is that, traditionally, up to 80% of service users with psychiatric disorders have their conditions diagnosed and managed by primary care physicians.[1] Consequently, a variety of collaborative care systems – in which psychiatrists not only provide consultation services, they also directly interact with primary physicians in a variety of contexts – have been set up in countries worldwide, including the U.S.,[2] the UK,[3,4] Germany,[5] Portugal,[6] Israel,[7] and Australia.[8,9,10,11]

Family practice service delivery models have definite strengths for managing individuals with SMI including accessibility, lack of associated stigma, possibility for long-term continuity of care, sensitivity to community and family issues, and the ability to provide integrated management of multiple problems. Unfortunately, they frequently consider themselves under-prepared to treat the more severe mental health problems.[12] Furthermore, they also feel inadequately supported by the health care system in this role, with problems involving communication and other issues being consistently reported in the relationships between family physicians and psychiatrists (*see* www.cpa-apc.org/browse/documents/38). Thus it becomes difficult to establish and maintain continuity of care, collaborative planning and a holistic approach. The resulting under-treatment of mental illness has a significant impact on the individuals' functional abilities and health care costs.[13,14]

The concept of shared mental health care, in which primary care physicians, psychiatrists and allied mental health providers form part of a single mental health care delivery system, was developed as a result of several issues. These are as follows: 1. The dissatisfaction experienced by service users, family members, family physicians and mental health service deliverers; 2. Problems with accessibility to psychiatric expertise; and 3. Political and economic efforts to reform the ways in which care is delivered.[15,16,17]

The focal point in most collaborative care models is the service user. The care is truly service-user centered, as it considers the service users' personal preferences, needs and values, family situations and their lifestyles. The model makes service users and their families an integral part of the decision-making process.[18]

Working Model

The first step involves transferring selected individuals with SMI from tertiary care mental health services into family practitioner-based collaborative care. A designated nurse associated with community mental health services actively identifies cases suitable for transfer, then engages with case managers and psychiatrists to support prospective individuals with SMI for transfer. These individuals have some insight, are clinically stable and have social supports. The model allows for onsite communication between primary care, psychiatry and the individual with SMI in a least-restrictive means with low stigma experience.

This above model requires completion of a referral form, demographic data instrument, the Threshold Assessment Grid (TAG),[19] and a baseline Global Assessment of Functioning score (GAF)[20] for each service user. The TAG is an instrument that is used to assess the severity of mental health problems in an individual along seven domains under three categories of risk, safety, and needs/disabilities. The nurse is responsible for identifying service users who are suitable for the clinical collaborative care program. Once a referral is determined to be appropriate, the preparation for transition and subsequent discharge into primary care practice begins.

The collaborative care clinical services include both direct consultation and indirect services through the following venues:

1. **Direct consultation** involves providing a transfer summary and a relapse signature plan[21] to simplify long-term management of individuals with SMI. The service user is officially transferred to the family physician at a face-to-face transition meeting. The meeting is conducted at the primary care practice site with the psychiatrist, mental health nurse, service user with some of the family members in attendance. The mental health nurse is responsible for inviting family members. The family members provide support to the service user and assist with the collection of collateral information that may help with relapse prevention and adherence to treatment. The relapse signature plan provides an early intervention strategy for the service user at high risk for relapse. The emphasis is on the total wellness of the service user, prevention of hospitalization and maintaining community integration.

A nurse with specialized mental health training visits the family physician at intervals of one to three months, and the psychiatrist visits at intervals of three to six months. The contacts are increased or decreased in frequency depending on the service user's need. During the visits, the service user's progress is reviewed and documented by the collaborative team and future management planning is done in a shared and collaborative manner; for example, the service user's symptoms, relapse signature list and medications are reviewed. In between the visits, the family physician monitors the service user's overall health status and consults the psychiatry services when issues related to medication adjustments, emergence of symptoms or additional support services are required. If access to other services is required, the nurse acts as the facilitator and assists the family physician and the service user in a timely manner.

2. **Indirect services** include telephone consultations with the psychiatrist and the mental health nurse, facilitation of access to community services, telephone support to service user as required, and a review of the service user's documentation at the family physician's office. The concept of the model is based on service user centeredness, community reintegration and accessible support services.[22,23]

Collaborative Care Systems in Canada

There have been efforts to create similar collaborative care systems within Canada, dating back at least to 1982.[24] The inception and advancement of these Collaborative Care efforts were pioneered by Dr. Nick Kates, who is now "Promoting Collaborative Care in Canada: the Canadian Collaborative Mental Health Initiative" (CCMHI) with his team.[25] This was funded through Health Canada's Primary Health Care Transitional Fund and comprises 12 national organizations. The CCMHI demonstrated the commitment to address collaborative mental health care nationally in Canada. They identified and described approximately 91 collaborative mental health care initiatives through a needs analysis and created a toolkit for implementation of these programs across the country in Pacific, Western, Central, Eastern and Northern Canada.[26] For a mapping of this, *see* Figures 5.1 and 5.2.

Examples of programs outside of Ontario with slight differences to ours as described above are found in the Pacific and Western regions. The Pacific Shared Care Program funded by the Fraser Health Authority was developed in 1999. This

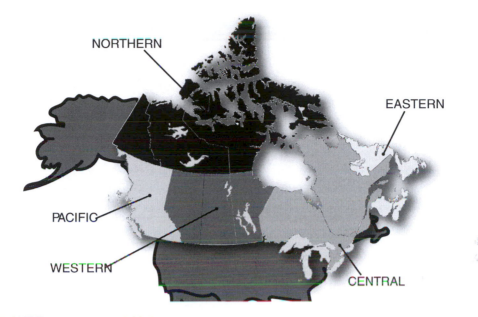

FIGURE 5.1 Canadian initiatives inventory map

Reproduced with permission from Pauze E, Gagne MA. *Collaborative Mental Health Care in Primary Health Care: a review of Canadian initiatives. Volume II: resource guide.* Mississauga, ON: Canadian Collaborative Mental Health Initiative; December 2005. Available at: www.ccmhi.ca (accessed 17 May 2011).

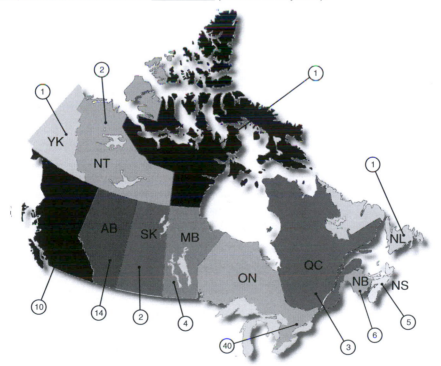

FIGURE 5.2 Geographical representation of canadian initiatives

Reproduced with permission from Pauze E, Gagne., op. cit.

program links the mental health clinicians with family physicians. The team consists of clinical psychologists, clinical counselors, psychiatric nurses and psychiatrists who are co-located in the family physician's office, providing direct and indirect care. Evaluation is integrated into the program.[27]

The Western shared program in Winnipeg under the Regional Health Authority is called the Shared Mental Health Care Program funded by the Primary Health Care Transitional Fund from Manitoba Health. This program services 10 different sites in the community, i.e. private practices, clinics and five alternate payment clinics. The family physician, the counselor and the psychiatrist collaborate on the care of the individual with SMI in a variety of ways. The mental health team provides consultation, psychosocial assessment and education to the family physician. Evaluation of the program is ongoing.[28]

The Northern program is unique from the remaining shared care programs. Started in February 2004, it is located and sponsored by Whitehorse General Hospital. The needs of the Northern and rural communities have revealed that there must be a collaborative approach to maximize resources and provide the highest quality of care. This program incorporates the principles and values of First Nation's culture and is integrated into the medical models within the hospital setting. The hospital is partnered closely with many community agencies. The model incorporates aboriginal holistic health values and beliefs, adding to it a spiritual and cultural context. A consulting psychiatrist visits the hospital for two hours each weekday to see individuals with SMI for consultation, education and support, both in person and via telephone. Individuals with SMI can also be referred to the psychiatrist at the consultation clinic. The team includes mental health nurses and psychiatrists, who work closely with family physicians that are often the first contact for the individual in crisis.[29]

In Ontario, Canada, service users receiving intensive mental health services are frequently transferred back to their family physician because of the province's mental health care reform. The goal of the reform is to develop a comprehensive continuum of services supporting a seamless transition between hospital and community-based care delivery.

In addition to more efficient use of resources, better coordination of services, easy access and community tenure found that family physicians can be an important part of shared mental health care models if systemic barriers such as poor communication, insufficient access to psychiatrists, and lack of continuity in mental health care are removed and collaborative practice is encouraged. The Canadian Psychiatric Association and the College of Family Physicians of Canada has identified shared mental health care as a solution to support both family physicians and psychiatrists, leading to better outcomes for service users.[30,31]

Few formal definitions exist for this type of service, but the broadest determination by Health Canada is that collaborative care requires a broad network of collaborative interactions among a variety of health service providers, service users, their families/caregivers and the community, with service users being focal points and full-fledged partners of the overall effort.[32]

Despite both longstanding and recent interest in collaborative care, there is paucity in the literature on implementing service user-centered care within these models from the service user's perspective.[33]

National and International Collaborative Care Models

Most national and international collaborative care models involve a team-based approach. The few models that exist for the SMI group of service users involve a team consisting of a mental health nurse with expertise in psychiatry and a psychiatrist, who both follow each person during the transition.[34,35,36,37] Services in the community, e.g. crisis intervention, psycho-education, short term psychotherapy, brokerage case management, vocational and occupational rehabilitation services, may also be utilized based on the needs of the service user.

An internationally recognized shared mental health care model for SMI, the Consultation-Liaison in Primary-Care Psychiatry (CLIPP) program has been successfully implemented in Australia.[38,39,40] The CLIPP program involves collaboration in consultation, liaison and continuing shared care, and it sets procedures to meet the needs of general practitioners, Area Mental Health Services (AMHS), and thereby those of service users and carers.[41,42]

In 1998, Meadows established a collaborative care program that included a component directed specifically at SMI individuals. This model provided consultation on any service users referred by family physicians, but in addition also identified individuals with SMI who were being cared for in a traditional outpatient setting who were stable for transfer to shared care. In this model specially trained psychiatric nurses reviewed each service user's file, prepared a detailed summary and a treatment plan, and then arranged for a bridging meeting for the individual with SMI, the family physician and the psychiatrist who would provide ongoing backup. SMI clients were reviewed every six to 12 months by the psychiatrist, with the family physician monitoring the service user's status in-between. The advantages of this model are that it addresses concerns that shared care tends to focus on the less severely ill;[43] it works actively to promote flow through the larger mental health system and it is better integrated into that system.

The role of the family physician in caring for the SMI group is an important one, but it remains ill-defined. The following is an example of a local model that has been implemented out of a tertiary care facility.

The Transition into Primary Care Psychiatry Program Model of Service User Centered Care

The Transition into Primary Care Psychiatry Program (TIPP) is a working example of Ontario mental health care reform, which was developed to enhance the collaborative relationship between family practitioners and psychiatrists (*see* Figure 5.3).

Its primary goal has been to streamline service users' access to mental health care by encouraging shared care models for service users with multiple service needs.[44,45]

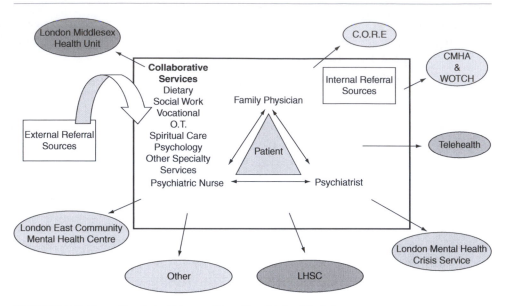

FIGURE 5.3 Transition into Primary Care Psychiatry Model

A modified version of Australia's CLIPP model,[46] TIPP is a "stepping down" service that facilitates the transition from tertiary or ambulatory care to care provided by a primary care physician for service users recovering from episodic or other types of mental health illness.[47] Service users can be enrolled in TIPP services if they have stable but persistent SMI and have maintained a period of wellness, as demonstrated by no requirement for significant medication adjustment or hospital-based care over the preceding year.

The TIPP team consists of the service user, the family physician, a psychiatrist and a nurse with mental health experience, with other community services available if needed. Ideally, service initiates with a face-to-face meeting of the entire team. The nurse and psychiatrist typically visit the family physician every one to three months and every three to six months respectively to discuss service user progress and to plan future management strategies; this frequency can be increased or decreased depending upon the service user's level of well-being. Between meetings, the family physician monitors and evaluates the service user's quality of life, symptoms, function, illness severity and perceived need of care, in addition to the team's level of satisfaction with service delivery.[48]

Evaluations within the Model

To the knowledge of the authors, TIPP is the only Canadian interdisciplinary collaborative health care program for tertiary care service users to systematically include outcome indicators consistent with the Canadian Institute for Health Information and the Advisory Network on Mental Health Framework. Evaluating this program offered a unique opportunity to investigate the fulfillment of Canadian Medical Education Directives for Specialists (CanMEDS) roles by family physicians working collaboratively with psychiatric providers. Consequently, we examined these roles by surveying the service users within the TIPP program. The purpose of the survey was to explore whether TIPP service users perceive that family physicians are fulfilling their CanMEDS roles in their delivery of care within the TIPP model. Our primary specific objective was to assess how service users seeing TIPP-associated physicians for mental health issues perceive the care they receive from their family physician, in terms of his or her levels of communication, "providerism," expertise, collaboration, advocacy and service user management.

Since the TIPP shared care model is in keeping with the system that existed before, we expected that the perceived effectiveness of care by a family physician would be high. More interesting, however, would be to identify specific aspects of care with which service users are less satisfied. We discovered that service users generally were satisfied with the TIPP service, compared to what they had received previously within the context of primary/specialty care models. Further, this was true in relation to all six CanMEDS domains, and there was no statistically significant difference in levels of satisfaction between the domains. However, the slightly lower rating for the roles of communicator and manager appears to be consistent with the literature.[49] This speaks to the need for further integrating CanMEDS roles at all levels of education and clinical practice (*see* Figure 5.4).

Fundamentally, TIPP is a service user-centered model of collaborative mental health care; consequently, the service user needs are an essential component of ongoing program evaluation.

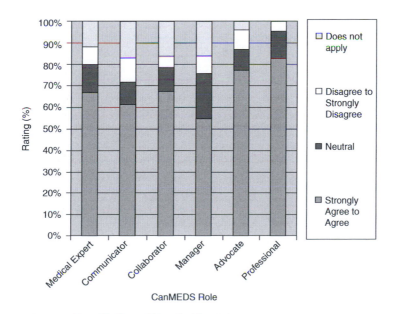

FIGURE 5.4 Service User Rating of Family Physician

Applying a Service User-Centered Approach within the Context of Transition into Primary Care Psychiatry Program

Example

The following is an illustration of how to provide care for a reluctant service user with the least restrictive means:

Margret is a 62-year-old woman who has been married three times in the past. The marital difficulties resulted from the emotional abuse that Margret was subjected to during her marriages. She has three children, ages 48, 46 and 43. The relationship with her daughter is very close, while with her sons it is dynamically turbulent. She is supported by Canada Pension Plan (CPP), inheritance and alimony, and she lives independently in the community and is socially well-engaged with the church and community agencies. She possesses excellent social skills.

Her diagnosis has been bipolar mood disorder over the years. There is a significant family history of psychiatric illness. She has had multiple admissions for this disorder in the past, but no suicidal attempts. The admissions have mostly been voluntary and she was successfully treated and maintained in the community for a number of years.

The medical history revealed a series of transient ischemic attacks (TIA) in the past, hypothyroid state, hypertension and high lipid levels, for which she received optimum care with medications.

Upon being accepted into TIPP her family doctor assumed her mental health care, with back-up psychiatric services from the TIPP team. Her inter-episodic functioning remained good, enabling her to work in several different volunteer positions. Her adherence to medications was relatively good in the past.

In the fourth year of treatment, she became increasingly involved in church activities and in the relationship of her family to this religious organization. She began to deteriorate slowly after this engagement with the church, as she found "God," became very religious, began to preach to others on the benefits of Christianity and became suspicious of other religious denominations. Her symptoms included delusions of persecution, overvalued ideas of obtaining justice, and advocating on behalf of others with mental illness. She firmly believed that she was wrongly diagnosed and treated in the past. She thought it was just a "little stress." She made a choice to go off all the medications for a period of eight months.

Several attempts were made in getting her to adhere with medications, such as a change in pharmacy to reduce the paranoia, blister packing the medications, having her consume the medication at another site with a TIPP nurse present or daily dispensing of the medications with the pharmacist. All of these attempts were unsuccessful, even with family engagement. Over time her mental status deteriorated to the point of her having clear delusions about people tampering with the medications/food, and a thought disorder was evident. She became very demanding, belligerent and intrusive. These symptoms impacted her excellent social graces and interpersonal style. Her mood became labile and irritable while her speech increased in volume and tone. She became impolite towards the care team.

In our attempts to remain objective and person-centered, we complied with her wishes and attempted to obtain a second opinion from a senior psychiatrist; however, Margret gradually disengaged from the TIPP team and her family doctor. In order to intervene in the least intrusive means, we declared her incompetent as an outpatient service user with support from the substitute decision maker. When this intervention failed, the team decided to admit her into hospital as an involuntary service user.

Once again to assist her in retaining dignity in the community and maintaining privacy, the TIPP nurse, along with Thames Valley Ambulance, worked collaboratively to ensure safety in transport to the emergency department as opposed to calling the police as in primary intervention. The TIPP nurse provided support and education regarding the process and remained with Margret in the emergency room until the next team was able to assume care. During this time regular communication and updates were provided to the family doctor and her family.

Example

This is an illustration of the transition from adolescent services to primary care psychiatry:

Tyler is a 21-year-old, single male who was referred to TIPP at the age of 18 years and is now living in the community with his mother. Tyler's past history dates back to age 12 years. The first symptoms noted were problems with behavior, academic delays, poor school attendance, short attention span, significant distractibility and inability to complete assigned schoolwork. An early elementary examination showed results consistent with attention-deficit hyperactivity disorder (ADHD), poor fine motor skills and some language difficulties, so Tyler was treated with stimulants. A few years later, symptoms of obsessive-compulsive disorder emerged along with insomnia, paranoia and aggressive behaviors. Subsequently, a diagnosis of early onset schizophrenia was made, and treatment with antipsychotic agents was initiated. Tyler was unable to complete any schooling but did some vocational training and worked part-time in sheltered employment. On his first visit, he was noted to have difficulties with attention, memory and information processing consistent with a borderline intellectual functioning.

Over the years, the course of his illness was complicated by depressive episodes, suicidality, poor impulse-control, and substance addiction. Care in the past included multiple antidepressants, antipsychotic and benzodiazepines, but no mood stabilizing agents. The diagnostic category was revised to schizoaffective disorder (mixed type) during adulthood. The addition of a mood stabilizing agent assisted in gaining stability in his overall state, i.e. his impulsivity, suicidality and mood instability, and adherence to follow-up appointments.

There was significant family history of psychiatric illnesses; his biological father suffered from depression and had attempted suicide. The mother as well has depression/substance abuse, while a maternal uncle has schizophrenia.

The social/developmental context in which this young man was raised was chaotic. The family dynamics were complex. Further complicating the situation was his borderline level of intellectual functioning, which had not been formally assessed. His development was delayed in terms of motor skills and academic performance; his social adaptation was limited.

Care for this service user was approached with an emphasis on integration and adaptation to his needs. A formal comprehensive psychological assessment was facilitated to develop a plan for community integration, housing, social adaptation and possible employment opportunities. Medication adjustments were made in consultation with the family doctor, the mother of the service user and the service user, along with the TIPP nurse and psychiatrist, so that a simplified balance of optimum care with greater concordance and minimal side effects could be instituted.

Tyler's goal of obtaining employment provided the opportunity to constructively address issues of hygiene, attire, attitude and behavior. Graduation from vocational training provided him with increased social exposure and prepared him for balancing the demands of working and his formerly neglected activities of daily living. Tyler began to take pride in himself and his accomplishments. He remains dedicated to his summer volunteer position at an amusement park, and his intent is to work toward meeting a girlfriend and eventual paid employment. Improvement took approximately two years to achieve with provision of continuity of care, emphasizing the relationship with family, service user and empowerment in the decision-making process and using concrete visually constructed, psychoeducational methods.

CONCLUSION: STRENGTHS, CHALLENGES AND THE FUTURE

The greatest benefit of the collaborative care approach between primary care and specialists is building the capacity of the family physician and the primary health care sector. The model itself can provide continuity of care, a comprehensive approach to complex mental health problems within a team-based setting.

The major challenge when models are based out of tertiary care is that disengagement between the service user and clinical staff can be difficult – a potential barrier to optimal service user independence. Development of training and expertise specific to the unique challenges of this transition is needed. Current funding models in primary care are "fee for service," and this can curtail effective communication between primary and secondary care.

A wonderful challenge and opportunity exist with the changing nature of primary care in Ontario and elsewhere. The emergence of primary care teams will bring a wider perspective, greater depth of knowledge and more team members to care for complex service users. This will require greater communication and may prove a challenge worth conquering to deliver better care.

The future involves the need for best practice models to help practitioners incorporate collaborative care principles into daily practice. More research is required into the evidence for the effectiveness of such models. The overall system needs to adopt incentives and payment schedules that support collaborative care models. It is essential to incorporate collaborative care methodologies in the training of health practitioners for expansion and sustainability of this model. In the future, supporting such quality care initiatives will become more important.

Authors' Note: We wish to thank Sandra Dunbar for her assistance in the preparation of this section.

REFERENCES

 1 Avant R. Psychiatric consultation and referral. *Med Clin North Am.* 1988; **72**(4): 929–35.
 2 Katon W, Gonzales J. A review of randomized trials of psychiatric consultation-liaison studies in primary care. *Psychosomatics.* 1994; **35**(3): 268–78.
 3 Bower P, Gask L. The changing nature of consultation-liaison in primary care: bridging the gap between research and practice. *Gen Hosp Psychiatry.* 2002; **24**(2): 63–70.
 4 Tyrer P, Ferguson B, Wadsworth J. Liaison psychiatry in general practice: the comprehensive collaborative model. *Acta Psychiatrica Scandinavica.* 1990; **81**(4): 359–63.
 5 Kremer G, Baune B, Driessen M, *et al.* Alcohol-related interventions in general hospitals in Germany: public health and consultation-liaison psychiatry perspectives. *Adv Psychosom Med.* 2007; **26**: 118–27.
 6 Botelho AM, Delgado MP. Psychiatry and primary care: a liaison experience. *Acta Med Port.* 1997; **10**(12): 917–20.
 7 Weingarten M, Granek M. Psychiatric liaison with a primary care clinic – 14 years' experience. *Isr J Psychiatry Relat Sci.* 1998; **35**(2): 81–8.
 8 Meadows GN. Overcoming barriers to reintegration of patients with schizophrenia: developing a best-practice model for discharge from specialist care. *Med J Aust.* 2003; **5**(Suppl.): S53–6.

9 Carr VJ, Donovan P. Psychiatry in general practice: a pilot scheme using the liaison-attachment model. *Med J Aust.* 1992; **156**(6): 379–82.

10 Carr VJ, Faehrmann C, Lewin TJ, *et al.* Determining the effect that consultation-liaison psychiatry in primary care has on family physicians' psychiatric knowledge and practice. *Psychosomatics.* 1997; **38**(3): 217–29.

11 Kisely S, Horton-Hausknecht J, Miller K, *et al.* Increased collaboration between primary care and psychiatric services: a survey of general practitioners' views and referrals. *Aust Fam Physician.* 2002; **31**(6): 587–9.

12 Craven MA, Cohen M, Campbell D, *et al.* Mental health practices of Ontario family physicians: a study using qualitative methodology. *Can J Psychiatry.* 1997; **42**(9): 943–9.

13 Simon G, Ormel J, VonKorff M, *et al.* Health care costs associated with depressive and anxiety disorders in primary care. *Am J Psychiatry.* 1995; **152**(3): 352–7.

14 Wells KB, Hays RD, Burnam MA, *et al.* Detection of depressive disorder for patients receiving prepaid or fee-for-service care: results from the Medical Outcomes Study. *JAMA.* 1989; **262**(23): 3298–302.

15 Burley J. Initiating and developing a shared care relationship in your community. *CPA Bulletin.* 2003; **35**(2): 34–6.

16 Kates N, Craven M, Crustolo AM, *et al.* Mental health services in the family physician's office: a Canadian experiment. *Isr J Psychiatry Relat Sci.* 1998; **35**(2): 104–13.

17 Royal College of Psychiatrists, Royal College of General Practitioners. Shared care of patients with mental health problems: report of a joint college working group. *Occ Pap R Coll Gen Pract.* 1993; **60**: 1–10.

18 Gagne MA. Advancing the agenda for collaborative mental health care. Available at: www.ccmhi.ca (accessed 9 May 2011).

19 Slade M, Powell R, Rosen A, *et al.* Threshold Assessment Grid (TAG): the development of a valid and brief scale to assess the severity of mental illness. *Soc Psychiatry Psychiatr Epidemiol.* 2000; **35**(2): 78–85.

20 Endicott J, Spitzer RL, Fleiss JL, *et al.* The global assessment scale. A procedure for measuring overall severity of psychiatric disturbance. *Arch Gen Psychiatry.* 1976; **33**(6): 766–71.

21 Meadows, 2003, op. cit.

22 Ibid.

23 Meadows GN, Joubert L, Donaghue J. *CLIPP (Consultation and Liaison in Primary Care Psychiatry) Manual.* 2000. Available at: www.health.vic.gov.au/mentalhealth/archive/clipp/index.htm (accessed 26 May 2011).

24 Links PS, Kates N, Gliva G, *et al.* A Canadian community mental health program: a clerkship experience. *General Hospital Psychiatry.* 1982; **4**(3): 245.

25 Kates N, Craven M, Bishop J, *et al. Shared Mental Health Care in Canada.* Ottawa, Ont: Canadian Psychiatric Association and College of Family Physicians of Canada; 1997.

26 Pauze E, Gagne MA. *Collaborative Mental Health Care in Primary Health Care: a review of Canadian Initiatives, Volume II: Resource Guide.* Mississauga, ON: Canadian Collaborative Mental Health Initiative; December 2005.

27 Ibid.

28 Ibid.

29 Ibid.

30 Bishop J, Lent B, Takhar J, *et al.* So you want to do a randomized, controlled clinical trial which involves equivalence, clustering and a combination of quantitative and qualitative measures? A feasibility study to prepare for a clinical trial of shared mental health care. In: *North American Primary Care Research Group Annual Meeting.* 2000; Florida, U.S.A.

31 Brown JB, Lent B, Stirling A, *et al.* Caring for seriously mentally ill patients: qualitative study of family physicians' experiences. *Can Fam Physician.* 2002; **48**: 915–20.

32 www.hc-sc.gc.ca/index-eng.php

33 Links, op. cit.

34 Brown, op. cit.

35 Haslam D, Haggarty J, McAuley L, *et al.* Maintaining and enhancing shared care relationships through the TIPP Clinical Model. *Families, Systems & Health.* 2006; **24**(4): 481–6.

36 Bindman J, Johnson S, Wright S, *et al.* Integration between primary and secondary services in the care of the severely mentally ill: patients' and general practitioners' views. *Br J Psychiatry.* 1997; **171**: 169–74.

37 Kendrick T, Sibbald B, Burns T, *et al.* Role of general practitioners in care of long term mentally ill patients. *BMJ.* 1991; **302**(2): 508–10.

38 Meadows, 2003, op. cit.

39 Meadows GN. Evaluating consultation-liaison in general practice. *Aust N Z J Psychiatry.* 1998; **32**(5): 728–30.

40 Meadows GN. Establishing a collaborative service model for primary mental health care. *Med J Aust.* 1998; **168**(4): 162–5.

41 Meadows GN, Gielewski H, Falconer B, *et al.* The pattern-of-care model: a tool for planning community mental health services. *Psychiatr Serv.* 1997; **48**(2): 218–23.

42 Meadows GN. Best Practices: the consultation-liaison in primary-care psychiatry program: a structured approach to long-term collaboration. *Psychiatr Serv.* 2007; **58**(8): 1036–8.

43 Low CB, Pullen I. Psychiatric clinics in different settings: a case register study. *Br J Psychiatry.* 1988; **153**: 243–5.

44 Bower, op. cit.

45 Haslam, op. cit.

46 Brown, op. cit.

47 Haslam, op. cit.

48 Ibid.

49 Brown, op. cit.

5.4 Serious Mental Illness of Special Populations

5.4.1 PERSON-CENTERED APPROACHES FOR ADOLESCENTS WITH SERIOUS MENTAL ILLNESS

Sandra Fisman

INTRODUCTION

SMI may infrequently manifest prepubertally, but with the onset of adolescence, the risk for a first episode of psychosis driven by an underlying schizophrenic or bipolar disorder increases markedly. Retrospectively, many adults with SMI recall their first episode beginning between 15 and 24 years of age. The effectiveness of early intervention programs in psychotic and mood disorders is being increasingly demonstrated.[1] Ideally, these programs should be delivered within a person-centered framework, not only because this enables a humanistic approach to care, but also because a person-centered approach is more likely to foster therapeutic engagement. In the first chapter of this book, the complex dimensions of PCC are described. In youth with these disorders, the potential risk for compromise of the multifaceted dimensions of PCC in SMI is further complicated, as these dimensions are overlaid by issues of cognitive, social and emotional development and the ethical challenges of young people's right to engage in their own treatment decisions. In addition, their perspectives on treatment may be in conflict with those of their parents and providers, who may interpret intended beneficence or non-maleficence quite differently than the youth. This section on PCC for special populations will focus on adolescents with SMI, reviewing the unique aspects for this age group. The chapter will begin with a review of normal adolescent development and will describe how each phase of adolescent development will differentially affect therapeutic engagement. The complex interplay between development, progression through adolescence, unanticipated onset of illness and family relationships as these relate to consent and person-centered treatment decisions will be explored. Note that other sections in this book address issues relevant to this section, such as Section 4.1, *Collaborating with Families of People with Serious Mental Illness*; hence the reader is referred to the section on family and to other sections as needed as complementary reading.

Subphases of Adolescent Development

In order to understand deviations from normal development, a brief discussion of the usual path will be provided so that all readers will have sufficient background knowledge. Broadly, adolescent development is divided into three subphases: the early adolescent (12–15 years), the mid-adolescent (14–18 years) and the late adolescent (17 years to maturity). Adolescence can be broadly defined as beginning with a physical event (puberty) and ending with a psychological event (the formation of a firm identity and the capacity [in Eriksonian terms] to establish an intimate relationship). The journey through adolescence requires mastery of developmental tasks in the cognitive, social-interactional and physical domains.

The characteristics of each subphase of adolescence influences the process of engagement in the therapeutic process.[2] Early adolescence brings a spurt in growth beginning in the extremities, with a rediscovery of the body that normally has not been a focus of the latency (middle childhood) years. This is accompanied by a shift in cognitive capacity from operational, concrete thinking to the formal-operational thinking of the adolescent, allowing a range of problem solving and hypothetico-deductive reasoning skills.[3] This newfound cognitive capacity generates the ability to project into the future and to manifest the sense of hopelessness that may be associated with post-latency suicidality. Beyond the physical and cognitive changes of early adolescence, the homeostasis of latency is also disrupted by the intense social pressures that pull toward peers and away from family in the service of beginning separation – individuation. The combined internal and external pressures of this adolescent stage often create some sense of inconsistency, confusion, moodiness and impulsivity, and frequently these feelings are acted out as rebellion toward adult figures. Many early adolescents begin to question beliefs and attitudes that previously were tenaciously held. At this stage, the early manifestations of SMI greatly amplify the vulnerability of an unstable personality.

Mid-adolescence at age 14 or 15 years brings about increasing feelings of self-control with the new growth and re-synthesis of the internalized self. New beliefs, ideals and values are taken in through representations of novel heroes (teachers, sports heroes, religious leaders, pop stars) in the youth's environment. Socially, there is increased investment in peers, who rather than family, become the new frame of reference. Teenagers at this stage typically like to argue and debate, activities which facilitate their sense of independence and separation, but also allow further incorporation of new ideas from adult figures. Tolerating ambivalent feelings as a mid-adolescent is difficult, so that one month's hero may shift a few months later with the fluctuation in idealization and devaluation that is part of normal personality development. At times, adolescents at this stage may become intensely introspective, manifesting a withdrawal to diary, poetry and journal writing, and to favorite music. These times of withdrawal may become extreme in the troubled teen, especially when his or her internal world is disintegrating with the onset of SMI.

Late adolescence, entered typically around the age of 17 or 18 years, brings a youth from the Eriksonian phases of identity vs. role confusion that had particularly characterized early adolescence, to the phase of intimacy versus isolation that heralds this stage.[4] Under usual circumstances, the late adolescent has a definitive sense of identity including sexual, moral, political and vocational aspects. Reciprocity with others both within and outside of the family and the ability to tolerate ambivalence become evident. Interference with mastery of the final task of adolescence that results from a severe depression or psychotic illness, affecting mood and/or thinking, will increase the sense of isolation; and interference with social and family connectedness escalates the risk for completed suicide in the late adolescent.

The subphases of development through adolescence shed light on the therapeutic relationship with adolescents and an understanding of these subphases will facilitate approaches to PCC in youth with SMI. Broadly speaking, treating the early adolescent requires the provider to be able to tolerate the apparent lack of empathy of the early adolescent, the neediness and repetitive making of demands, and the sense of giving on the part of the provider with no sense of obligation from the young service user. The stability and consistency of the provider who is unflappable, warm and "permanent" is key to engagement of the early adolescent in the treatment process.

Treating the mid-adolescent requires the provider to be a much more active participant in the therapeutic process, willing to share ideas, values and beliefs of his or her own, and understanding the process of identification with others as central to this developmental phase. This requires the provider to, at times, challenge the omnipotent, often aggressive stance of the mid-adolescent, while maintaining a sense of empathy for the internal distress of the young service user. The provider must respect the service user's developing uniqueness but be willing to maintain and share his own aspects of individuality and separateness as a provider.

The approach to the late adolescent is increasingly akin to the therapeutic engagement of the adult. However, the potential challenge in this developmental phase is the tendency for these individuals, faced with the regressive effects of a SMI on the stability of the personality, to oscillate between the more dependent stance of earlier adolescence and the independence of the adult. Approaches that are developmentally sensitive remain very important in these individuals, often referred to as "transitional age youth," both in terms of an overall therapeutic alliance as well as the incorporation of person-centered approaches within this alliance.

Example

Tina is a 17-year-old beginning her final year of high school. She presented (with her parents) to the emergency room with poor sleep, pressured speech, psychomotor agitation and religious preoccupations. Family history revealed the presence of lithium-responsive bipolar disorder in a paternal aunt. Tina was reading the Bible constantly and wanting to speak with her parents exclusively about her religious beliefs, which had become extreme. Although her affect was labile, her mood was predominantly elevated. Always an outstanding student, her ability to focus on schoolwork had deteriorated, and her grades had declined. She had not used alcohol or street drugs. Tina was an excellent athlete and enjoyed a strong relationship with her 14-year-old brother, who was upset and perplexed at the changes in his sister. Tina had minimal insight into the fact that she was ill and was convinced that her parents and others were plotting to have her lose her virginity; she accused her parents of orchestrating her hospitalization to accomplish this.

Tina responded well to lithium as a mood stabilizer with an accompanying atypical antipsychotic, but as she became well, she was reluctant to be on any medication. With her psychotic symptoms resolved, her antipsychotic medication was tapered and discontinued. She became significantly depressed and slowed down and was willing to entertain the addition of a small dose of antidepressant. Tina, with the support of her parents, was involved in making each treatment decision, and a compromise was reached in maintaining her at the low end of the therapeutic range for her lithium.

Tina's sense is that she was consulted and respected in her treatment decisions and well-informed about her illness by the treatment team, while her parents remained supportive and involved in her care, enhancing the likelihood of her treatment concordance and successful outcome.

Developmental Concepts of Consent and Capacity

Assessment of the adolescent's competence to consent to treatment is central to opportunities for a young person to be involved in his/her own care decisions (for both medical and physical treatments).[5] In considering the broad concepts of consent, there are generally four categories:

➤ **implied consent** where a service user presents for diagnosis and/or treatment involving minimal harm
➤ **presumed consent** in the case of the need for emergency treatment in an unconscious service user
➤ **substitute consent** in an individual deemed incapable of consenting where a parent, guardian or health care proxy consents on behalf of that individual
➤ **voluntary, competent, informed consent** in an individual who understands his/her illness and is fully informed of the risks and benefits of treatment and the implications of remaining untreated.

Adults are presumed to be competent and the burden of proof is on the treater to demonstrate the presence of incompetence. However, unlike adults who are presumed competent to consent to treatment unless otherwise demonstrated, adolescents, defined as minors by age (younger than 16 years of age in Canada and younger than 18 years of age in the U.S.), have historically – at least with the establishment of the first juvenile justice system at the turn of the twentieth century – not had the right to consent to or refuse medical treatment until reaching the age of majority.[6,7] In a landmark case involving involuntary hospitalization (Parham v. J.R., 1979), Chief Justice Warren Berger wrote: "The law's concept of the family rests on a presumption that parents possess what a child lacks in maturity, experience and capacity for judgment for making life's decisions." This presumption is somewhat in conflict with the fundamental engagement of the adolescent in his or her own care decisions.[8]

Over the past decade, congruent with the consumer (service user) rights movement, there has been a shift in thinking toward ways, other than a blunt age cut-off, that would focus more on cognitive development and emotional maturity as determinants of the adolescent's ability to understand and appreciate information relevant to a treatment decision.[9] There is also evidence that acquisition of reading skills correlates with objective measures of competency to consent to treatment.[10] There is an awareness of the adolescent's right to autonomy in decision-making, in so far as is possible, as well as the importance of decision-making that is not driven by coercion and is derived freely and voluntarily. The need to respect confidentiality for the adolescent service user may also complicate the consent process.[11]

Four ethical principles have been defined that underpin assessment of the young person's competence to consent to treatment and which resonate with the principles of competence to consent in adults.[12] These principles include respect for autonomy of the young person, which may be regarded as fundamental in the ethical rights of youth in their own treatment decisions. The right to autonomy, using this ethical framework, may even override the second and third principles of beneficence and non-maleficence, both of which are intended to ensure that decision-making is in the best interest of the young service user. The fourth principle involves assurance that the principles of justice are maintained in the treatment consent process, while fairness is ensured for all involved.[13]

In applying these principles to clinical decision-making in person-centered treatment of youth with SMI, there are a number of important considerations that must still be kept in mind to ensure that with the primacy of autonomy, the best interest of the young person is not compromised. To do so can, at times, be detrimental to the ultimate prognosis for treatment outcome and success for that individual. One must also bear in mind that the developmental factors contributing to cognitive capacity to make an informed decision about one's treatment, while not presently tied specifically to age, still correlate with the approximate onset of middle adolescence. There remains a consensus in the literature that it is around 14 years of age when the cognitive ability to understand the information necessary for consent is attained. This approximates the age at which the risk for onset of major mental illness begins to increase.

Another important consideration in treatment decisions is the need to remain respectful of parental authority and the family context of the early and mid-adolescent.[14] In addition, SMI may particularly limit the insight of the young person into the reality of his or her deteriorating mindset and ability to function. There is significant risk for tension between the need to hear and address parental concerns and at the same time optimize the adolescent's right to autonomy and participation in decision-making. The therapeutic team can become caught between the opposing needs and perspectives of the adolescent and his or her parent(s) or legal guardians. While much of the existing literature addressing these dilemmas focuses on medical decision-making with physical illness,[15] extrapolation to mental illness is helpful. These challenges do not preclude efforts that respect person-centered solutions.

Example

The following is an illustration of the aforementioned tension that may arise and a person-centered compromise:

Alex is 15 years of age, living with his single parent widowed father and an 11-year-old sister. Over a 12-month period, he had become increasingly socially isolated, spending most of his time withdrawn to his room. He had not attended school for six months. He was troubled by multiple auditory hallucinations and was convinced that there was a plot to poison the water in his home. This resulted in his refusal to drink and then eat because of a fear that the water had contaminated his food. He was hospitalized because of a deteriorating physical state with weight loss and dehydration.

In the initial phase of treatment, Alex's right to autonomy in the treatment decision-making process was very difficult to maintain. His refusal to allow rehydration and/or nutritional rehabilitation resulted in a life-threatening medical situation, and substitute consent was required with his father as decision-maker. Once physically more stable, Alex was willing to entertain antipsychotic treatment provided this was not orally administered because of his fear of oral contamination. He was treated with a depot antipsychotic with gradual improvement in his mental status. Thus, although it was not possible for this young man to retain his decision-making autonomy, a person-centered approach allowed a compromise in treatment that was more palatable in the presence of his mental state.

A Solution-Focused Lens to Person-Centered Treatment

Solution-focused approach to treatment of service users in mental health services has been well-described and successfully utilized.

Originally described and utilized by de Shazer[16] in family therapy and with challenging and difficult service users, de Shazer utilized a philosophical framework to develop the technique. Fundamental to this approach is its atheoretical nature with an emphasis on listening to service users, their lived experience and a focus on assisting individuals and families to reach therapeutic goals and derive life satisfaction in spite of continued symptoms. More recently, similar approaches have been utilized in the treatment interventions for young people with long-term mental health treatment needs.[17] Such approaches are person-centered to a very significant extent in that they help people focus on what the service user wants rather than focusing on what he or she does not want. This is particularly helpful in establishing a therapeutic alliance with youth rather than negatively engaging in counter-therapeutic power struggles.

CONCLUSION

While the clinical phenomenology of a psychiatric illness, be it bipolar disorder, schizophrenia or another mental illness, is similar across individuals, the disease experience for each individual is unique. Each person's context – cultural, personal, interactional and developmental – is different. Understanding this context facilitates a strength-based, less pathologizing, more recovery-oriented and consequently person-centered approach to treatment. At the same time, there is a need for pragmatism in balancing an extreme "liberationist" approach to care delivery that considers autonomy in treatment decisions by the adolescent as an over-riding consideration versus a "protectionistic" approach, which risks alienating and marginalizing the adolescent service user.[18]

REFERENCES

1 Melle I, Larsen TK, Haahr U, *et al.* Prevention of negative symptom psychopathologies in first episode schizophrenia. *Arch Gen Psychiatry.* 2008; **65**(6): 634–40.

2 Geertjens L, Waaldijk O. Client-centered therapy for adolescents: an interactional point of view. In: Thorne B, Lambers E. *Person-Centered Therapy: a European perspective.* Thousand Oaks, CA: Sage Publications, 1988. pp. 159–74.

3 Piaget J. *The Language and Thought of the Child.* London: Routledge & Kegan Paul; 1952.

4 Erikson EH. *Childhood and Society.* 2nd ed. New York, NY: Norton, 1963.

5 Forehand L, Ciccone R. The competence of adolescents to consent to treatment. *Adolescent Psychiatry.* 2004; **28**: 5–27.

6 Billick SB. Developmental competency. *Bull Am Acad Psychiatry Law.* 1986; **14**(4): 301–9.

7 Broome ME, Stieglitz KA. The consent process and children. *Research in Nursing and Health.* 1992: **15**(2): 147–52.

8 Harrison L, Hunt B. Adolescent involvement in the medical decision making process. *Journal of Applied Rehabilitation Counselling.* 1999; **30**(4): 3–9.

9 Schachter D, Kleinman I, Harvey W. Informed consent and adolescents. *Canadian Journal of Psychiatry.* 2005; **50**(9): 534–40.

10 Billick SB, Burgert III W, Friberg G, *et al.* A clinical study of competency to consent to treatment in pediatrics. *J Am Acad Psychiatry Law.* 2001; **29**(3): 298–302.

11 Tan JOA, Passerine GE, Steward A. Consent and confidentiality in clinical work with young people. *Clinical Child Psychology & Psychiatry.* 2007; **12**(2): 191–210.

12 Spencer GE. Children's competency to consent: an ethical dilemma. *Journal of Child Health.* 2000; **4**(3): 117–22.

13 Harrison C, Kenny NP, Sidarous M, *et al.* Bioethics for clinicians: involving children in medical decisions. *Can Med Assoc J.* 1997; **156**(6): 825–8.

14 Foreman DM. The family rule: a framework for obtaining ethical consent for medical interventions from children. *Journal of Medical Ethics.* 1999; **25**(6): 4916.

15 Hagger L. Some implications of the Human Rights Act 1998 for the medical treatment of children. *Med Law Int.* 2003; **6**(1): 25–51.

16 de Shazer S, Berg L, Lipchick E, *et al.* Brief therapy: focused solution development. *Family Process.* 1986; **25**(2): 207–22.

17 Simon JK, Nelson TS. *Solution-Focused Brief Practice with Long-Term Clients in Mental Health Services: "I am more than my label."* New York: Haworth Press; 2007.

18 Ibid.

5.4.2 DUAL DIAGNOSIS: AN INDIVIDUALIZED APPROACH

Jay Rao

INTRODUCTION

In planning individualized interventions, often the first step is to define the problem clearly. Only then can one proceed to find solutions. When one applies established interventional approaches to a set of problems, the assumption is that valid diagnostic schemes have been utilized.

In considering individualized approaches to supporting, treating and rehabilitating cognitively disabled individuals with significant psychiatric or behavioral issues, one is struck by the "enormous problems in applying established diagnostic systems" to persons with dual diagnosis. "Establishing validity in an area such as behavioral/psychiatric diagnosis in mental retardation where no gold standard already exists is of concern."[1]

It becomes difficult for the service provider to apply evidence-based interventions to treating an individual with dual diagnosis when there is such variability in assessment and treatment. To assist with this, this section will consider some of the relevant issues of definition and of prevalence and will discuss whether treatment approaches could be based on formulating hypotheses that take into account multiple influences, such as neurodevelopmental influences, psychiatric influences and environmental/social influences. Although this section addresses a special population, issues addressed by other sections in this book are relevant as well, such as issues addressed by Section 4.1, *Collaborating with Families of People with Serious Mental Illness*, and Section 6.2, *Person-Centered Approaches to Psychopharmacology for People with Serious Mental Illness*.

Issues of Definition

Dual diagnosis is a term used, especially in Canada, to designate conditions in which individuals who are cognitively disabled may experience the additional handicaps of psychiatric illnesses and/or significant behavioral disturbances. Unfortunately, dual diagnosis in some jurisdictions may also refer to the co-occurrence of mental illness and substance abuse. DSM-IV[2] and ICD-10[3] do not include dual diagnosis as a separate category in their classification systems. However, in Ontario and several Canadian provinces, the term dual diagnosis is accepted widely by policymakers, service providers and academics as indicating the co-occurrence of life-long developmental disabilities and mental health problems. The position paper on dual diagnosis published by the National Coalition of Dual Diagnosis in Canada defines the term similarly and provides support to such usage.[4]

The term "developmental disability" is used to describe impairment in cognitive abilities that renders individuals unable to *adapt* their behaviors to societal demands. The function of *adaptation* involves a number of abilities in many areas of daily living. It includes such abilities as communicational skills, motivational skills and other skills necessary for self-care, maintaining health and safety, adequate social skills, and reasonable motivation, to name but a few.[4,5,6,7] However, there is as yet no international consensus on the use of a term that is acceptable in all countries. In the UK, the term "learning disabilities" is used, and in the U.S., "mental retardation" is acceptable. Unfortunately, such terminology only serves to provide a cross-sectional, current view of an individual's functioning based on either specific measurements or arbitrary inferences, and may or may not have predictive value in terms of the individual's future adaptation to societal demands, which are themselves constantly changing.[8]

"Intelligence" is a collection of various cognitive and regulatory functions and abilities in several domains of brain activity. Pre-fixed terms such as "mental," "developmental," and "learning" do not accurately depict such activity. They can even be misleading. Intelligence is a product of neurobiologically based sequences that are invariant and universal followed by the establishment of higher cognitive functions that are modulated and shaped by "experience."[9] Thus 'intelligence' is a dynamic ability. Intellectual impairment or disability may, therefore, be a more accurate term than developmental disability.

Such issues of definition become important when one considers that often, our approach to these individuals, whether in public policy development or in providing education, medical care or social support, is ad hoc. For instance, the educational needs of a child with autism differ from that of a hyper active child with poor attentional focus. The funding requirements and support needs for the children and their families vary considerably. It is imperative, therefore, to provide descriptions of these individuals in terms that specifically identify their vulnerabilities, rather than seeing them as belonging to certain general categories. Such an individualized approach takes into account the heterogeneity inherent in this population.

Prevalence of Developmental Disability and Dual Diagnosis

Mental retardation or developmental disability is not a discrete illness or condition but a heterogeneous group of genetic syndromes, metabolic deficiencies, and neurological morbidities, affecting each individual differently.[10,11]

Unfortunately, there is considerable variability in prevalence estimates of developmental disabilities. Several methodological difficulties contribute to this. Some of these include different terminologies that are used (mental handicap, deficiency, developmental disability, retardation) to define this population, as well as differing methods of data collection. The inter-rater reliability and reliability over time have been unsatisfactory.[12,13,14] Harris[15] highlights three approaches that have been used to define cases. The statistical model looks at the normal distribution of intelligence and defines those who are two standard deviations below the mean as having developmental disability. The pathological model refers to studies that examine the prevalence of specific genetic or metabolic syndromes. The administrative model collects cases from the registers of institutions such as the school boards, hospitals and service provider organizations. Depending on the models used, the prevalence estimates vary.[16,17,18] It is generally accepted that approximately 3% of the population can be classified as having a developmental disability (or mental retardation).

Prevalence studies of individuals with a dual diagnosis are even more challenging. For example, diagnosing conditions such as schizophrenia in the cognitively disabled is problematic, given the significant cognitive, language and communicational disabilities in this population. However, most prevalence studies have highlighted the very high rates of psychiatric disorders in those identified as cognitively disabled. These have varied from 30–70%.[19] The Classic Isle of Wight studies by Rutter[20] identified 40% of children with "mental deficiency" as having a psychiatric disorder. Several Swedish and British studies have also shown rates of psychiatric disorders in the cognitively disabled as high as 60%.[21,22,23] Schizophrenia and anxiety disorders have also been found to occur at a higher rate in this population than in the general population.

There are wide variations in the reported rates of even such a clearly identifiable behavior as "aggression" in this population. It has been found to vary from 2–60%. This variability has been seen as a function of the targeted population, the definition of *aggression*, the instruments used, the time surveyed and the geographical location.[24,25]

Verbal ability is an important determinant for the robustness of psychiatric diagnosis. Most literature on assessment of dually diagnosed individuals indicates that in the "verbally" able, diagnoses such as schizophrenia, depression, obsessive compulsion, phobias, anxiety disorders, and bipolar disorders can be made. However, ability to use verbal language does not necessarily imply that many of such individuals are cognitively mature enough to be able to understand such terms as "voices," "thoughts," "depression" or "anxiety." In clinical situations, one frequently encounters individuals who are unable to understand these concepts, who nevertheless answer in the affirmative when leading questions are asked. Many questionnaires and inventories that are useful in the non-cognitively disabled may not be applicable to this population. Clinical skill and experience may have an important bearing on accurately diagnosing psychiatric disorder in this population. Even then, it is a clinically challenging task.[26,27]

In the non-verbal population, diagnosing psychiatric disorder is even more challenging. There are many behavioral equivalents of mood and psychotic symptoms and of anxiety and phobias. However, these are neither specific nor sensitive and seem to have the limited utility, in so far as they raise certain diagnostic possibilities. For instance, aggression or self-injury may be the common mode of expressing distress, and may not specifically indicate depression, anxiety or psychosis. In fact, "aggressive behavior" is one of the most common reasons for seeking admission in this population.[28,29] The prevalence rates for aggression in this population vary, as stated earlier, from 2–60%.[30,31] Mood swings, frustration and personality disorders are often considered to be correlated with aggression.[32,33] Diagnosis in such individuals, if a DSM/ICD-based diagnosis is sought, becomes speculative and may have little inter-rater reliability and test-retest reliability (consistency over time).[34,35] Another confounding factor is that physical/medical factors often significantly contribute to distress among these individuals as well, and the final mode of expression may be aggression or self-injury. Thus, reliance on a certain profile of behavioral symptoms for making psychiatric diagnoses is fraught with difficulties.

Diagnostic decisions are also based on obtaining relevant information from the individual, from the informant, and on observational data. If the individual is either non-verbal or his/her ability to express mental experiences or emotional distress is impaired, the clinician has to rely largely on observation or on the informant's account. However, caregiver opinions are not always reliable. Poling,[36] in discussing the use of medications in individuals with behavioral challenges, emphasized the pitfalls in total reliance on caregiver opinions. Gadow and Poling[37,38] emphasized that "care givers often lacked adequate information and training and poorly informed care providers are apt to form opinions concerning drug usage on the basis of limited and idiosyncratic personal experience." Unfortunately, in gathering evidence for making diagnostic decisions, one not only relies on caregivers' personal opinions and observations based on, sometimes, biased perceptions, but even the clinicians' observations can be unreliable, both on account of insufficient observations and because of the fact that clinicians may observe such individuals through the filter of preformed opinions. This includes the phenomenon of diagnostic overshadowing, in which the predominant perception of "mental retardation" overshadows all other diagnostic possibilities.

Aman,[39] in his review of available instruments for assessing psychopathology and behavioral problems in this population, states that such considerations seem to challenge the routine application of traditional taxonomic psychiatric systems across the spectrum of mental retardation.

A Theoretical Framework

The question arises: why are behavioral dyscontrol and emotional dysregulation the common modes of expression of distress in such heterogeneous psychiatric and neurodevelopmental conditions? The answer could be that many dually diagnosed individuals experience a significant failure in their ability to "adapt" to their intrapersonal and interpersonal environment. For example, auditory hallucinations (intrapersonal) and conflict with others (interpersonal) may provoke dysregulated behaviors, resulting in self-injury or aggression.

Adaptation is dependent on efficient processing of information. Gathering (through correct perception) of information, evaluating such information, and taking decisions based on such processing, lead to the next steps of action: evaluating results and the storage of these experiential patterns.

Information Is Processed Highly Individually

Information processing is influenced by many factors, such as the motivation to avoid pain, discomfort, distress, manipulation to gain results, and activation of past patterns. It is also dependent on such factors as varied experience, problem-solving skills, and the ability to predict personal outcomes. In a cognitively disabled individual, there are several problems in such a process.

Perceiving and integrating experiences are affected by selective or poor attention, sensory deficits, absence of prior knowledge or experience, poor problem-solving skills, and lack of ability to generalize. Therefore, processing of information is *faulty*, given the *faulty input*. There is no flexibility, given the difficulty in "shifting mental sets" in these individuals. There are difficulties with sequencing and in logical operations. This leads to disorganized behavior and perseveration.

Some of the signs and symptoms of such a failure in executive functions would be:

➤ perseveration
➤ inflexibility
➤ catastrophic anxiety
➤ emotional dysregulation
➤ working memory deficits
➤ poor judgment
➤ low threshold for frustration
➤ impulse control difficulties.

Example

Joe was admitted with a history of aggressive behaviors, sexual acting out, disinhibition and explosive anger. He had been hospitalized several times and had received various diagnoses including schizophrenia, bipolar disorder, anxiety disorder and personality disorder. He had not responded to psychotropic medications or mood stabilizers. When examined and tested over a number of sessions, he was found to have significant difficulties in shifting mental sets, poor judgment, impaired working memory, and poor problem-solving skills. Consequently Joe had difficulty in retaining information, would become very stuck with certain themes and demands, unable to consider alternatives, and would become highly anxious. This would lead to explosive anger and aggression.

Joe was unable to deal with even simple day-to-day issues and required support and guidance. Much of his "maladjustment" was because of his executive deficits rather than a psychiatric disorder. His past history revealed childhood encephalitis with frontotemporal ischemia.

Neurodevelopmental Influences

What are the neurodevelopmental deficits that predispose individuals to significantly dysregulated behaviors that are often the presenting symptoms of many biomedical, psychiatric and emotional disorders? To answer this we have to understand the concept of executive dysfunction.

"Executive function" is an umbrella construct that includes such interrelated functions as behavioral regulation and meta-cognitive abilities that enable the individual to express purposeful, goal-directed behaviors.[40] The executive system in the frontal lobe develops and matures very much later into fetal life, and into infancy and early childhood. Any disruption to this process may result in deficits in the development of emotional control, problem-solving and attention control.[41,42]

Executive dysfunction is a concept that describes an individual who, because of neuro-developmental problems, has significant deficits in control of behavior and emotions, as well as in problem-solving abilities. Such an individual, when he/she has to deal with the additional burden of symptoms related to mental illness, physical distress or environmental stress, becomes dysregulated. Aggression, self-injury, perseveration and anxiety may be the consequences.

Executive "dysfunction" has been studied in many specific syndromes such as autism, ADHD, and Tourette's, and in a heterogeneous group of dually diagnosed individuals.[43,44] In a significant proportion of these individuals, deficits have been noted in various domains of behavioral regulation or in the domains of metacognitive ability. The domains of inhibition (of impulses, etc.) and "shift" (which enables flexibility), emotional regulation and self-monitoring are significantly impaired. As well, such metacognitive skills as working memory, prediction and problem-solving abilities are also impaired.

Sensory Modulation Disorders

Sensory processing difficulties are often a significant factor in initiating and maintaining disorganized behaviors. Individuals with sensory modulation difficulties are at a higher risk of experiencing poor confidence, anxiety, depression and are likely to exhibit aggressive behaviors.[45] Schoen, Miller, *et al.*[46] describe three subtypes of sensory modulation disorders:

➤ sensory over-responsivity
➤ sensory under-responsivity
➤ sensory seeking/craving.

Those with sensory over-responsivity have extreme emotional reactions to typically non-aversive sensory stimuli (touch, sound, bright lights). These individuals are over-aroused and manifest attention problems, disorganized behaviors and poor adaptive environmental interactions. Those with sensory under-responsivity ignore or appear oblivious to their environment. They are under-aroused physiologically and have decreased awareness of environmental stimuli, and they lack the inner drive to seek social and environmental stimulation. They fail in their ability to function independently. Those with sensory-seeking/craving profiles are hyper active, reckless and behave "dangerously." These children may be misdiagnosed as having ADHD disorders or anxiety disorders.

This highlights the importance of understanding sensory processing difficulties in the cognitively disabled, in order to avoid misdiagnoses and wrong pharmacological and behavioral interventions.

Speech and Language Impairment

Stringer and Lozano[47] studied speech and language impairment in children who had emotional and behavioral disorders. They found a high incidence of language impairment in these children. Many behaviors exhibited by these children were misinterpreted as non-adherence, inattention, lack of self-control, etc. These children had difficulties in forming social relationships and fell into a negative spiral that reduced their ability to cope in class and social situations, resulting in behavioral difficulties. In such individuals a misattribution of these behaviors to psychiatric diagnoses will lead to inappropriate pharmacological and behavioral interventions.

Example

John is a young man with autism. He was referred for self-injurious and aggressive behaviors. He had a long history of extremely disruptive behaviors both at school and at home. He was unable to sit for more than a few minutes and would constantly rock, bounce and jog around the room on tiptoes. He would hit his head with his closed fist, bang his head violently against the wall, and was very intolerant of anyone approaching his personal space. He would stand in one spot and bounce up and down for hours. He could not engage in any activity for longer than a few seconds.

He had received a diagnosis of ADHD but had not responded to any stimulants or atomoxetine, the standard pharmacological approaches to ADHD. Sensory evaluations revealed significant problems in sensory processing. He had problems with modulating proprioceptive information, which is necessary for spatial orientation; he also had a low threshold for touch, noise and bright lights. In addition, he had significant expressive language dysfunction.

In John's case, his constant "motion" and sensory seeking were driven by his poor modulation of proprioceptive information and his low threshold for auditory, tactile and visual sensations. He was successfully managed in a carefully designed sensory environment, by helping him filter sensations that he could not tolerate, and by providing other safe ways of satisfying his need for movement (swings, hammocks, rocking chairs). All medications were successfully withdrawn.

Psychiatric Influences

There is sufficient epidemiologically derived evidence to enable one to conclude that the cognitively disabled person is at a higher risk for suffering from mental disorders and emotional difficulties.[48] Lund,[49] and more recently, Smith and O'Brien,[50] have found that the rates of emotional and psychiatric disorders in this population are higher than in the general population. Lund found a range of psychiatric disorders including schizophrenia, affective disorders and anxiety disorders at a higher rate in the cognitively disabled population than in the general Danish population. The more severe the developmental disability, the higher were the rates of psychiatric disorders.[51] Schizophrenia has a prevalence that is three times that of the general population.[52]

Johnstone *et al.*[53] found higher rates of schizophrenia-related psychopathology in people with intellectual disability. This would suggest a schizophrenic phenotype in these individuals. Despite such compelling evidence, psychiatric disorders often go unrecognized in this population because of the phenomenon of "diagnostic overshadowing"[54] that was mentioned earlier.

Additional disabilities, including those of poor mobility, speech impediment, visual and hearing deficits, epilepsy and multiple organ deficits are more commonly found in the cognitively disabled. As Harris[55] states, these disabilities are not simply additive, but rather multiplicative in their effects, especially when considered with the psychiatric vulnerabilities.

Social-Environmental Influences

The association between social disadvantage and a variety of health problems is well-established. In the dually diagnosed, there is some evidence that disadvantaged families with low morale had children who revealed very low adaptive behaviors, high maladaptive behaviors and low self-esteem. The families of these children were not only financially impoverished, they were emotionally impoverished as well.[56] However, more recently, the emphasis has not been so much on social disadvantage as on social and environmental "experiences" as determining an individual's adaptation to the environment. The cognitively disabled person may not experience an optimal communicative environment for the acquisition of social cognition. Beveridge and Conti-Ramsden[57] describe the individual's social world as "a baffling and problem strewn battle ground" to which the person reacts maladaptively.

The cognitively disabled child is more likely to experience stresses such as early separations through hospitalizations, illnesses and failed communication through aberrant crying; the experience of being unable to communicate pain and discomfort; disequilibrium of circadian rhythms (sleep, etc.); and negative social experiences at school.[58]

All of these developmental disadvantages intertwined with neurobiological and psychiatric problems lead to a massive failure in the ability of individuals to cope with their lives adaptively.

Interventional Approaches

In discussing the multiple vulnerabilities to which the cognitively disabled person is subjected, it is inevitable that one concludes that the most effective approaches address all or most of these adverse factors.

Such biopsychosocial factors may act as:

➤ instigating conditions
➤ vulnerabilities/risk influences
➤ maintaining conditions for the behaviors.[59]

Harris[60] makes an eloquent case for the need to pull together an interdisciplinary team to deliver comprehensive and effective care. "In the future, better methods of assessment are needed that highlight the interface between environmental and neurobiological mechanisms involved in both affective and behavioral disturbances."[61] The "biopsychosocial" approach proposed by Griffiths and Garder[62] addresses some of these concerns.

Typically, such a biopsychosocial assessment is person-centered. The individual becomes the focus rather than the "diagnosis," the approach becomes "specific" rather than "generic" and "individual" rather than "collective." In each individual, a different factor may be of predominant concern and have the most powerful influence, but all other factors contribute to maintaining the illness and preventing recovery.

Understanding Biopsychosocial Influences:
the Multi-Factor Approach

Every individual exists and functions in the context of his/her environment. The family, the school, the workplace, the social network, biomedical status and temperament are all components of this environment, with multiple functions. The cognitively disabled individual is, to a significant extent, shaped in his/her behaviors by the complexities of these systems and their inter-relationship. All of these sub-systems are in turn influenced by the behaviors/dysfunction of the individual. Adaptive behaviors, recovery from physical and psychiatric illnesses and cognitive functions are all affected by the interplay of the many variables in this complex system. However, it has to be kept in mind that while any or all of these factors show a consistent and substantial statistical association with dysfunction/disorder, these are associations only, and not etiological.

While such "intra-personal" vulnerabilities, i.e. the combination of cognitive immaturity, psychiatric issues, neurodevelopmental and medical problems, may underlie a person's dysfunctional behaviors, environmental and social factors often trigger, modify and maintain such nonadaptive responses.

Garber[63] stated that: "If the nature of interaction among possible sources of environmental and genetic influence were better understood, we would increasingly be able to predict individual differences in cognitive behavioral outcome."

In assessing dually diagnosed individuals, the clinician may assess several factors that instigate and maintain maladaptive behaviors with a view to developing specific, individually tailored care plans in a truly multi-modal fashion.

Example

Joan had severe self-injurious behaviors. She was taken to the local hospital frequently for behaving aggressively. When asked once during a visit if she heard voices, she replied "yes." A diagnosis of schizophrenia followed her for several years. Antipsychotic medications were unsuccessful.

A multi-factor assessment was done and its results were as follows:

- Biomedical: epilepsy, spasmodic malabsorption syndrome
- Psychiatric: panic disorder
- Developmental: severe autistic rigidity, poor expressive language ability
- Environmental: intolerance to noise and crowds, changes and transitions
- Self-Care: totally dependent for self-care
- Motivation: selectively motivated
- Emotional: parental neglect and abuse
- Risk: aggression, self-injury

The burden of such a constellation of adverse influences always leads to a breakdown in adaptive functioning. This failure is reflected in the emotional sphere; it affects interpersonal behaviors. Coping with environmental demands becomes difficult, and adjusting to intrapersonal difficulties becomes a challenge (mental illness, physical discomfort).

CONCLUSION

Identification of the specific adverse factors that affect an individual's functioning is important, as it leads to the development of multi-faceted treatment approaches. For instance, enhancing communication skills and teaching social skills enables the individual to adapt to his/her school environment more effectively. Individuals with verbal skills deficits may have good visual-spatial skills, and they often benefit from using visual forms of communication. Self-care skills can be improved with specific behavioral programs using shaping, reinforcers and extinction procedures. At the same time, social interventions designed to provide support, guidance and advocacy for the individual and his/her caregivers significantly influences recovery and positive outcomes.

Interventional strategies should, therefore, take a multi-pronged approach. One does not place all of one's emphasis on psychopharmacological or behavioral or social interventions alone. A systematic multi-factor approach, with careful assessment of neurodevelopmental, psychiatric and environmental vulnerabilities, will not only result in the development of more rational, thoughtful and scientific clinical approaches, but will also lead to productive inter-professional collaboration. Such a state-of-the-art assessment and collaborative treatment strategy would replace the speculative, fragmented approach that has unfortunately dominated our conceptualization and management of dysfunction in the dually diagnosed.[64]

REFERENCES

1 Aman MG. *Assessing Psychopathology and Behavior Problems in Persons with Mental Retardation: a review of available instruments*. Rockville, MD: DHHS Publication; 1991. pp. 91–1712.

2 American Psychiatric Association. *Diagnostic and Statistical Manual of Mental Disorders, 4th Edition*. Washington, DC: American Psychiatric Association; 1994.

3 Organization WH. *The ICD-10 Classification of Mental and Behavioral Disorders: clinical descriptions and diagnostic guidelines*. Geneva: World Health Organization; 1992.

4 American Psychiatric Association, Committee on Nomenclature and Statistics, op. cit.

5 Organization WH, op. cit.

6 National Coalition on Dual Diagnosis. *Position Paper on Dual Diagnosis*. 2009. Available at: www.camh.net/Public_policy/Public_policy_papers/Position%20statement.pdf (accessed 10 May 2011).

7 Grossman H. *Manual on Terminology and Classification of Mental Retardation*. Washington, DC: American Association of Mental Deficiency; 1973.

8 Clarke AM, Clarke ADB. *Mental Deficiency: the changing outlook*. 3rd ed. New York, NY: Free Press; 1974.

9 Hodapp. One road or many? Issues in similar-sequence hypothesis. In: Hodapp RM, Burack JA, Zeigler E, editors. *Developmental Approach to Mental Retardation*. New York, NY: Cambridge University Press; 1990.

10 Clarke AM, Clarke DB, Berg JM. *Mental Deficiency: the changing outlook*. 4th ed. New York, NY: Free Press; 1985.

11 Harris JC. *Developmental Neuropsychiatry*. New York, NY: Oxford University Press; 1998. p. 91.

12 Holmes N, Shah A, Wing L. The Disability Assessment Schedule: a brief screening device for use with the mentally retarded. *Psychol Med*. 1982; **12**(4): 879–90.

13 Isett R, Roszkowski M, Spreat S, *et al*. Tolerance for deviance: subjective evaluation of the social validity of the focus of treatment in mental retardation. *Am J Ment Defic*. 1983; **87**(4): 458–61.

14 Jacobson JW. Problem behavior and psychiatric impairment within a developmentally disabled population I: behavior frequency. *Appl Res Ment Retard*. 1982; **3**(2): 121–39.

15 Harris, 1998, op. cit.

16 Baird PA, Sadovnick AD. Mental retardation in over half-a-million consecutive live-births: an epidemiological study. *Am J Ment Defic*. 1985; **89**(4): 323–30.

17 Gillberg C, Persson E, Grufman M, *et al*. Psychiatric disorders in mildly and severely mentally retarded urban children and adolescents: epidemiological aspects. *Br J Psychiatry*. 1986; **149**: 68–74.

18 Hagberg B, Hagberg G, Lewerth A, *et al*. Mild mental retardation in Swedish school children. I. Prevalence. *Acta Paediatr Scand*. 1981; **70**(4): 441–4.

19 Harris JC. *Developmental Neuropsychiatry*. New York, NY: Oxford University Press; 1999. p. 114.

20 Rutter M, Tizard J, Whitmore K, editors. *Education, Health and Behavior.* London: Longman; 1970.

21 Isett, op. cit.

22 Gillberg, op. cit.

23 Lund J. The prevalence of psychiatric morbidity in mentally retarded adults. *Acta Paediatr Scand.* 1985; **72**(6): 563–70.

24 Crocker AG, Mercier C, Allaire J, *et al.* Profiles and correlates of aggressive behaviour among adults with intellectual disabilities. *J Intellect Disabil Res.* 2007; **51**(Pt. 10): 786–801.

25 McClintock K, Hall S, Oliver C. Risk markers associated with challenging behaviours in people with intellectual disabilities: a meta-analytic study. *J Intellect Disabil Res.* 2003; **47**(Pt. 6): 405–16.

26 Fraser WI, Leudar I, Gray J, *et al.* Psychiatric and behaviour disturbance in mental handicap. *J Ment Defic Res.* 1985; **30**(Pt. 1): 49–57.

27 Senatore V, Matson JL, Kazdin AE. An inventory to assess psychopathology of mentally retarded adults. *Am J Ment Defic.* 1985; **89**(5): 459–66.

28 Cowie VA, Rao JM. Reasons for admission to a hospital for the mentally handicapped: preliminary report of a 10-year survey. *British Journal of Clinical and Social Psychiatry.* 1985; **3**: 77–80.

29 Rao JM. Trends in short term and long term care admission to a hospital of the mentally handicapped and the influence of socio-economic, familial and clinical factors. *Social Psychiatry.* 1987; **22**(2): 118–22.

30 Emerson E, Kiernan C, Alborz A, *et al.* The prevalence of challenging behaviors: a total population study. *Res Dev Disabil.* 2001; **22**(1): 77–93.

31 Crocker AG, Mercier C, Lachapelle Y, *et al.* Prevalence and types of aggressive behaviour among adults with intellectual disabilities. *J Intellect Disabil Res.* 2006; **50**(Pt. 9): 652–61.

32 Tyrer F, McGrother CW, Thorp CF, *et al.* Physical aggression towards others in adults with learning disabilities: prevalence and associated factors. *J Intellect Disabil Res.* 2006; **50**(Pt. 4): 295–304.

33 Novaco RW, Taylor JL. Assessment of anger and aggression in male offenders with developmental disabilities. *Psychol Assess.* 2004; **16**(1): 42–50.

34 Fraser, op. cit.

35 Wing L, Gould J. Severe impairments of social interaction and associated abnormalities in children: epidemiology and classification. *J Autism Dev Disord.* 1979; **9**(1): 11–29.

36 Poling A, Bradshaw L. *Psychopharmacology.* In: Hersen M, Bellack A, editors. *Handbook of Behavior Therapy in the Psychiatric Setting.* New York, NY: Plenum Press; 1993. pp. 113–32.

37 Gadow KD, Poling A. *Pharmacotherapy and Mental Retardation.* Boston, MA: College-Hill Press; 1988.

38 Aman MG, Singh NN, White AJ. Caregiver perceptions of psychotropic medication in residential facilities. *Research in developmental disabilities.* 1987; **8**(3): 449–65.

39 Aman MG. Review and evaluation of instruments for assessing emotional and behavioural disorders. *Australia and New Zealand Journal of Developmental Disabilities.* 1991; **17**(2): 127–45.

40 Gioia GA, Isquith PK, Guy SC. *Behavior Rating Inventory of Executive Function-Self Report Version.* Lutz, FL: Psychological Assessment Resources, Inc.; 1996.

41 Diamond A, Goldman-Rakic PS. Comparison of human infants and rhesus monkeys on Piaget's AB task: evidence for dependence on dorsolateral prefrontal cortex. *Exp Brain Res.* 1989; **74**(1): 24–40.

42 Fletcher JM, Ewing-Cobbs L, Miner ME, *et al.* Behavioral changes after closed head injury in children. *J Consult Clin Psychol.* 1990; **58**(1): 93–8.

43 Gioia, op. cit.

44 Rao JM, Hall M. Reconceptualizing diagnosis for the dually diagnosised [presentation]. *Ontario Association of Developmental Disabilities Annual Conference.* Barry, ON; 2009.

45 Schoen SA, Miller LJ, Brett-Green BH, *et al.* Physiological and behavioural differences in sensory processing: a comparison of children with autism spectrum disorder and sensory modulation disorder. *Front Integr Neurosci.* 2009; **3**: 29. Epub 2009 Nov 3.

46 Ibid.

47 Stringer H, Lozano S. Under identification of speech and language impairment in children attending a special school for children with emotional and behavioural disorders. *Educational and Child Psychology.* 2007; **24**(4): 9–19.

48 Menolascino FJ, Levitas A, Greiner C. The nature and types of mental illness in the mentally retarded. *Psychopharmacol Bull.* 1986; **22**(4): 1060–71.

49 Lund, op. cit.

50 Smith AH, O'Brien G. Treatment of developmentally disabled offenders with dual diagnosis. In: Lindsay WR, Taylor JL, Sturmey P, editors. *Offenders with Developmental Disabilities.* Chichester: Wiley; 2004. pp. 241–64.

51 Gostason R. Psychiatric illness among the mentally retarded. A swedish population study. *Acta Psychiatr Scand Suppl.* 1985; **318**: 1–117.

52 Turner TH. Schizophrenia and mental handicap: an historical review, with implications for further research. *Psychol Med.* 1989; **19**(2): 301–14.

53 Johnstone EC, Owens DG, Hoare P, *et al.* Schizotypal cognitions as a predictor of psychopathology in adolescents with mild intellectual impairment. *Br J Psychiatry.* 2007; **191**: 484–92.

54 Reiss S, Levitan GW, Szyszko J. Emotional disturbance and mental retardation: diagnostic overshadowing. *Am J Ment Defic.* 1982; **86**(6): 567–74.

55 Harris, op. cit.

56 Mink IT, Nihira K, Meyers CE. Taxonomy of family life styles: I. Homes with TMR children. *Am J Ment Defic.* 1983; **87**(5): 484–97.

57 Beveridge M, Conti-Ramsden G. Social cognition and problem-solving in persons with mental retardation. *Australia and New Zealand Journal of Developmental Disabilities.* 1987; **13**: 99–106.

58 Fraser WI, Rao JM. Recent studies of mentally handicapped young people's behaviour. *J Child Psychol Psychiatry.* 1991; **32**(1): 79–108.

59 Griffiths D, Garder WI. An integrated biopsychosocial model: state of the art. In: Griffiths DM, Stavrakaki C, Summer J, editors. *An Introduction to the Mental Health Needs of Persons with Developmental Disabilities.* Sudbury, ON: Habilitative Mental Health Resource Network; 2002. pp. 81–114.

60 Harris, 1999, op. cit.

61 Harris, 1998, op. cit.

62 Garber HL. *The Milwaukee Project.* Washington, DC: American Association on Mental Retardation; 1988.

63 Ibid.

64 Harris, 1998, op. cit.

5.4.3 SERIOUS MENTAL ILLNESS: PERSON-CENTERED APPROACHES IN FORENSIC PSYCHIATRY

Jose Mejia and Janice Vandevooren

INTRODUCTION

In this section, we intend to illustrate how person-centered approaches apply to the rehabilitation of individuals who suffer from a mental disorder and who have also come into conflict with the law. In Canada, such individuals are served in the forensic system. While this section will focus on the Canadian context, the discussion may be relevant to other jurisdictions as well. With that purpose we have included a description of the mental health and justice interface as it relates to forensic psychiatry, two clinical vignettes to illustrate the application of person-centered approaches in forensic settings, and a discussion of some of the unique challenges in applying person-centered approaches in the forensic context. Note that although this section addresses a special population, many issues addressed by other sections in this book are relevant, such as the issues addressed by Section 6.2, *Person-Centered Approaches to Psychopharmacology for People with Serious Mental Illness*, Section 6.3, *Person-Centered Individual Psychotherapy for Adults with Serious Mental Illness*, and Section 6.4, *Cognitive and Psychiatric Rehabilitation: person-centered ingredients for success*.

Person-Centered Approaches in Forensic Settings

Person-centered approaches in mental health have the objective of addressing the complex and multiple needs that an individual has when he or she finds him/herself in contact with psychiatric services. These approaches are relevant and beneficial to the individual, given that the organ being compromised, the brain, is also the one involved in decision-making processes that define lifestyle, habits, behaviors, etc., and in turn determine the individual's health status as a whole. As would be expected, the presence of a mental health disorder is likely to negatively impact those processes by which the person defines him/herself as an individual and as part of his/her community, family and environment. Socialization and social interactions are often disturbed. Notwithstanding this fact, those behaviors affected by a mental disorder are usually contained sufficiently to avoid impinging on the personal rights of others. However, on occasion, the person affected by an SMI may violate societal rules and engage in criminal activities that range in severity from a minor transgression to loss of life.

Congruent with PCC, many systems have been developed in which mental health issues take precedence over criminal offending. There has been a shift within the criminal justice system from the traditional punitive/corrective model towards a model of therapeutic jurisprudence, in which it is recognized that individuals who come in contact with the law as a direct result of mental illness must be diverted towards a therapeutic/rehabilitation-oriented system. The increased emergence of mental health courts across Canada exemplifies this shift. Such courts aim to divert individuals away from the justice system towards the necessary mental health services. These courts also have access to professional expertise that assists in determining when such individuals require involvement of forensic providers.

Forensic psychiatry programs are mandated to comprehensively address disorders affecting the minds of individuals that find themselves in trouble with the law by virtue of their mental disorder. The ultimate objective is to reintegrate the person into society as soon as the mental health condition is improved to the point where the risk of recidivism is manageable in the community.[1] Of course, there are situations in which the mental disorder affecting the individual may not be related to their trouble with the law. For instance, in the course of serving a sentence a person may feel depressed, anxious or become psychotic. Notwithstanding that these are mental disorders as well, they are usually dealt with by the correctional system if the person is in custody, or by the general mental health system when the sentence is being served in the community. Not infrequently though, these individuals may find themselves in a vacuum of lack of services due to the stigmatizing effect of their criminal offenses. In this section we will not address such a complex situation given that it is our objective to focus on forensic systems. Consequently, the reader should keep in mind that the types of individuals dealt with by forensic systems are those in which the mental disorder has a causal or etiological effect in the criminal actions they commit.

According to the Forensic Mental Health Services Expert Advisory Panel,[2] a forensic service user is a person with a serious mental disorder who is involved in the criminal justice system under the Mental Disorders Provision (Section XX.1) of the Criminal Code of Canada.[3] However, not all serious mental health conditions confer a *not criminally responsible* (NCR) status to the individual who suffers them. For a mental health condition to be considered as a defense against criminal responsibility (as established in Section 16 of the Criminal Code of Canada),[4,5] such a condition has to impair the capacity of the individual "of appreciating the nature and quality of the act or omission or of knowing that it was wrong." It is also widely accepted in forensic psychiatry that the mental health condition has to have caused such an effect on the individual at the time of the offense. Henceforth, if a subject is affected by a mental disorder, but at the time of the offense the disorder was in remission – allowing the individual to appreciate the nature and quality of the act or omission and knowing that it was wrong – then the subject will be considered criminally responsible and the mental health condition will be managed in the correctional system. Exempt from the categorization of disorders that are considered as a cause for loss of criminal responsibility are: 1. Disorders that are pervasive in nature and only affect those aspects of mental function related to personality (personality disorders); 2. Conditions in which the individual voluntarily enters a state of intoxication that impairs his/her capacity of analysis and judgment; and 3. Situations in which the individual presents with symptoms of a psychiatric condition that are conveniently evident in order to avoid responsibility for their actions or for the purposes of benefiting from the role of being sick (malingering).[6]

Although most individuals entering the forensic psychiatric system are not responsible for their criminal actions (NCR), some of them may find themselves unfit to stand trial, even before an analysis of criminal responsibility is made. In Canadian law (Criminal Code of Canada S2), this determination is based on an assessment of the individual's ability to:

➤ Understand the nature of object of proceedings
➤ Understand the possible consequences of the proceedings
➤ Communicate with counsel.

When the above factors are suspected not to be present by virtue of a mental disorder, the person may be deemed to be unfit to stand trial. This may be followed by a court order for assessment as an inpatient in a forensic psychiatric facility. Once the unfit status is confirmed, the individual could be voluntarily or involuntarily treated in order to regain fitness, usually by means of pharmacological care. Once recovered and fit, the individual will be brought back to court to continue with the judicial process. Meanwhile, the courts may also request that the individual be returned to the forensic psychiatric unit to maintain fitness as the trial progresses.[7]

Once integrated into the forensic system, forensic service users fall under the auspices of a judicial body regulated by the Criminal Code of Canada, which in Ontario is known as the Ontario Review Board (ORB). This is an independent tribunal whose role is to make dispositions for each individual that are the "least onerous and restrictive," taking into consideration the following four factors:

1 the need to protect the public from dangerous persons
2 the mental condition of the accused
3 the reintegration of the accused into society
4 the other needs of the accused.

Forensic services thus have a unique challenge of balancing the need to protect the public from criminal acts committed by individuals with a mental illness, the service users' rights to freedom and their rehabilitation and community reintegration needs.

While the commission of a criminal offense differentiates forensic service users from those service users in the general mental health system, there are many more similarities than differences. According to data published by the Department of Justice, the three most frequent primary diagnoses of those individuals in the Canadian Forensic System are schizophrenia (51.7%), affective disorders (26.6%) and delusional disorders (4.6%).[8] Data on primary diagnoses at discharge from specialty mental health facilities in Ontario show schizophrenia, schizotypal and delusional disorders as the most frequent diagnostic categories, followed by mood disorders and mental and behavioral disorders due to psychoactive substance use.[9]

It is easy then to understand that forensic service users exhibit similar psychiatric symptoms and functional deficits as other individuals with mental illness in non-forensic settings, and thus require similar approaches to care, rehabilitation and support – all of which aim to facilitate the service user's recovery.[10] Anthony, Cohen and Farkas, *et al.*[11] define the recovery concept as follows:

> Recovery is a deeply personal, unique process of changing one's attitudes, values, feelings, goals, skills, and/or roles. It is a way of living a satisfying, hopeful, and contributing life, with or without limitations caused by the illness. Recovery involves the development of new meaning and purpose in one's life as one grows beyond the catastrophic effects of a mental illness.12, p. 31

A recovery-oriented, person-centered PSR approach that focuses on role recovery and the development of skills and supports necessary to be successful and satisfied in the community is highly applicable to forensic psychiatry. Implementation of such a person-centered approach within a forensic setting is, however, often met with some unique challenges related to organizational culture, security constraints, excessive reliance on behavioral control and providers who may perceive themselves more as "jailers than rehabilitation practitioners."[13, p. 74]

While the daily attention to assessment and monitoring of risk is central to forensic services, *positive risk management*, as articulated by the *Best Practices in Managing Risk* document prepared for the Department of Health in the UK,[14] is based on the following fundamental components:
➤ a trusting therapeutic relationship
➤ a spirit of collaboration between provider and service user
➤ recognition of the service user's strengths and protective factors
➤ an emphasis on recovery
➤ awareness of the capacity for risk levels to change over time
➤ recognition of the need for individualized approaches
➤ a multidisciplinary approach.

Forensic programs are thus challenged to adopt such best practices and move away from what has traditionally been a "negative risk management cycle."[15, p. 17]

Example

This is an illustration of the application of a person-centered PSR approach to the recovery of mentally disordered individuals in a forensic setting:

Jacob is a 20-year-old male referred by the courts for assessment of criminal responsibility for charges of attempted murder, possession of a weapon, assault with a weapon and aggravated assault. With no previous psychiatric history and responding to hallucinations and delusions focused on the voice of the victim, Jacob found himself in the forensic psychiatry system. His crime received significant media attention, and victim support groups clamored for punishment. Jacob was diagnosed with schizophrenia complicated by the use of street drugs. He was found NCR on account of his mental disorder.

Jacob's involvement with the law also represented his introduction to the mental health system. He was floridly psychotic and tortured by voices in his head that he thought belonged to his victim. He showed no insight into his mental health status nor his offense. He was reclusive and difficult to engage in any kind of activity or relationship. Despite taking antipsychotic medication that eliminated Jacob's hallucinations, he remained in bed most of the day, lacked motivation and struggled with self-care.

At that time the forensic program was implementing a PSR approach based on the work and research of William Anthony and colleagues at Boston University.[16] A rehabilitation readiness tool was used to gather information by evaluating the service user's readiness to engage in rehabilitation activities. The instrument addresses five key areas: Need for Change, Commitment to Change, Environmental Awareness, Self-Awareness and Personal Closeness.[17] Jacob's results indicated that he was not ready for rehabilitation, but the information gleaned was instrumental in enabling the team to connect with Jacob and focus his subsequent care. A pivotal finding in the assessment was Jacob's love of guitar playing. His care plan was formulated around individual interactions with a nurse who shared his guitar interest. Jacob's family also identified his fondness for playing cards – an activity which was also built into his care plan. Through these interactions, providers were able to engage with Jacob, and therapeutic relationships began to emerge. He became aware of his mental illness and its horrible consequences.

In addition to coping with the anxiety of his psychotherapeutic process, Jacob experienced significant stress related to his ORB hearings. While staff work closely with each person to understand their needs and individualize their goals, the reports to the ORB also require the team make a determination of level of risk the individual presents. The two processes may appear antagonistic in that while trying to facilitate a service user's recovery, the team may also need to recommend that the process be delayed or otherwise stalled due to the risk that releasing, or increasing an individual's privileges, represents. Equally important, the duty to report truthfully positive and negative events may hinder the therapeutic relationship. It is thus crucial that staff maintain open and honest communication with all service users such that the relationship can be sustained and recovery can continue while managing the risk of recidivism appropriately.

As Jacob's care progressed the focus shifted to relapse prevention and a more detailed assessment of Jacob's leisure and vocational needs. Psychotherapy interventions assisted him in coping with the impact of his offense and were a critical component of his care. Throughout his rehabilitation Jacob was an active partner and participant in his care planning. Once the possibility of living in the community emerged, Jacob had a second assessment of his readiness for rehabilitation. He was able to identify a need for change in several areas of his life including housing, education and work. In collaboration with the team he set realistic goals and identified supports he would need in order to succeed. He identified three residential options, and evaluated the advantages and disadvantages of each. Jacob chose to move to a group residence and return to school to complete his Grade 12 education. The team worked with Jacob to identify the skills needed to achieve his goals, e.g. meal planning and preparation and management of finances. Jacob also demonstrated many skill strengths including taking his medication regularly, caring for himself and engaging in leisure activities.

Critical to Jacob's recovery was involvement of his family. Jacob's parents joined a support group and became "approved persons" to facilitate Jacob's access to the community. Once in the community he was provided care by the forensic outreach team. Jacob attended school and met with the outreach team regularly to provide direct skills teaching in the area of activities of daily living, e.g. making healthy meal choices and comparison-shopping skills, as well as skills programming, e.g. use of a structured form to assist in budgeting. Psychotherapeutic sessions addressed some of Jacob's fears around returning to the community and establishing new relationships.

An important part of risk management in the community is to identify an individual's protective factors that contribute to mitigating risk. These resources can be people, places, activities, or things that support the individual's success.[18] In addition to pursuing his education and maintaining close connections with the forensic team, many critical resources were identified to be of assistance in ensuring Jacob's ongoing wellness. These included his nuclear and extended family, the outreach team, his psychologist and other members of staff. Being close to a music studio and other amenities such as the grocery store was important for Jacob. Jacob engaged in regular activities including walking, bike-riding, music lessons and guitar playing. The team also ensured that Jacob's living environment had a television and video games so he had activities at home. All of these resources were identified within Jacobs's care plan.

Today Jacob has received an absolute discharge from the forensic system. He lives independently in his own apartment and continues to study music. He has completed his high school education and has a girlfriend. Though he is not required to, Jacob remains in contact with a number of the forensic team members – a testimony to the strength of those relationships. Jacob continues to have hope for his future and is working toward competitive employment.

Although in Jacob's case there were no psychiatric antecedents of relevance, in other cases the individual may have been affected by a mental disorder for a long period of time and entered the revolving door of adherence-improvement/non-adherence-relapse, whereby the criminal offense brings the individual to the doors of the justice and mental health systems. This is such a frequent occurrence that many authors have maintained that the growth of the forensic system is a result of a failure of the civil mental health system.[19,20]

As with non-forensic settings, the acute phase of an individual's illness that often presents upon admission to hospital provides a challenge to care providers with respect to PCC. Cognitive deficits may compound other symptoms, making it difficult and sometimes impossible for the individual to make decisions for him or herself. In a forensic setting, the challenge of having individuals arrive to assessment units often untreated and having languished, sometimes for long periods, in jail, can present an additional risk factor. Historically, these programs have tended to manage the risk of violence through heightened controls and seclusion in order to ensure the safety of all. Such approaches often have a negative effect, eliciting oppositional behaviors from individuals experiencing mental illness who resist the controls being placed upon them.

The introduction of person-focused approaches has led to a shift away from the need for restrictive measures applied indiscriminately to all persons to a more individualized approach that provides the least amount of restriction necessary to ensure safety. This approach demands increased skill and expertise of providers, as it is crucial to conduct a comprehensive assessment and get to know the individual in order to ensure that the appropriate security measures are in place. This is likely to remain a bit of a tightrope walk for forensic teams as they shift to a new paradigm while maintaining accountability for safety. For the same reasons explained above, individuals entering the forensic system usually do so in the context of a medium secure environment, which necessarily limits autonomy and self-determination. While this indeed seems to be in opposition to a person-centered approach, from a broader perspective this is an approach required within forensic services in order to ensure a safe environment for every individual residing in the forensic facility. The introduction of person-centered PSR practices implemented within the legal limitations placed on individuals in a forensic system, including an emphasis on the protection of public safety, is supported in the literature by Linhorst.[21] While individuals will necessarily have a narrower array of options to choose from relative to those in non-forensic settings, there remains substantial opportunity for choice and self-determination within the parameters of such constraints. As an example, an individual may be required, as part of the conditions of his or her disposition order, to reside in accommodation approved by the hospital. Through the use of psychiatric rehabilitation techniques that match skill levels of an individual to the demands of a given environment, it is quite conceivable that individuals can come to reside in housing that is acceptable to them and to the care team.

Example

Jonathan is a 38-year-old man who was discharged from the forensic program, had been living in a group home in the community for several years and was receiving care from the forensic outreach team. He has a long history of mental health problems, and his index offense was criminal in nature but did not involve harm to another person. The focus of the clinical team had always been to have Jonathan achieve a level of stability in the community so that he would eventually be able to receive an absolute discharge. The quandary in this case was that Jonathan continued to have brief episodes where he would threaten someone in the community with minor theft or other minor nuisance behaviors. These events caused a revolving door trend with periodic readmissions and ensured that he remained a significant threat to the community and thus within the forensic system.

With the newly adopted psychosocial, rehabilitation, recovery-oriented approach to care, the team began to approach their work with Jonathan in a different manner. The next time Jonathan required admission to hospital the team completed a rehabilitation readiness assessment. The main realization that came from this assessment was that while the team viewed Jonathan's tenure in the group home as successful stabilization, Jonathan viewed it as stagnation. Jonathan was living his life in a group home in the community with the view that, at best, every tomorrow would be the same as today. By staff engaging Jonathan in the process of the rehabilitation readiness assessment it was easy to ascertain that, while this client did not possess much self-confidence, he did have hopes and dreams that were in no way satisfied by his current situation – a situation that staff had inadvertently strived to maintain.

Assessment findings revealed that Jonathan very much wanted to live in his own apartment and be able to do things for himself. Staff who had been working with him said he would voice this from time to time, but since he lacked the drive to be able to do it there seemed to be no point in trying. With the new model of care, staff now began to view this as an opportunity. A mini-team comprised of a social worker, an occupational therapist, a registered nurse and a registered practical nurse began meeting with Jonathan as a group to see how best to support him in achieving his goals. Staff clearly conveyed a belief that Jonathan's goal was achievable. It appeared that the client's lack of belief in himself had been supported to a great extent by the fact that staff believed he was not capable of further progress.

With a clear goal established, the team, including Jonathan, was able to identify two key barriers – potential for loneliness and certain deficits in skills required for independent living. Jonathan required support in reconnecting to people who now lived in the community – people he had befriended while in hospital. In terms of skill development, one of the first things that Jonathan would need to do would be to find himself an apartment, including consideration of all relevant factors, e.g. affordability, proximity to services, etc. Jonathan engaged in skill development around setting up and maintaining an apartment, getting to the grocery store, menu planning, shopping and meal preparation. He also learned how to do his own laundry. Staff would initially accompany and assist him in the tasks and gradually withdraw as his skills and confidence developed. Team members with a more traditional view were concerned about the time investment this required and still doubted the outcome would be any different over time.

Eventually, Jonathan was gradually more social and confident in himself. The periodic returns to the hospital or challenging periods of implied risk faded away. Jonathan has since received an absolute discharge and has returned to his home city to live. The future is open to him, and every tomorrow will certainly not be a monotonous repetition of yesterday and today but something new and unique. When the tools and values of PSR were applied to Jonathan's care the direction of care shifted entirely and the client was actively engaged in a partnership. Client and staff became entirely focused on the client achieving his goals. It would seem that the energy that had previously fueled risk was being produced largely from the client's frustration over being stuck in a life that in no way represented his hopes and dreams.

CONCLUSION

In summary, and as illustrated by Jacob and Jonathan's stories, we maintain that it is both possible – and indeed desirable – to adopt person-centered approaches within forensic psychiatry. As Menditto states: "it is incumbent upon care providers, program directors, and administrators to offer the care and rehabilitation services most likely to effectively address the clinical problems and needs of people with mental illnesses residing in such facilities. This requires changing the philosophy and culture and shifting provider perceptions of rehabilitation experiences for service users within the constraints posed by security policies and physical setting limitations."[22, p. 74]

As discussed in the introduction of this book, the person-focused dimension of PCC for individuals with mental illness may seem to conflict with the principle of *justice*, which seeks to maintain a balance between health care for an individual and the interests of other parties. This is precisely the delicate balance dealt with on a daily basis in the provision of forensic psychiatry services. As is also pointed out in Section 1.1, *Foundations and Ethics of Person-Centered Approaches to Individuals with*

Serious Mental Illness, while this particular aspect of PCC may at times be compromised, other aspects need not be. The ongoing emphasis on the unique needs of each individual and the person-contextualized dimensions can continue to be the cornerstone of rehabilitation. Despite the challenges, our experiences have shown that through a recovery-focused PSR approach many individuals can progress through the forensic system to achieve successful and satisfying lives within the community.

Davenport, Holloway, Roberts and Tattan[23] proposed that given the very nature of serious mental illnesses, there might be times when providers need to employ compulsory interventions in order to protect the greater good (and ultimately the individual him/herself). If done in the context of a therapeutic relationship, good communication – including with family and/or substitute decision-makers – with the intent to move as quickly as possible to a situation where the individual can regain control and decision-making abilities is likely to remain an essential component of effective psychiatric care in both forensic and non-forensic settings.

REFERENCES

1 Weinstock R, Leong GB, Silva A. Defining forensic psychiatry: roles and responsibilities. In: Rosner R, editor. *Principles and Practice of Forensic Psychiatry.* New York, NY: Oxford University Press Inc.; 1998. pp. 7–12.

2 Ontario Ministry of Health and Long-Term Care. *Assessment, Treatment and Community Re-Integration of the Mentally Disordered Offender: final report of the forensic mental health services expert advisory panel.* Toronto, ON: Ministry of Health and Long-Term Care; 2002.

3 Criminal Code of Canada. R.S., 1985, c. C-46. Available at: www.canlii.org/ca/sta/c-46 (accessed 1 Dec 2009).

4 Weinstock, op. cit.

5 Bloom H, Schneider RD, editors. *Mental Disorder and the Law: a primer for legal and mental health professionals.* Toronto, ON: Irwin Law; 2006. pp. 121–4.

6 Ibid.

7 Bloom H, op. cit. pp. 61–97.

8 Latimer J, Lawrence A. *The Review Board Systems in Canada: overview of results from the mentally disordered accused data collection study.* Ottawa, ON: Department of Justice; 2006.

9 Ontario Ministry of Health and Long-Term Care. *Mental Health and Addictions in Ontario LHINs: health systems intelligence project.* Toronto, ON: Ministry of Health and Long-Term Care; 2008.

10 Menditto AA. A social learning approach to the rehabilitation of individuals with severe mental disorders who reside in forensic facilities. *Psychiatric Rehabilitation Skills.* 2002; **6**: 73–93.

11 Anthony WA, Cohen M, Farkas M, *et al. Psychiatric Rehabilitation.* 2nd ed. Boston, MA: Boston University Center for Psychiatric Rehabilitation; 2002.

12 Ibid.

13 Menditto, op. cit.

14 Department of Health, National Risk Management Programme. *Best Practice in Managing Risk: principles and evidence for best practice in the assessment and management of risk to self and others in mental health services.* London, UK: Department of Health; 2007.

15 Ibid.

16 Anthony, op. cit.

17 Farkas M, Sullivan-Soydan AP, Gagne C. *Introduction to Rehabilitation Readiness.* Boston, MA: Center for Psychiatric Rehabilitation; 2000.

18 Anthony, op. cit.

19 Schneider RD, Bloom H, Heerema M. *Mental Health Courts: decriminalizing the mentally ill.* Toronto, ON: Irwin Law; 2007.

20 Torrey EF. *Criminalizing the Seriously Mentally Ill: the abuse of jails as mental hospitals.* Washington, DC: Health Research Group and National Alliance for the Mentally Ill; 1992.

21 Linhorst DM. Implementing psychosocial rehabilitation in long-term inpatient psychiatric facilities. *The Journal of Mental Health Administration.* 1995; **22**: 58–67.

22 Menditto, op. cit.

23 Roberts G, Davenport S, Holloway F, *et al.*, editors. *Enabling Recovery: the principles and practice of rehabilitation psychiatry.* London, UK: Gaskell; 2006.

5.4.4 TREATMENT OF CO-OCCURRING SUBSTANCE USE DISORDERS USING SHARED DECISION-MAKING AND ELECTRONIC DECISION-SUPPORT SYSTEMS

Kim T. Mueser and Robert E. Drake

INTRODUCTION

Substance use disorders (SUDs), including substance abuse and dependence, are characterized by the repeated use of psychoactive substances to the point where it interferes with functioning and dominates one's life. Commonly abused substances include alcohol; cannabis; stimulants, e.g. cocaine, amphetamines; narcotics, e.g. heroin; hallucinogens, e.g. LSD, ecstasy; and sedatives, e.g. benzodiazepines. *Substance abuse* is defined by substance use that interferes with day-to-day functioning or an illness (such as a medical or psychiatric disorder), or that places the person or others at increased risk for harm, e.g. driving while intoxicated.[1] *Substance dependence* is defined in terms of either physical dependence or psychological dependence. *Physical dependence* is substance use that leads to either tolerance, i.e. requiring greater amounts of a substance to achieve the same effects, or withdrawal symptoms. *Psychological dependence* is a pattern of substance use in which the person spends inordinate amounts of time using or trying to obtain substances, gives up important activities in order to use substances, and/or has made repeated unsuccessful attempts to cut down or stop using. Although nicotine use has mild psychoactive effects and serious health consequences and is common in people with SMI,[2] we do not address it in this section as it does not appear to interact significantly with the symptoms or course of mental illness. This section will focus on PCC for people with co-occurring disorders (SMI with SUDs), with some special emphasis on a particularly innovative aspect of such PCC: electronic decision-support systems.

In the general population, the lifetime prevalence of SUD is approximately 15%.[3,4] In contrast, for people with SMIs, SUDs are common, with more than half of such individuals affected by this comorbidity over their lifetime.[4,5] Many of the adverse outcomes related to SMI, such as relapse,[6] homelessness[7,8] and incarceration,[9] are strongly associated with SUDs. Further, addiction tends to be a persistent, relapsing condition for this population, as for others.[10] Even when people appear to achieve stable remissions, returning to dangerous levels of abuse and dependence is common.[11,12,13,14]

The problem of the poor outcomes of many people with comorbid, or co-occurring, disorders is compounded by the lack of engagement of service users in treatment planning and treatment itself. Electronic decision-support systems have the potential to make treatment more person-centered by involving service users in treatment planning, treatment selection and monitoring outcomes. In this chapter we consider person-centered treatment of co-occurring substance disorders from the service user's perspective. What does "recovery" really mean? How does a person with mental illness learn to manage this persistent disorder? How can active participation in treatment make a difference? We briefly consider the chronic disease management model, the relatively new model of shared decision-making (SDM), and the evidence regarding treatment and recovery. Finally, we offer guidelines for current clinical programs.

Principles of Treating Long-Term Illness: the Disease Management Model

From the service provider's perspective, treatment of long-term illnesses follows the chronic illness care model.[15] Numerous disease management systems have been developed on the basis of this broad approach to address three targets: 1. Service users' needs for education and self-management skills; 2. Providers' needs for knowledge, skills and task facilitators; and 3. Practice systems' need for redesign to promote multi-component interventions.[16] Using the example of diabetes, service users can learn to monitor their blood sugars and report them from home; providers can be prompted to obtain regular blood tests, eye exams and other measures to optimize care; and computerized information systems can be used to monitor tests and clinical status, and to match these parameters with evidence-based guidelines.

The Service User's Response to Persistent Illness: the recovery model

From the service user's perspective, responding to a long-term illness involves a complex educational, psychological, social and behavioral process that in recent times has been termed *recovery*.[17] Although phenomenological response to long-term illness has been an artistic theme for centuries, e.g. see Thomas Mann's *The Magic Mountain*, in mental health the recovery movement is emergent, highly variable and even more highly politicized.[18] Various service users emphasize that the experience of recovery spans a broad range of attributes, including awareness, acceptance, hope, respect, personal responsibility, education, self-help, peer support, personal goals, moving beyond illness, belonging to a community and sense of agency.[19,20,21,22] Similarly, numerous service providers have proposed their own definitions of "recovery outcomes" and "recovery-oriented services."[23,24,2526]

For the person with a mental illness, learning to manage symptoms so that they interfere as little as possible with one's life and goals is complicated, often takes years and extends beyond traditional treatments.[27] For example, Deegan[28] conceptualizes "personal medicine" as comprising all of the activities that allow one to pursue personal goals, such as friendship, exercise, work, self-help and hobbies.

Collaborative Care: shared decision making

How can the service provider's approach to evidence-based treatment guidelines and the service user's perspective on personal recovery be combined? The Institute of Medicine,[29] the U.S. Surgeon General's Report[30] and the President's New Freedom Commission[31] all call for involving service users more actively in the care process, as is discussed in greater length in Section 9.1, *Implications of Person-Centered Care for Evidence-Based Practice*. Similarly, the evidence-based medicine paradigm asserts that the inclusion of service user preferences, along with scientific evidence and service provider skills, should be a pillar of medical decision-making.[32] The question is, how can this be practically accomplished?

As health care systems have attempted to incorporate service users' values, goals and preferences into daily operations, the model of SDM, which is described in Section 5.2, *Clinical Communication with Persons Who Have Serious Mental Illness*, has emerged as a central operational approach.[33,34,35] In this model, two partners – the health care service provider and the service user – share their respective areas of expertise (scientific knowledge and personal experience and preferences) and then negotiate and commit to a collaborative agreement regarding major health care decisions.[36,37] The reality of modern health care is that the treatment of most disorders involves multiple reasonable choices with complex tradeoffs, which are sensitive to service users' preferences, rather than a single treatment clearly representing the best choice.[38] SDM has been adopted in manifold forms in physical health care settings, but limited work has been extended to the mental health field.[39,40,41] In one early test of collaborative goal setting, Priebe and colleagues[42] demonstrated that SDM improved satisfaction with care and decreased unmet needs.

Electronic Decision Support Systems

Practice system re-engineering has great potential to improve all of the components of care for persistent disorders, including shared decision-making, through the advances in modern information technology. Six components are generally addressed in re-engineering care, but are usually lacking in mental health programs, although they could all be provided within an electronic decision support system.[43]

1 *Identification* – Almost any clinical population can be screened and assessed to identify cases automatically and inexpensively, because nearly all service users can interact with the computer system directly, by reading or by listening to questions with earphones and by touching the screen to self-identify problems and needs.[44]

2 *Guidelines* – Service users and service providers can each be exposed directly to EBP guidelines through electronic decision support systems. The challenge is to make the guidelines brief, relevant, understandable and accessible.

3 *Collaborative care* – Interactive models ensure that service providers and service users share their perspectives and negotiate an action plan, such as by considering the evidence base for treatment options and arriving at a decision together.

4 *Self-management* – Computerized systems can not only provide education but also prompts to take medications, remember diets, enter lab tests, use cognitive-behavioral techniques and so forth.

5 *Measurement, evaluation and management* – Data on processes and outcomes can be entered by service users, service providers and labs, and can be collated,

assembled longitudinally and displayed by the computer to aid decision-making in treatment encounters, program evaluation and management of systems of care.

6 *Routine reporting/feedback loop* – Service users can be reinforced for self-care, service providers for concordance with guidelines, and clinics and systems for quality improvements by routine feedback of synthesized data.

We next suggest how electronic decision support systems within a comprehensive electronic medical record might be used to enhance care of co-occurring SUDs.

Shared Decision-Making and Co-Occurring Substance Use Disorders

SDM is ideal for persistent conditions where progress, options and decisions need to be revisited repeatedly,[45] such as co-occurring substance use problems and SMI. The treatment of substance use problems can be organized into a series of five steps, including screening, education, personal preferences, treatment planning, and monitoring participation and outcomes. We briefly describe each of these steps below, including the use of electronic decision support systems. We illustrate each step with a brief clinical vignette, alternating between examples that use an electronic support system and examples that do not. We then discuss the issue of service user motivation for change and the stages of treatment and recovery, which can inform the SDM approach by ensuring that the information provided to the service user and potential treatment options are consonant with the person's desire to make changes in his or her life. Finally, we consider the advantages of a SDM approach to co-occurring disorders to both the service user and the service provider.

Step 1: Screening, diagnosis and risk assessment

The purpose of screening is to use a brief tool capable of identifying most people with a particular disorder in as efficient a manner as possible, while missing as few people with the disorder as possible. Thus, "casting a wide net" at the screening stage is desirable, as there is a presumed lower cost of incorrectly identifying someone as having an SUD when he/she does not than incorrectly identifying someone as not having such a disorder when in fact he/she does.[46] A variety of brief screening instruments for SUD have been shown to be valid for persons with SMI,[47,48] which can be administered either in person or electronically as part of routine intake or periodic assessment procedures. In addition, urinalysis can be very useful for detecting substance use that service users may fail to report using on self-report measures or during interviews.

The results of a urinalysis test provide information about recent drug use, whereas positive scores on a screening test are indicative of a probable SUD. However, additional assessment is required to confirm a diagnosis. Critical information for establishing a diagnosis includes: the amount and frequency of substance use; social, occupational, self-care, medical and legal consequences; development of tolerance to substance effects; withdrawal symptoms; using more than intended; and unsuccessful attempts to cut down or stop. Standard and reliable instruments exist for obtaining this information, such as the Alcohol Use and Drug Use Scales[49] and the Timeline Followback Calendar.[50] However, since denial and minimization are common features of SUDs, the most valid information about a service user's substance use behavior can usually be obtained by tapping a combination of sources, including the service user, the service provider and significant others, such as family members. This information can be obtained through either in-person interviews, electronic methods or a combination of the two. There may be some advantages to using computer-based assessments for service users, since there is evidence that people are more willing to admit to engaging in socially disapproved behaviors, e.g. drug abuse, homosexual behavior or engaging in unprotected sex, when the evaluation is administered by computer than in person.[51,52]

Example

Luis, a 30-year-old man with schizoaffective disorder, was admitted to a psychiatric hospital for treatment of an acute exacerbation of his psychiatric symptoms. As part of the standard admission procedure at the hospital, Luis was administered a computer-based screening measure of substance abuse, the Dartmouth Assessment of Lifestyle Instrument.[53] The results of this screen indicated that Luis probably had recent alcohol and cocaine use disorders. Based on these results, Luis's inpatient social worker interviewed him about his substance use and completed a Timeline Followback Calendar to understand his pattern of alcohol and cocaine use over the past six months, and the situations in which he most frequently used. In order to get as complete a picture as possible of Luis's substance use, she also met with Luis's mother, with whom he lived, and his case manager at his local community mental health center. Based on all of this information, and additional input from his inpatient treatment team, Luis's social worker completed the Alcohol Use Scale and Drug Use scale[54] and concluded that over the past six months Luis had met diagnostic criteria for alcohol dependence and cocaine abuse.

Step 2: Education

Service users with SMI often have a limited understanding of their psychiatric disorder, how it interacts with the environment, and the principles of its treatment. Electronic decision supports are an ideal technology for providing service users with basic information about their psychiatric illness, e.g. diagnosis, symptoms, onset, causes; the effects of social factors on the illness, e.g. stress, social support; and the influence of biological factors, e.g., medication, substance use. Explaining that psychiatric disorders have a biological basis,[55] and are no one's fault, can reduce feelings of guilt and shame many service users have about their condition, and increase their interest in learning how to better manage their disorder. Of particular relevance to co-occurring disorders, service users are often surprised to learn that their psychiatric disorder increases their vulnerability to experiencing negative consequences from alcohol and drug use compared to people without such a disorder.[56] This helps many service users who used substances before they became ill understand why they have had so many more problems with their use since developing their illness.

Education about psychiatric disorders leads naturally to providing similar information about alcohol and drug use problems. Although most people are familiar with some of the negative consequences of substance use, they are usually not aware of the specific symptoms of a SUD, as defined by standard diagnostic systems such as the DSM-IV.[57] For example, describing the symptoms of *substance abuse* and *substance dependence* can help service users recognize when their use is not normative and constitutes a treatable disorder.

A key goal of education is to mobilize hope for an improved quality of life and recovery from substance use problems. Service users with co-occurring disorders frequently suffer from depression, demoralization and suicidal thinking.[58] Developing a sense of hope for the service user and for everyone involved with him or her, including the belief in every person's inherent ability to recover, can instill hope in people who have given up. Electronic decision-making supports can be very helpful for creating hope by providing service users with information about treatment options and recovery, and through the use of service user testimonials that chronicle the recovery experiences of others with co-occurring disorders who have gotten better and improved their lives.

Example

Ruth, a 41-year-old woman with bipolar disorder who was receiving services at her local community mental health center, was identified by routine screening and substance use assessment to have a current alcohol abuse diagnosis. In order to provide Ruth with more information about her alcohol use problems, her clinician explored with her whether she would prefer participating in an educational group about co-occurring disorders or meeting individually with her clinician to learn more about these types of problems and their treatments. Ruth was surprised to hear that many people with serious psychiatric disorders have problems related to substance use, and she elected to participate in the group education program in order to hear about others' experiences. Ruth found that the educational program, which lasted for eight sessions over a one-month period, was informative and hopeful, and she was encouraged to learn that there are effective treatments for overcoming her alcohol use problems and regaining control of her life.

Step 3: Personal preferences

Educating service users about co-occurring disorders can be a delicate matter, since they can be easily put off by providing more information than they want or can assimilate at one point in time, leading to confusion, disengagement or denial. Attention to personal preferences for more information on environmental, social, psychological and biological risk factors for SUDs can help service users understand the nature of their problems and generate hope for recovery without overwhelming them. Electronic decision support systems can be especially useful for attending to service users' preferences by giving them control over the information they want in a timely fashion, provided in manageable chunks with the option to take a break, review, continue with more information or stop at any point. Providing service users with the option of learning more about common reasons for using substances, and identifying their own motives for using, can help them balance the information about negative consequences of use and give them a more complete understanding of their own circumstances. Electronic decision supports can also be used to help service users weigh information about the positive and negative effects of substance use, as well as the expected benefits and costs of sobriety, i.e. decisional balance, to facilitate making a personal decision about whether to change their substance use habits.[59]

Personal preferences are also critical to the process of learning about different treatment options. After understanding more about co-occurring disorders, and weighing the pros and cons of using vs. sobriety, service users often become interested in addressing their substance use problems. Electronic decision supports can be used to provide service users with information about their treatment options. Our experience is that service users take different paths to recovery and express strong preferences for different treatments, such as medications, e.g. naltrexone, disulfiram, group interventions, self-help groups, individual work and residential treatment. Supporting these preferences enhances service users' motivation and adherence to the treatments they choose and fosters the therapeutic alliance with the service provider.

Example

Isaac had a severe major depression that was complicated by a poly-substance use disorder that included at various times abusing alcohol, cocaine, marijuana and heroin. After Isaac's SUD was identified, his clinician introduced him to an electronic decision support system to learn more about his substance use problems and different treatment options. Isaac liked the electronic decision support system because it gave him the freedom to learn more and explore about his use of substances at his own leisure and that he could review information whenever he wanted, without feeling under any pressure from someone else. Isaac still met with his clinician regularly, when they would touch on the material covered in the electronic decision support system and address questions that Isaac had. Isaac liked learning more about his own reasons for using substances, which included trying to escape his depressive feelings, having something to do when he felt bored and using when he hung out with friends. Understanding that other people use substances for similar reasons made Isaac feel more "normal," and he was encouraged to hear that he could learn new strategies to deal with his depression and to find fun things to do with other people aside from using substances. When Isaac reviewed his different options, he decided that he would like to learn more about participating in a group on coping with co-occurring disorders at the mental health center. He also expressed an interest in learning more about a local self-help group in the community for people with an addiction.

Step 4: Treatment planning

Effective intervention for co-occurring disorders requires the integrated treatment of mental health and SUDs at the clinical level in order to maintain engagement in treatment and avoid the fragmentation of service delivery.[60] A wide range of different treatment options are now available for people with co-occurring disorders.[61] Although the exact services available to service users may differ from one agency to another, a growing list of interventions is gaining support, including a variety of group interventions,[62] individual motivational interviewing and cognitive-behavioral therapy,[63] pharmacological treatment,[64] residential treatment[65] and contingent reinforcement.[66] Electronic decision supports can be used to familiarize service users with the different treatment options available to them, without obligating them to a particular course of action before they are ready. The use of these supports can further facilitate collaborative treatment planning when they are reviewed jointly by the service user and service provider, and also when they are evaluated in the context of the service user's overall personal treatment goals, which are often unrelated to substance abuse per se, e.g. getting a job, independent living, being a better parent and having a rewarding relationship.

Example

Allison recently developed a schizophreniform disorder during her first year of college at the age of 20, which interfered with her studies and led her to drop out and return home to receive treatment. Before her psychotic episode, Allison smoked cannabis with her friends, which she continued to do after her episode, and which tended to interfere with the stabilization of her symptoms and efforts to resume her studies at a local community college. After Alice's cannabis use was detected, she was provided with information about the interactions between psycho-sis and substance use, and then about different treatment options for changing her cannabis use habits and achieving her goals. After considering a variety of treatment options, Allison decided to try a family psychoeducation program first because she lived with her parents and she said that her cannabis use was a source of conflict with them; she felt that they were supportive of her goal of returning to college.[67]

Step 5: Monitoring participation and outcomes

Once a treatment plan has been agreed upon, ongoing monitoring is needed to determine whether the service user is participating in it as intended, and whether outcomes are improving. Although such monitoring is critical even in the absence of computer technology, electronic decision-making systems have particular advantages over traditional monitoring methods. These systems can be designed to track participation in treatment and to incorporate routine outcome data based on inputs from both the service user and service provider. Collaborative review of involvement in treatment and substance abuse and mental health outcomes can be facilitated by programming the electronic decision-making system to periodically summarize the relevant data. This review can be used by the service provider and service user to evaluate whether the treatment plan is working or if any changes in course are called for.

Example

Fred had bipolar disorder, alcohol dependence and abused cannabis. After receiving information about his co-occurring disorders from his mental health treatment providers, and learning about and exploring different treatment options, Fred decided to participate in a group specifically for people with bipolar disorder and addiction.[68] Fred's participation in this group and his substance use were monitored regularly with an electronic decision support system, which he periodically reviewed, as did his treatment team. A review of Fred's progress at six months indicated that he had been regularly participating in the group and that over the past few months he had reduced and then stopped using cocaine completely. However, although he attempted to stop drinking several times over these months, each time he quickly relapsed and returned to his former level of drinking. Fred was helped to use the electronic decision support system to consider other possible treatments for his alcohol dependence. After reviewing the different options, Fred elected to talk to the psychiatrist about trying naltrexone, a medication that has been shown to reduce relapses in people with alcohol dependence and psychiatric disorders.[69]

Stages of Treatment and Recovery

How do people change unhealthy habits and behaviors to healthier ones? Or in the case of people faced with a persistent illness or illnesses, such as co-occurring disorders, how do they learn how to manage their disorders in order to pursue their own meaning of recovery, and what is the role of the service provider in this process? Over 20 years ago the *stages of change* concept was proposed to describe a series of discrete motivational states people pass through in the process of changing their behavior, including *precontemplation, contemplation* of change, *preparation* for change, *action*, and *maintenance* of change.[70,71] The concept of stages of change has been adapted to describe similar motivational states that people pass through in the process of recovery from co-occurring disorders, or the *stages of treatment.*[72,73] The heuristic value of the stages of treatment is that it addresses how treatment providers can optimize their effectiveness by recognizing the service user's motivational stage of change and providing intervention that is appropriately geared to helping the service user move onto the next stage.

A core feature of the stages of treatment concept is that motivation to address substance use behaviors is most effectively harnessed by working with service users on areas that they most want to change, such as housing, work, social relationships, illness management and health. As service users are helped to make improvements in these important areas of their lives, awareness of the negative effects of substance use grows, and with it motivation of work on their substance use problems. Electronic decision-making systems can be designed to facilitate the change process based on the stages of treatment. We describe the stages of treatment below, focusing on SUDs, although the same principles apply to helping service users learn how to manage their psychiatric disorder. We illustrate each stage with a brief demonstration based on the example of "Jerome."

The first stage of treatment is the *engagement stage*, which assumes that a therapeutic relationship or working alliance must first be established before the service provider can help the service user change his or her life. The goal of this stage can be pragmatically set as the service provider seeing the service user on a regular basis, which can be accomplished through a variety of strategies, such as assertive outreach, providing practical assistance, social network support, exploring with the service user his or her concept of recovery, and personal recovery goals.

Example

Jerome had an SMI, complicated by polysubstance abuse that had led to him losing his housing and becoming homeless. Although Jerome was a client at a local community mental health center, he rarely attended the center and had infrequent contact with his treatment team. In order to reengage Jerome in treatment, his case manager began to visit him on the street or in homeless shelters, listen to his concerns and help him get some of this needs met. For example, she arranged for Jerome to see a dentist in order to replace his dentures, which he had lost, and she began to identify possible apartments where he could live and receive supported housing services.[74] After several weeks, Jerome and his case manager were meeting regularly, once or twice per week.

The *persuasion stage* follows, which assumes that actually helping a person change first requires the person to *want* to change. The goal of this stage is to instill motivation for recovery from co-occurring disorders before attempting to change any behaviors, through the use of strategies such as education about dual disorders, motivational interviewing, i.e. developing discrepancy between the person's values and goals and their continued use of substances and poor mental illness self-management; decisional balance, i.e. weighing the pros and cons of using substances versus sobriety; and rehabilitation to teach coping and other adaptive skills that reduce service users' reliance on using substances for getting their needs met. Persuasion-stage interventions are most effective when they are provided in the context of helping the service user pursue and attain personally meaningful recovery goals. A wide range of treatment modalities are useful at this stage, including individual, group and family approaches, and electronic decision-making systems can be used as one means of educating service users about their disorders and facilitating exploration of different treatment options.

When Jerome was engaged in treatment and his living situation had been stabilized, his case manager arranged for him to meet with his psychiatrist again to evaluate his medication needs. This psychiatrist prescribed Jerome an antipsychotic medication; this reduced his distressing auditory hallucinations, which he often used substances to cope with, and which improved his attention span. Jerome's case manager began to provide him with information about his mental illness and how it interacted with substance abuse. In the case manager's meetings with Jerome, she also continued to use motivational interviewing techniques begun in the engagement stage,[75] with an initial emphasis on demonstrating empathy and seeking to understand Jerome's world, before moving onto exploring some of his personal goals or unfulfilled desires. One particular desire to which Jerome resonated especially strongly was wanting to reconnect with his 12-year-old son, whom he had not seen for five years. Further exploration with Jerome led him to begin to see that his continued substance abuse was interfering with his goal of reconnecting with his son, i.e. "developing discrepancy," a motivational interviewing technique, since he wanted to present himself as a good role model to his son, and this included living stably, taking care of himself and having a job. Jerome started to contemplate cutting down on his substance use. Jerome's case manager explored some of his ambivalence about changing his substance use and worked with him to address some of his concerns. For example, she taught him some sleep hygiene skills so that he could get to sleep without drinking until he passed out, and she supported his self-efficacy that he was capable of reducing or stopping his use of substances in order to reconnect with his son. Over a period of several weeks, Jerome began to cut down on his substance use.

When service users are motivated to reduce their substance use, as indicated by efforts to do so, they enter the *active treatment stage*, in which the goal shifts to helping them make the desired changes while maintaining the focus on the person's recovery goals. Achieving such changes may involve a host of activities focused directly on reducing or stopping substance use, preventing relapses and coping with cravings, as well as other efforts aimed at helping the person develop a rewarding and sober lifestyle necessary to achieve personal goals, such as SE, safe housing and satisfying social relationships. As a multitude of treatment options exist at this stage, electronic decision-making systems can be useful in helping service users and service providers sort out the different options together, establish treatment plans, and monitor their success or change them as needed.

As Jerome began to reduce his substance use, his case manager gradually shifted attention to helping him change his substance use behavior. She reviewed with Jerome a variety of treatment options for helping him gain control over his substance use, thereby helping him achieve his personal goals. Based on these discussions, Jerome chose three options. First, he began to participate in a group at the center for service users with a co-occurring disorder who shared the goal of reducing or stopping their use of substances. Second, Jerome chose to participate in the IMR program in order to learn how to manage his psychiatric illness more effectively, including developing new coping strategies for dealing with symptoms that he sometimes attempt to "self-medicate." Third, Jerome decided to start looking for a job because it would give him something to do with his time instead of using substances, and it would make him feel proud of himself when he reconnected with his son. To achieve this goal, Jerome enrolled in an SE program.[76] Over the next several months Jerome continued to work on reducing his substance use. At first he did not want to stop using substances completely and only wanted to "control" his use. However, Jerome experienced great difficulty limiting his substance use and eventually concluded that the only way for him to control his use was to stop using altogether.

The *relapse prevention stage* follows after the service user has succeeded in changing his or her substance use behavior, in which the focus shifts to maintaining the gains the service user has made. This is accomplished through a combination of developing relapse prevention plans, e.g. identifying high-risk situations, dealing with offers or urges to use; ensuring ample social supports for sobriety, e.g. involvement in self-help groups for addiction or co-occurring disorders; and continued work towards the service user's personal recovery goals. As in the active treatment stage, electronic decision supports can play an important role in helping service providers collaborate with service users in weighing the different treatment options, selecting interventions and monitoring their outcomes.

Jerome continued to participate in the three programs that he began in the active treatment stage. When he stopped using substances, his case manager helped him develop a relapse prevention plan. Jerome was also successful in obtaining a job with the help of his SE specialist. Based on his progress in achieving sobriety and getting a job, Jerome felt ready to meet his son again. Jerome's case manager offered to contact his ex-partner to arrange a meeting.

Advantages for the Service User

The use of electronic decision supports affords a number of advantages to providing PCC to service users. As computers become an increasingly established technology used in all walks of life, service users are often comfortable interacting with computers and using them to obtain information and achieve goals. Electronic decision support systems can facilitate the provision of PCC, because service users can more readily access information and self-management tools on their own terms from computers as compared to clinicians, and service users can review these materials whenever they want. This may have particular relevance for service users with SMI, who are often anxious around other people and lack interpersonal skills, which can lead to feeling uncomfortable interacting with service providers, or avoiding them altogether. For this reason, service users report high satisfaction when completing computer-based assessments compared to in-person interviews.[77] Furthermore, using electronic decision supports collaboratively with a service provider may foster the development of a trusting, therapeutic relationship by mutually engaging through a technology designed to be used together for the service user's benefit, providing a shared focus of attention on tasks of agreed importance.[78]

Another advantage of electronic decision supports is that they make it easy for service users to access and review information about their disorders, treatment options and progress on an as-needed basis, without solely relying on their service provider. Service users with SMI often have information-processing limitations that make it difficult for them to absorb and integrate large amounts of information. Providing them with the ability to pace their own learning and to review information whenever necessary gives them greater control over their own treatment and may contribute to better self-efficacy. Similarly, teaching service users how to track their own participation in planned treatment and progress towards personal goals can serve to better invest them in their own recovery process, and to view service providers as functioning in a more collaborative and less hierarchical or coercive fashion.

Electronic decision support systems can also be changed and updated as new information becomes available. For example, in the future individualized risk-benefit information about different treatment options and expected outcomes could be provided to service users based on personal information such as their substance use pattern and factors related to their psychological functioning, social relationships, environment and even genetic profile. Thus, electronic decision support systems are well-suited for reducing the lag between scientific progress and access to new and personally relevant information for service users.

Advantages for the Service Provider

Many of the same advantages to service users of using electronic decision supports have similar benefits to service providers. For example, computers can be used to facilitate development of the therapeutic relationship, to reduce reliance of service users on service providers as the primary source of information about co-occurring disorders, and to ensure collaboration with the service user in treatment planning and monitoring progress towards personal goals, enabling the service provider to share the tasks of treatment rather than shouldering most of the responsibility alone. Obtaining data directly from service users through these systems can alleviate the burden of data collection on service providers, freeing up their time for more meaningful discussions with service users about their goals and treatment options.

Service providers also benefit from receiving feedback about service users' participation in treatment and outcomes. While such feedback can be obtained in the absence of a decision support system, the use of an electronic support system can facilitate the routine collection and review of data by programming the necessary prompts to both service user and service provider to input relevant data, summarizing the data and prompting regular review of treatment participation and outcome. These are advantages for mental health administrators as well, since they permit the aggregation of data across multiple service users and the evaluation of the effectiveness of programming for co-occurring disorders. Using computers to help prompt and collect relevant information may also result in more reliable information and reduce interpersonal tension related to feelings of shame and guilt service users may experience when they do not follow through on treatment plans or make expected progress towards goals, since the information is not obtained directly from the service user by the service provider.

Finally, decision support systems can be programmed to ensure that service providers are aware of, and review with service users, the full range of treatment options available at their particular stage of treatment. Since decision-making is shared, service users need to know what their options are, yet service providers are not always aware of all the options. In addition to ensuring that service users are informed about different treatment options, electronic decision support systems can be programmed to incorporate new information and treatment options as they become available. This permits the service provider (and service user) to remain abreast of new treatment developments as they become available, minimizing the traditionally slow "trickle down" of new information from research to the treatment agency to the service provider and service user.

CONCLUSION

Co-occurring substance use and serious psychiatric disorders present multiple challenges to service users and service providers alike. Service providers often do not take a person-centered, recovery-based approach to working with service users that is aimed at addressing their own priorities and helping them achieve their own goals. Service providers are unaware of or fail to provide EBP for treating co-occurring disorders, and service users are not given information about the nature of their disorders and different treatment options. As a result of these deficiencies, clinical decision-making is typically not person-centered and shared with service users, it varies widely between different service providers, and service users often have minimal investment and follow-through on their own treatment plans. Advances in information technology have the potential to overcome all of these problems through the development of electronic decision support systems.[79]

Providing information to service users with SMI about substance use problems, different treatment options, testimonials from other service users, and likely outcomes can ensure a more person-centered approach to care by instilling hope for recovery in service users and invest them in their own treatment. Electronic decision support systems can also foster a more person-centered approach to treatment (by providing service users with ready access to a broad range of information about the nature of co-occurring disorders and their treatment) than has traditionally been available and provide a venue for service users to express their personal preferences, while not eliminating traditional in-person approaches that some service users may prefer over computer-based systems. The sharing of decision-making between the service user and service provider, facilitated through electronic decision supports, acknowledges the complexities inherent in treating and recovering from co-occurring disorders, and the necessity of establishing a collaborative approach to treatment, which is part of PCC.

REFERENCES

1 American Psychiatric Association. Diagnostic and Statistical Manual of Mental Disorders, 4th Edition. Washington, DC: American Psychiatric Association; 1994.

2 Dixon L, Medoff DR, Wohlheiter K, *et al.* Correlates of severity of smoking among persons with severe mental illness. *American Journal on Addictions.* 2007; **16**: 101–10.

3 Kessler RC, Bergland P, Demler O, *et al.* Lifetime prevalence and age-of-onset distributions of DSM-IV disorders in the National Comorbidity Survey Replication. *Archives of General Psychiatry.* 2005; **62**: 593–602.

4 Regier DA, Farmer ME, Rae DS, *et al.* Comorbidity of mental disorders with alcohol and other drug abuse: results from the Epidemiologic Catchment Area (ECA) study. *Journal of the American Medical Association.* 1990; **264**(19): 2511–18.

5 Teeson M, Hall W, Lynskey M, *et al.* Alcohol and drug use disorders in Australia: implications of the National Survey of Mental Health and Wellbeing. *Australian and New Zealand Journal of Psychiatry.* 2000; **34**: 206–13.

6 Linszen D, Dingemans P, Lenior M. Cannabis abuse and the course of recent onset schizophrenic disorders. *Arch Gen Psych.* 1994; **51**(4): 273–9.

7 Drake RE, Osher FC, Wallach MA. Homelessness and dual diagnosis. *Am Psychol.* 1991; **46**(11): 1149–58.

8 Susser E, Struening EL, Conover S. Psychiatric problems in homeless men: lifetime psychosis, substance use, and current distress in new arrivals at New York City shelters. *Arch Gen Psych.* 1989; **46**(9): 845–50.

9 Peters RH, Greenbaum PE, Edens JF, *et al.* Prevalence of DSM-IV substance abuse and dependence disorders among prison inmates. *American Journal of Drug and Alcohol Abuse.* 1998; **24**(4): 573–87.

10 McLellan AT, Lewis DC, O'Brien CP, *et al.* Drug dependence, a chronic medical illness: implications for treatment, insurance, and outcomes evaluation. *JAMA.* 2000; **284**(13): 1689–95.

11 Harris M, Fallot RD, Berley RW. Qualitative interviews on substance abuse relapse and prevention among female trauma survivors. *Psychiatr Servs.* 2005; **56**(10): 1292–5.

12 McGovern MP, Wrisley BR. Relapse of substance use disorder and its prevention among persons with co-occurring disorders. *Psychiatr Serv.* 2005; **56**(10): 1270–3.

13 Rollins AL, O'Neill SJ, Davis KE, *et al.* Substance abuse relapse and factors associated with relapse in an inner-city sample of patients with dual diagnoses. *Psychiatr Serv.* 2005; **56**(10): 1274–81.

14 Xie H, McHugo GJ, Fox MB, *et al.* Substance abuse relapse in a ten-year prospective follow-up of clients with mental and substance use disorders. *Psychiatr Serv.* 2005; **56**(10): 182–97.

15 Wagner EH, Bennett SM, Austin BT, *et al.* Finding common ground: patient centeredness and evidence-based chronic illness care. *J Altern Complement Med.* 2005; **11**(Suppl. 1): S7–15.

16 Coleman K, Mattke S, Perrault PJ, *et al.* Untangling practice redesign from disease management: how do we best care for the chronically ill? *Annu Rev Public Health.* 2009; **30**: 385–408.

17 17. Deegan PE. Recovery: the lived experience of rehabilitation. *Psychosocial Rehabilitation Journal.* 1988; **11**: 11–19.

18 Jacobson N, Greenley D. What is recovery? A conceptual model and explication. *Psychiatr Serv.* 2001; **52**(4): 482–5.

19 Fisher DB. Health care reform based on an empowerment model of recovery by people with psychiatric disabilities. *Hosp Community Psychiatry.* 1994; **45**(9): 913–15.

20 Frese FJI. Self-help activities. In: Mueser KT, Jeste DV, editors. *Clinical Handbook of Schizophrenia.* New York, NY: Guilford Press; 2008. pp. 298–305.

21 Mead S, Copeland ME. What recovery means to us: consumers' perspectives. *Community Ment Health J.* 2000; **36**(3): 315–28.

22 Ralph RO, Kidder K, Phillips D. *Can We Measure Recovery? A Compendium of Recovery and Recovery-Related Instruments.* Cambridge, MA: The Evaluation Center at Human Services Research Institute; 2000.

23 Anthony WA. A recovery-oriented service system: setting some system level standards. *Journal of Psychiatric Rehabilitation.* 2000; **24**: 159–68.

24 Davidson L, Tondora J, Lawless MS, *et al. A Practical Guide to Recovery-Oriented Practice: tools for transforming mental health care.* New York, NY: Oxford University Press; 2009.

25 Liberman RP, Kopelowicz A, Ventura J, *et al.* Operational criteria and factors related to recovery from schizophrenia. *International Review of Psychiatry.* 2002; **14**: 256–72.

26 Noordsy DL, Torrey WC, Mueser KT, *et al.* Recovery from severe mental illness: an interpersonal and functional outcome definition. *International Review of Psychiatry.* 2002; **14**: 318–26.

27 Leete E. How I perceive and manage my illness. *Schizophr Bull.* 1989; **15**(2): 197–200.

28 Deegan PE, Rapp CA, Holter M, *et al.* Best practices: a program to support shared decision making in an outpatient psychiatric medication clinic. *Psychiatr Serv.* 2008; **59**(6): 603–5.

29 Institute of Medicine. *Crossing the Quality Chasm: a new health system for the 21st century.* Washington, DC: National Academy Press; 2001.

30 US Surgeon General. *Mental Health: a report of the Surgeon General.* Rockville, MD: U.S. Department of Health and Human Services; 1999.

31 President's New Freedom Commission on Mental Health. *Achieving the Promise: Transforming Mental Health Care in America: Final Report.* Rockville, MD: Substance Abuse and Mental Health Services Administration; 2003.

32 Sackett DL, Richardson WS, Rosenberg W, *et al. Evidence-Based Medicine.* New York, NY: Churchill Livingstone; 1997.

33 O'Connor AM, Stacey D, Entwistle V, *et al.* Decision aids for people facing health treatment or screening decisions. *Cochrane Database of Systematic Reviews.* 2003; **2**: CD001431.

34 O'Connor AM, Wennberg JE, Legare F, *et al.* Toward the "tipping point": decision aids and informed patient choice. *Health Affairs.* 2007; **26**: 16–25.

35 Wennberg JE, O'Connor AM, Collins ED, *et al.* Extending the P4P Agenda, Part 1: how Medicare can improve patient decision making and reduce unnecessary care. *Health Affairs.* 2007; **26**: 1564–7.

36 Charles C, Gafni A, Whelan T. Shared decision-making in the medical encounter: what does it mean? (or it takes at least two to tango). *Soc Sci Med.* 1997; **44**(5): 681–92.

37 Charles C, Gafni A, Whelan T. Decision-making in the physician-patient encounter: revisiting the shared treatment decision-making model. *Soc Sci Med.* 1999; **49**(5): 651–61.

38 Wennberg JE, O'Connor AM, Collins ED, *et al.*, op. cit.

39 Adams JR, Drake RE. Shared decision-making and evidence-based practice. *Community Ment Health J.* 2006; **42**(1): 87–105.

40 Fenton WS. Shared decision making: a model for the physician-patient relationship in the 21st century? *Acta Psychiatr Scand.* 2003; **107**(6): 401–2.

41 Hamann J, Leucht S, Kissling W. Shared decision making in psychiatry. *Acta Psychiatr Scand.* 2003; **107**(6): 403–9.

42 Priebe S, Broker M, Gunkel S. Involuntary admission and posttraumatic stress disorder symptoms in schizophrenia patients. *Compr Psychiatry.* 1998; **39**(4): 220–4.

43 Dietrich AJ, Oxman TE, Williams JWJ, *et al.* Re-engineering systems for the primary care treatment of depression: a cluster randomized controlled trial. *BMJ.* 2004; **329**: 602–5.

44 Wolford G, Rosenberg SD, Rosenberg HJ, *et al.* A clinical trial comparing interviewer and computer-assisted assessment in clients with severe mental illness. *Psychiatr Serv.* 2008; **59**(7): 769–75.

45 Montori VM, Gafni A, Charles C. A shared treatment decision-making approach between patients with chronic conditions and their clinicians: the case of diabetes. *Health Expectations.* 2006; **9**: 25–36.

46 Mueser KT, Noordsy DL, Drake RE, *et al. Integrated Treatment for Dual Disorders: a guide to effective practice.* New York, NY: Guilford Press; 2003.

47 Maisto SA, Carey MP, Carey KB, *et al.* Use of the AUDIT and the DAST-10 to identify alcohol and drug use disorders among adults with a severe and persistent mental illness. *Psychological Assessment.* 2000; **12**: 186–92.

48 Rosenberg SD, Drake RE, Wolford GL, *et al.* The Dartmouth Assessment of Lifestyle Instrument (DALI): a substance use disorder screen for people with severe mental illness. *Am J Psychiatry.* 1998; **155**: 232–8.

49 Mueser, Noordsy, Drake, *et al.*, 2003, op. cit.

50 Carey KB, Carey MP, Maisto SA, *et al.* Temporal stability of the Timeline Followback Interview for alcohol and drug use with psychiatric outpatients. *J Stud Alcohol.* 2004; **65**(6): 774–81.

51 Turner CF, Ku L, Rogers SM, *et al.* Adolescent sexual behavior, drug use, and violence: increased reporting with computer technology. *Science.* 1998; **280**: 86–73.

52 Waterton JJ, Duffy JC. A comparison of computer interviewing techniques and traditional methods in the collection of self-report alcohol consumption data in a field survey. *International Statistical Review.* 1984; **52**: 173–82.

53 Rosenberg, Drake, Wolford, *et al.*, op. cit.

54 Mueser, Noordsy, Drake, *et al.*, 2003, op. cit.

55 Zubin J, Spring B. Vulnerability: a new view of schizophrenia. *Journal of Abnormal Psychology.* 1977; **86**: 103–26.

56 Mueser KT, Drake RE, Wallach MA. Dual diagnosis: a review of etiological theories. *Addictive Behaviors.* 1998; **23**: 717–34.

57 American Psychiatric Association, op. cit.

58 Bartels SJ, Drake RE, McHugo G. Alcohol use, depression, and suicidal behavior in schizophrenia. *Am J Psych.* 1992; **149**(3): 394–5.

59 Mueser, Noordsy, Drake, *et al.*, 2003, op. cit.

60 Ibid.

61 Drake RE, O'Neal E, Wallach MA. A systematic review of psychosocial interventions for people with co-occurring severe mental and substance use disorders. *J Subst Abuse Treat.* 2008; **34**(1): 123–38.

62 Mueser KT, Drake RE, Sigmon SC, *et al.* Psychosocial interventions for adults with severe mental illnesses and co-occurring substance use disorders: a review of specific interventions. *J Dual Diagn.* 2009; **1**: 57–82.

63 Barrowclough C, Haddock G, Tarrier N, *et al.* Randomized controlled trial of motivational interviewing, cognitive behavior therapy, and family intervention for patients with comorbid schizophrenia and substance use disorders. *Am J Psychiatry.* 2001; **158**(10): 1706–13.

64 Green AI, Noordsy DL, Brunette MF, *et al.* Substance abuse and schizophrenia: pharmacotherapeutic intervention. *Am J Psychiatry.* 2001; **158**: 1706–13.

65 Brunette MF, Mueser KT, Drake RE. A review of research on residential programs for people with severe mental illness and co-occurring substance use disorders. *Drug Alcohol Rev.* 2004; **23**(4): 471–81.

66 Sigmon SC, Higgins ST. Voucher-based contingent reinforcement of marijuana abstinence among individuals with serious mental illness. *J Subst Abuse Treat.* 2006; **30**(4): 291–5.

67 Mueser KT, Fox L. A family intervention program for dual disorders. *Community Ment Health J.* 2002; **38**(3): 253–70.

68 Weiss RD, Connery HS. *Integrated Group Therapy for Bipolar Disorder and Substance Abuse.* New York, NY: Guilford Press; 2011.

69 Petrakis IL, Nich C, Ralevski E. Psychotic spectrum disorders and alcohol abuse: a review of pharmacotherapeutic strategies and a report on the effectiveness of naltrexone and disulfiram. *Schizophr Bull.* 2006; **32**(4): 644–54.

70 DiClemente CC, Prochaska JO. Toward a comprehensive, transtheoretical model of change: stages of change and addictive behaviors. In: Miller WR, Heather N, editors. *Treating Addictive Behaviors.* 2nd ed. New York: Plenum Press; 1998. pp. 3–24.

71 Prochaska JO, DiClemente CC. *The Transtheoretical Approach: crossing the traditional boundaries of therapy.* Homewood, IL: Dow-Jones/Irwin; 1984.

72 Mueser, Noordsy, Drake, *et al.*, 2003, op. cit.

73 Osher FC, Kofoed LL. Treatment of patients with psychiatric and psychoactive substance use disorders. *Hospital and Community Psychiatry.* 1989; **40**(10): 1025–30.

74 Kloos B, Zimmerman SO, Scrimenti K, *et al.* Landlords as partners for promoting success in supported housing: "it takes more than a lease and a key." *Psychiatr Rehabil J.* 2002; **25**(3): 235–44.

75 Miller WR, Rollnick S, editors. *Motivational Interviewing: preparing people for change.* 2nd ed. New York, NY: Guilford Press; 2002.

76 Becker DR, Drake RE, Naughton WJ Jr. Supported employment for people with co-occurring disorders. *Psychiatr Rehabil J.* 2005; **28**(4): 332–8.

77 Wolford, Rosenberg, Rosenberg, *et al.*, 2008, op. cit.

78 Horvath AO, Greenberg LS. Development and validation of the Working Alliance Inventory. *Journal of Counseling Psychology.* 1989; **36**(2): 223–33.

79 Drake RE, Deegan PE, Woltmann EM, *et al.* Comprehensive electronic decision support systems. *Psychiatr Serv.* 2010; **61**: 714–17.

CHAPTER 6

Management and Finding Common Ground

This (sixth) chapter of the book addresses clinical procedures – assessments and interventions – in relation to people with SMI. It is related to other chapters of this book, such as Chapter 2, Magnitude of the Problem; Chapter 3, The Person's Experience of the Illness; Chapter 4, Understanding the Context of the Individual; and Chapter 5, The Person/Patient-Provider/Clinician Relationship. This is because providing care for people with SMI from a PCC perspective has to be compatible with knowledge of the disorder, with subjective illness experiences, with relevant environmental factors, with processes of care, and with special populations that may require some PCC modifications due to their particular challenges. Also, finding common ground with service users in relation to the management of their SMI may be more or less challenging from a PCC perspective, depending on personal and environmental factors such as cultural differences between service users and providers, which can be addressed and accommodated. This is an illustration that clinical aspects of PCC are closely linked to other aspects of PCC.

Section 6.1, *Person-Centered Assessment of People with Serious Mental Illness,* argues for PCA as an important component of PCC, as it is one of the important first steps in the development of a PCC plan, and notes that there is limited systematic information in the literature regarding this important component. The section focuses on what and how can be utilized in a PCA and the challenges providers face when conducting a PCA with persons with SMI. Section 6.2, *Person-Centered Approaches to Psychopharmacology for People with Serious Mental Illness,* addresses psychotropic medications as well as other biological interventions such as ECT in relation to PCC for people with SMI. The section also addresses adherence to (or concordance with) medications and capacity to consent to or refuse treatment. Section 6.3, *Person-Centered Individual Psychotherapy for Adults with Serious Mental Illness,* explores one way of conceptualizing a person-centered approach to individual psychotherapy for persons with SMI. The section focuses on the subjective experience of a diminished sense of self and how to try to improve that experience; it also suggests principles and outcome assessment in relation to such a psychotherapy. Section 6.4, *Cognitive and Psychiatric Rehabilitation: person-centered ingredients for success,* describes cognitive and PSR interventions to improve functioning and quality of life of people with SMI. The section highlights three key elements that center on the person and that are thought to contribute to the success of these interventions: readiness, cognitive remediation and peer support.

6.1 Person-Centered Assessment of People with Serious Mental Illness

Parmjit Sanghera, Abraham Rudnick and Deborah J. Corring

INTRODUCTION: THE ROLES OF ASSESSMENT IN PERSON-CENTERED CARE

The primary purpose of assessment in PCC for people with SMI is to assist with care planning. During the assessment, goals are formulated and interventions are planned. Assessments can also monitor the person's responsiveness to the care provided, which in turn may lead to the modification of goals to ensure their continued appropriateness. Assessments can also include the administration of measures to aid program evaluation and research. Specific services that may necessitate increased resources and equipment can thus continue to be funded. In this section we explore how a PCA differs from more traditional biomedical assessments usually employed in clinical settings. We then discuss how PCAs can be classified, and this is followed by an analysis of the various components and processes which underlie a PCA. Note that many other sections in this book are relevant to this section, such as Section 6.2, *Person-Centered Approaches to Psychopharmacology for People with Serious Mental Illness*, Section 6.3, *Person-Centered Individual Psychotherapy for Adults with Serious Mental Illness* and Section 6.4, *Cognitive and Psychiatric Rehabilitation: person-centered ingredients for success* (which assessment serves); hence the reader is referred to those sections for complementary reading.

Person-Centered Approach versus Biomedical Assessment

The biomedical model, also referred to as the disease model, is the traditional and dominant approach adopted in many clinical settings. This approach minimizes the human element and focuses on accurate diagnoses and completing the agenda of the health care provider. In contrast, PCA highlights the humanistic characteristics of the person and involves them in the assessment process. The health care provider attempts to set the agenda and goals collaboratively with the person,[1] to tailor the assessment to the person's goals and circumstances, e.g. assessing areas of daily functioning that are relevant to the person's actual and planned living situation, rather than all areas of daily functioning. Levenstein *et al.*[2] add that at the basis of the PCA are characteristics and skills that each health care provider must possess and convey during the assessment process. These include: empathy, genuineness, a non-judgmental manner, listening skills, forming a rapport and asking pertinent questions.

A PCA provides persons with SMI opportunities to discuss their beliefs and experiences in relation to their illness. A study by Fiscella[3] found that a person's trust was associated with the exploration of the person's perception of the illness by the health care provider. In general, a PCA aligns with a recovery approach, which focuses on the personal meaning and valued social roles of individuals with SMI.[4] It should be noted that both PCA and the more biomedical approach to assessment of people with SMI are faced with the fact that mental health-related assessment is still mostly based on symptoms, i.e. subjective reports (and in the case of SMI, these would include reports of mental health challenges). This is in contrast to assessment in most other areas of health, which is largely based on laboratory and other test results and signs, i.e. systematic examination by physicians and other clinicians, which is presumably more objective and hence purportedly more valid. Although subjectivity may be considered a constraint on mental health-related assessment, it should be recognized that such subjective information is no less important than so-called objective information for mental health-related assessment and care based on it. It should also be recognized that some mental health-related assessment is not subjective, in that it is conducted by physicians or other clinicians, as in some clinician-rated standardized questionnaires and interviews, and that some mental health-related assessment, such as neurocognitive testing, is akin to validated and normalized laboratory tests more than to subjective reports. A balance of more and less subjective mental health-related assessments may be optimal for people with SMI.

Classification of Person-Centered Approach

Any assessment or evaluation can be viewed as consisting of a structure and a process. The structure consists of the variables, or more generally the issues, that are assessed, and the values of those variables, or more generally the data, that are found as a result of the assessment. The process has some aspects that are generic, such as obtaining voluntary informed consent, and some aspects that are specific to particular assessments, such as standardization of assessment conditions in psychological testing. Process will be addressed later in this section.

PCA (particularly person-reported outcomes) in relation to SMI such as schizophrenia can be classified as evaluation of illness and of benefit from care – pertaining to need for care, satisfaction from care, experience of the therapeutic relationship, experience of mental health and attitudes towards care – and evaluation of resilience of the self – pertaining to empowerment, self-esteem, sense of coherence and recovery.[5] PCA can also be classified according to the type and extent of involvement of the assessed person. Type of involvement addresses involvement in variables/issues and/or in values/data. Extent of involvement addresses involvement by informing or by determining variables/issues and/or values/data. This classification generates a matrix, as presented in Table 6.1 (in which specific assessments are used for illustration). Note that assessments in which the assessed person informs the values/data are *clinician-rated*, or more generally, *other-rated*, as the assessed person provides information about himself or herself, and the clinician uses that information with other

TABLE 6.1 Classification of PCA

	Variables/Issues	Values/Data
Informing	Hypothetical (service user informs the variables/issues with or without determining the values/data)	BPRS* (clinician-rated/other-rated, i.e. information is obtained from the service user during PCA)
Determining	GAS** (service user determines the variables/issues)	BDI***; GAS** (self-report/self-rated, i.e. the service user determines the values/data)

* Brief Psychiatric Rating Scale (BPRS); ** Goal Attainment Scaling (GAS); *** Beck Depression Inventory (BDI).[52]

information to determine the values/data. Assessments in which the assessed person determines the values/data but not the variables/issues are *self-report* or *self-rated*. Assessments in which the assessed person determines the values/data as well as the variables/issues are *self-generated*. Assessments in which the assessed person determines the variables/issues but not the values/data are hypothetical, at least at this stage, as are assessments in which the assessed person informs the variables/issues with or without determining the values/data. This classification may be helpful to understand in what way, if at all, an assessment is a PCA, and to select it (or not) accordingly.

Components of Person-Centered Approach

Clinical Interview

Personal Goals and Strengths: In traditional or biomedical assessment, goals are predetermined, e.g. to cure an infection in physical health care, or to alleviate symptoms in mental health care. A PCA approach does not assume that goals for care are known in advance, but rather explores the specific person's goals for care. It is important to note that as a result a PCA assessment process will be multi-dimensional as the clinician is exploring goals related to several areas of an individual's life. This is further illustrated in psychiatric rehabilitation, where setting of a goal with the psychiatrically disabled person comes first, and drives the assessment (of what challenges, strengths and opportunities should be addressed in order for that person to achieve and/or maintain that goal); if such a personal goal is not clear or not feasible, a rehabilitation readiness assessment and development process can be used to reach a clear and feasible personal goal.[6] A caveat is risk assessment, which will be discussed later in this chapter. Note that a PCA assesses personal strengths that can facilitate achieving and maintaining personal goals, such as sense of humor.

Psychopathology: The current gold standard for a diagnostic semi-structured interview is the Structured Clinical Interview for DSM Disorders (SCID),[7] which both determines existence and severity of psychopathology. To complement a SCID, PCA adds an unstructured or semi-structured interview to explore personal aspects of the presentation of psychopathology that a structured interview does not address. This includes the influence of culture, e.g. depressive symptoms present as more cognitive (such as guilt) in Western cultures, and as more somatic (such as abdominal pain or discomfort) in other cultures.[8]

Physical Health: Medical problems and risks are commonly relevant to mental health care, e.g. in relation to adverse effects of psychiatric medications, to lifestyle (such as sedentary habits), and more.[9,10] Depth of interviewing about physical health depends on level of medical expertise, as well as on the goal of the person interviewed in PCA. At a minimum, medical problems and risks that may pose a health risk or a serious challenge to achieving and/or maintaining a person's goals need to be briefly explored, and a plan for further investigation should be established with the person's voluntary, informed consent.

Functioning: When assessing activities of daily living, as well as vocational, educational, social and leisure functioning, the provider must ensure that he/she is clear regarding what issues within these large areas are important to the person. Included in that is ensuring that what the provider determines as issues within these areas is in keeping with what the person determines the issues are. For example, Rowan[11] found the people she talked to defined self-care as health practices that dealt with hygiene but also with coping mechanisms, responsibility and routines, enjoyment and solitude. Willis[12] found that the importance of an individual working related to the individual's self-esteem, self-confidence and to the benefits of structuring his or her day, as well as to socialization in the workplace and a sense of contribution to society. These areas are multifaceted and highly individualized. They can be assessed through standardized tests, but a thorough understanding of their meanings and importance to the individuals is necessary if the results of the assessments are to be meaningful in the recovery process.

Emotions: During the assessment, efforts are undertaken to assess the emotional functioning of the person. For example, how does he or she feel in general and about his or her supports (or lack thereof) in particular? Smith[13] cautions health care providers to only explore emotion after assessing the person's readiness to the assessment process thus far. A therapeutic alliance is conducive to the person disclosing personal information, especially with regards to negative emotions such as fear and frustration. In a PCA, the health care provider focuses on building rapport and explores emotions empathically and non-judgmentally according to the service user's goals and level of comfort.

Cognition: This is an important area to assess, as research links neurocognitive abilities to success in social and occupational functioning.[14,15] Cognition can be assessed in a clinical interview and also during formal psychological testing. For example, cognition can be assessed by paying attention to the person's language abilities, organization of responses, problem-solving abilities, i.e. how they have sought assistance with the presenting problem, and attention and memory processes. During the assessment, if cognitive impairments of a person with SMI are identified, a PCA approach is expected to explore the person's lived experience of his or her cognitive impairments.

Supports: One of the most common types of support needed by individuals with SMI is social, i.e. people who provide them both emotional and practical support,[16] e.g., encouragement at school, individualized job coaching at work and more. In addition, cognitive and other accommodations are sometimes required, such as visual cues and prompts, and flexible time schedules. In a PCA of an individual with SMI, the need for such supports and accommodations is examined according to the goals the person wants to achieve, addressing the existence (or not) of needed supports as well as the extent of their utilization.[17]

Process: In PCA, if the person is capable of deciding on his or her assessment, he or she determines which issues or areas should be assessed, e.g. a depressed person may decide that he or she does not want some of his or her physiological symptoms assessed (such as constipation), but rather only his or her emotions and cognition. Also, PCA accommodates for impairments of SMI, such as short attention span (common in SMI), e.g. by chunking the assessment into small enough bits of time as much as possible.[18] PCA fits well with qualitative assessment, which can help increase the depth of understanding the human experience of becoming ill, coping with a lifelong illness and recovering from illness, so as to better understand how to contribute to desired outcomes.[19]

When conducting a PCA it is important to pay attention to the person's individual needs and identify what is most appropriate for the person in order to obtain quality information and optimize the person's performance during the assessment.[20] This includes meeting in a subjectively safe place as identified by the person and pacing the assessment to his or her needs. Furthermore, paying particular attention to process variables provides valuable qualitative information to assist with care planning. This includes observing how the person approaches the assessment and his or her behavior during the assessment. Care plans need to be individualized and flexible to accommodate changing needs. Reviewing the collaborative goals that comprise the care plan with the person after the assessment allows for the instillation of hope prior to the termination of the assessment process.

The Person as a Historian: Numerous researchers have called for the use of strategies in the assessment phase that seek to understand the importance of individual context, meaning, influence of relationships, influence of culture and other variables.[21,22] The importance of listening to the person's story, exploring the subjective experience of the person experiencing the illness, and not making premature assumptions about the individual's world should be a part of our everyday work, says psychiatrist John Strauss.[23]

The initial meeting focuses on getting to know the individual and beginning to understand his or her story as well as his or her perspective on the reason for

Example

The following is an illustration of a challenge with PCA:

During the discharge planning for Scott, a middle-aged man with SMI, it was noted that he appeared to underestimate his abilities in that he identified a preference for residence in a group home where many tasks would be done for him, e.g. medication management, meal preparation, laundry and more. However, the clinical team, based on their clinical assessment, believed that he was higher functioning and therefore capable of completing these activities. Thus, there was a discrepancy in assessment and care goals between the service user and his mental health service providers, in this case with the service user subjectively underestimating his ability as compared to the providers' supposedly more objective estimation. This presented a challenge that will be discussed and illustrated below.

meeting with the clinician. The discussion includes present and historical information and focuses on strengths as well as challenges.[24]

A PCA recognizes that the service user has priorities that may take precedence over what others think they should be doing. In order to do this, we as service providers have to give up the traditional control/authority of providers.[25] The achievement of a balance of authority is central to PCC but is difficult to accomplish.[26] In large part, this is about finding common ground between the service user and the provider, which can be achieved by defining together the problem, i.e. the discrepancy between the client's perceived abilities and needs and the treatment team's evaluation of the client and goals for discharge, which included independent living, establishing together the goals and priorities of the management (specifically assessment in this case), and identifying together the roles to be assumed by both the service user and the provider.[27] We need to look for creative ways for individuals to tell us what they know and what they want.

In relation to Scott, the service user described above, his priority could be summarized as acclimatization into the community and stability, as his history revealed years of instability where he moved from one treatment facility to another with brief periods of unsuccessful community living. Therefore, by developing an interpretive ear to evaluate our service users' expressions of wants and needs, the service user in this case was saying "not yet" to independent living (the goal promoted by the treatment team). It probably does not mean "never," and this feeling can be explored with the service user. In this example, the service user and the clinical team agreed to evaluate the living arrangement after six months (which allowed for a degree of stability) to explore if priorities, wants and needs were modified after that. As Nagle et al.[28] reported, participants in their study wanted service providers to be supportive and hopeful, but they also wanted them to trust that they will do more when they can.

In summary, listening closely to a service user's story will inform the assessment process and ensure the development of goals and action plans that are more likely to succeed since they have been part of the development of the plan. Increasingly, researchers are accepting service users' self-report as valid and reliable, which facilitates finding common ground between service users and providers.

Other Sources of Information

Rose *et al.*[29] advocated for a multiple-perspective paradigm in mental health, one focused towards service delivery and the evaluation of research, i.e. with respect to evidence-based research, deciding what information constitutes "evidence." A PCA considers the service user as the central source of information when beginning the process of assessing his or her strengths, needs and challenges. However, this assessment also appreciates that other sources of information assist in gaining as full an understanding as possible of the person and his/her circumstances. Furthermore, by obtaining multiple perspectives during a PCA and integrating these varied sources of information, a unified care plan and direction can be created, which will reduce tensions and contradictions.[30] One such measure that attempts to reconcile the perspective of persons with SMI, their caregivers and staff is the Camberwell Assessment of Need.[31] This tool recognizes the multiple perspectives obtained during assessments and attempts to explore these in as comprehensive and objective a manner as possible, with the goal of reconciling these perspectives.

Other sources of information include: 1. Significant others such as family and friends; 2. Other institutions and health care teams; and 3. Health care records. A PCA would elicit not just these people's observations about the person, but also their impression of the person's beliefs and desires. For instance, a family's impression of a person's beliefs and desires is very valuable, as many times the family knows the person better than anyone else. In addition, a PCA assessment should include an assessment of the caregivers themselves, as their ability to cope will impact the well-being of the person with the SMI. For example, family's EE is predictive of relapse in a person with an SMI.[32]

Standardized Assessment Tools

Symptom Ratings: Assessment of the existence and severity of psychiatric symptoms is most commonly done in the mental health field by standardized measures, using either clinician-rated or self-report tools, most of which are quantitative questionnaires.[33] Such tools are usually either generic, such as the Symptom Check-List-90-Revised (SCL-90-R) for a variety of psychiatric symptoms; or disorder/syndrome specific, such as the Beck Depression Inventory (BDI) for depression and the PANSS for schizophrenia.[34] While self-report measures are apparently more person-centered, when cognition or illness awareness (insight) are severely impaired, clinician-rated measures may be more valid than self-rated measures. In such situations, a person-centered approach may be used both to assess a symptom or a set of symptoms, in order to better understand the extent of discrepancy (if any) between the individual's experience of his or her symptoms and the clinician's evaluation. If a large discrepancy exists, a discussion could be attempted with the assessed individual, in order to try to reach common ground and to agree on what not to agree. This is particularly important as person-centered treatment of symptoms can then be based on such a discussion.

Psychological Assessment: A major advantage of psychological testing within a PCA is the objectivity of the data that the assessment provides, particularly when evaluating cognitive abilities. As mentioned earlier in this section, PCA elicits information from the person with an SMI with regards to any difficulties they are encountering. However, poor insight may interfere with the person's ability to accurately assess their abilities. Also, there are now evidence-based interventions to reduce or overcome impairments such as cognitive deficits typically seen in persons with SMI. This includes research by Hogarty *et al.*[35] on cognitive enhancement therapy and the Neuropsychological Educational Approach to Remediation (NEAR) program by Medalia *et al.*[36] It is therefore no longer best practice to document the deficits that interfere with goal planning and goal achievement, as best practice particularly in a PCA can identify the remediation of these abilities as collaborative goals. Assessment tools utilized in this regard focus on evaluating various cognitive domains including attention, memory and executive functioning (such as planning and problem solving), which enable independent functioning. A PCA should accommodate for the person's impairments, such as testing in small bits of time as much as possible within test standardization. It should also engage the person in interactive feedback about his or her cognitive and other tested impairments, as well as use other strategies of collaborative (neuro)psychological assessment.[37]

Risk Measures: Perhaps the most controversial aspect of PCC for people with SMI relates to the risk to self or others. Such risk can be intentional or not, in which (latter) case the issue can be more clearly viewed as safety, and will be addressed elsewhere in this section in relation to functional assessment. As for intentional risk (also termed dangerousness), aggression such as violence – and even more so, self-harm such as suicidality – are more prevalent in people with SMI such as schizophrenia than in the general population.[38,39] Yet the person may not want to disclose his or her dangerous intention, or his or her dangerous behavior may be impulsive and therefore unpredictable, even by himself or herself. Hence a person-centered approach to risk assessment may have to include others' assessment of the risk; indeed, most common violence and suicidality assessments in the mental health field have an other-rated component or version, with or without a self-report component version.[40,41] As with the assessment of other domains, such as psychiatric symptoms, a PCA may use both other-rated and self-report assessment to assess intentional risk. If a large discrepancy exists, a discussion could be attempted with the assessed individual, in order to try to reach common ground within legal requirements and to agree on what not to agree. This is particularly important, as person-centered reduction of risk to self or others can then be based on such a discussion.

Readiness and Functional Assessments: "Rehabilitation readiness" is defined as the process used to prepare an individual for engaging in a rehabilitation plan.[42] It is thought to increase the willingness of the person to be engaged in the process with a view to establishing goals that are important and meaningful to him or her and likely increasing the potential for success in achieving these goals. There is an established process for assessing and developing rehabilitation readiness that clinicians can easily access.[43] Five domains are assessed, including: perceived need or satisfaction with the individual's current environment, commitment to change, personal closeness, self-awareness and environmental awareness. The completion of these activities helps the person to set his/her goals for rehabilitation and directs the focus of the functional assessments to follow. Common barriers to achieving rehabilitation readiness include: lack of understanding of self, of the possibility of recovery and of options available for individuals; and lack of support from others for participation in the rehabilitation process. Service providers who aspire to work in a person-centered approach must act as facilitators to this process, not as barriers. Corring[44] found in her exploration of what PCC means to persons living with mental illness that these individuals have experienced many service providers who have been barriers to their recovery.

Researchers experienced in PSR approaches note that there are current limitations of functional assessments. Focusing on individual deficits before getting to know a person as an individual is problematic. It does not allow the service provider to hear the person's perspective on how the functions to be assessed relate to the individual's own vision of recovery, and what a meaningful life might look like for him or her. Using standardized assessments with little regard to their meaningfulness or relevance to the individual does not fit with person-centered practice. The use of PSR techniques fits with person-centered practice, as they are designed to help individuals set an overall goal and provide interventions that build skills and supports to achieve their recovery vision.[45] Personalizing the activities within the assessment, based on the rehabilitation goals set by the person, will further assist in ensuring that it is person-centered. For example, if the person is moving into an environment where he/she will be using a microwave to heat already prepared meals, then the assessment must be focused on the use of the microwave – not preparing a full-course meal utilizing a stove. In this case, safety assessment of using a stove is not relevant, while other safety assessments may be pertinent, such as assessment of locking the front door.

Quality of Life, Recovery and Stages of Change: Assessment of these very important areas is relatively new but of growing importance in an environment where person-centered practice is valued. It is important to ensure that the measures used for quality of life assessment are constructed with the benefit of the input of persons with the illness perspective.[46] Recovery measures are available to obtain perspectives of the persons with the illness and family members as well as clinicians.[47,48] Finally, the stages of change model will help providers understand the process of making changes that they can expect service users to experience.[49]

Service Use Satisfaction: This is the domain of assessment that is perhaps most clearly person-centered in health care in general. It addresses the satisfaction of the person with SMI regarding the mental health services he or she has been provided. Although most, if not all, existing tools in this domain are not self-generated, many are self-report,[50] and hence are at least minimally person-centered. Note that assessment of service user satisfaction, even if self-generated, is necessary but not sufficient for a person-centered approach to comprehensive assessment.

Documentation

Although documentation is not specific to assessment, we will highlight person-centered aspects of it here in relation to assessment, recognizing that the discussion may be relevant to documentation of other aspects of PCC, as addressed in other sections of this book – particularly in Section 6.2, *Person-Centered Approaches to Psychopharmacology for People with Serious Mental Illness*, Section 6.3, *Person-Centered Individual Psychotherapy for Adults with Serious Mental Illness* and Section 6.4, *Cognitive and Psychiatric Rehabilitation: person-centered ingredients for success*. Assessments should be documented in order to preserve their valuable information for communication with the service user, other health care providers and other relevant parties, and for legal reasons. There are various formats of assessment documentation, which traditionally depend on the type of assessment, on the assessor, and on other factors that are not necessarily related to the service user personally. Person-centered documentation of assessments can be facilitated in various ways. For instance, verbatim statements of the service user can be documented, thus illustrating the service user's personal experiences in relation to or as part of the assessment. Another approach is to provide feedback to the service user about the assessment, and then to document his or her input on that assessment. Additionally, the service user can be asked to document his or her impression of the assessment. These approaches are neither mutually exclusive nor exhaustive.

A person-centered approach would require a documented assessment to be easily accessible to the service user. Access is required by law in most Western jurisdictions, but this may not suffice. For instance, a documented assessment is not easily accessible if it is not easily comprehensible to the service user in terms of language, organization, and more. It is also not easily accessible if access is conditioned on considerable payment by the service user, as required by some health records departments. A person-centered approach would minimize these barriers as much as possible within cultural, financial and other constraints. Note that these suggestions about a person-centered approach to documentation of assessments are not exclusive to assessment and may apply, possibly with some modifications, to clinical documentation in general.

Example

Ken was a 32-year-old, single, Caucasian man who was an inpatient in a long-term psychiatric unit. He was diagnosed with schizophrenia, disorganized type, since his late teens. His symptoms of schizophrenia, mainly severe thought disorganization such as incoherent thinking at times, were persistent in spite of evidence-based treatment for refractory schizophrenia in the form of clozapine (within a therapeutic and safe range based on blood levels). It was considered by the mental health care team impossible to discharge him to the community, even to sheltered housing, due to his thought disorganization, which led to severe challenges in maintaining a daily routine without frequent reminders and hands-on support. On the unit, care for Ken consisted for a long while mainly of medication maintenance, addressing physical health issues when they arose, and occasional recreation.

When a new service provider who was particularly interested in PSR joined Ken's team, that provider started focusing with Ken on Ken's goals and what could help him achieve them. Ken was unclear about this initially, but over a few months, using a rehabilitation readiness assessment approach that focuses on clarifying personal goals, it became clear to Ken and to his team that he wanted to have more friends. The team then engaged Ken in an assessment focused on what may be making it difficult for him to have more friends, as well as relevant strengths (the question of why he wanted more friends was not explored in-depth, nor was the value judgment of whether he had enough friends or not considered, as PCC – and PCA as part of it – do not usually question goals of service users, so long as they do not pose serious harm to the service user or to others and are achievable, even if only in the long term).

The team observed that Ken did not attend many of the social gatherings on the unit, as he seemed to forget them. Therefore, the assessment included unstructured observation by the nursing staff of his social behavior when possible, a clinical interview with his psychiatrist to rule out or confirm social anxiety, and a structured assessment by his psychologist of his cognitive abilities and challenges, using the Wisconsin Card Sorting Test for executive functioning and the Wechsler Adult Intelligence Scale (WAIS) to assess various other cognitive abilities, including a measure to evaluate social cognition. Thus, his assessment was fully clinician-rated and partly informed directly by him; a larger role for him in his own assessment was difficult if not impossible to achieve, due to partial collaboration related to his severe thought disorganization. These assessments demonstrated that when he was with others, he was polite and friendly but mostly passive; that he did not have social anxiety; and that he had some severe cognitive impairments, particularly in sustained attention and in working memory.

The assessment results were shared with Ken, and a plan based on these results was established with him to try to address these challenges and build on his relevant strengths. The plan consisted primarily of basic social skills training and of compensatory cognitive remediation (see Section 6.4, Cognitive and Psychiatric Rehabilitation: person-centered ingredients for success). The team evaluated this and its outcomes with Ken on a monthly basis, and after a few months they agreed that it was effective and that social skills training could be ended but that compensatory cognitive remediation should continue indefinitely. Ken had more friends and started considering steps towards discharge, such as using compensatory cognitive remediation to facilitate activities of daily living.

CONCLUSION

PCA makes individuals with SMI the so-called drivers of their own assessments as much as possible. Its principles can be incorporated into most if not all areas of assessment of individuals with SMI, e.g. in interviewing, in standardized testing, in collateral history gathering and in documentation of assessments. There are challenges to PCA with individuals who have SMI that can be addressed within PCA or with additional frameworks, e.g. cognitive impairments may require tailored accommodations for the assessment, and legal constraints may require risk assessment that is not fully person-centered. Overall, there is an emerging agreement that PCA and related approaches are needed in mental health care and that PCA can considerably influence the care provided to individuals with SMI.[51]

REFERENCES

1 Stewart M, Brown JB, Weston WW, *et al. Patient-Centered Medicine: transforming the clinical method.* 2nd ed. Oxford: Radcliffe Publishing; 2003.

2 Ibid.

3 Fiscella K, Meldrum S, Franks P, *et al.* Patient trust: is it related to patient-centered behavior of primary care physicians? *Med Care.* 2004; **42**(11): 1049–56.

4 Anthony W, Cohen M, Farkas M, *et al. Psychiatric Rehabilitation.* 2nd ed. Boston, MA: Center for Psychiatric Rehabilitation; 2002.

5 McCabe R, Saidi M, Priebe S. Patient-reported outcomes in schizophrenia. *Brit J Psychiat.* 2007; **191**(Suppl. 50): S21–8.

6 Anthony, Cohen, Farkas, *et al.*, op. cit.

7 First MB, Spitzer RL, Gibbon M, *et al. Structured Clinical Interview for DSM-IV Axis I Disorders (SCID I), Clinical Version.* Washington, DC: American Psychiatric Association; 1997.

8 Tseng WS, Streltzer J, editors. *Cultural Competence in Clinical Psychiatry.* Washington, DC: American Psychiatric Publishing; 2004.

9 Leucht S, Burkard T, Henderson JH, *et al. Physical Illness and Schizophrenia: a review of the evidence.* Cambridge: Cambridge University Press; 2007.

10 Haddad P, Dursun S, Deakin B, editors. *Adverse Syndromes and Psychiatric Drugs: a clinical guide.* Oxford: Oxford University Press; 2004.

11 Rowan R. An examination of the self-care needs of individuals with schizophrenia. *First Annual Conference Presenting Individual Studies in Evidence-Based Practice.* London, ON: University of Western Ontario; 1999.

12 Willis A. *The Role of Work for Individuals with Chronic Mental Illness.* London, ON: The University of Western Ontario; 2000.

13 Smith RC. *Patient-Centered Interviewing: an evidence-based method.* Philadelphia, PA: Lippincott Williams & Wilkins; 2002.

14 Hogarty GE, Flesher S, Ulrich R, *et al.* Cognitive enhancement therapy for schizophrenia. *Arch Gen Psychiatry.* 2004; **61**(9): 866–76.

15 Matza LS, Buchanan R, Purdon S, *et al.* Measuring changes in functional status among patients with schizophrenia: the link with cognitive impairment. *Schizophrenia Bull.* 2006; **32**(4): 666–78.

16 Lohman A, Bar L, Carter G, *et al.* PSR/RPS Ontario Develops and Promotes Equation: "PSR = People Supporting Recovery". *PSR/RPS Express.* 2008; **4**(2): 27–8.

17 Anthony, Cohen, Farkas, *et al.*, op. cit.

18 Rudnick A, Roe D. Diagnostic interviewing. In: Mueser KT, Jeste DV, editors. *Clinical Handbook of Schizophrenia*. New York, NY: Guilford; 2008. pp. 117–24.

19 Madjar I, Walton JA. What is problematic about evidence? In: Morse JM, Swanson JM, Kuzel AJ, editors. *The Nature of Qualitative Evidence*. Thousand Oaks, CA: Sage Publications; 2001. pp. 28–45.

20 Groth-Marnat G. *Handbook of Psychological Assessment*. 3rd ed. New York, NY: John Wiley & Sons Inc.; 1999.

21 Joyce CRB, Hickey A, McGee HM, *et al.* A theory- based method for the evaluation of individual quality of life: the SEIQoL. *Qual Life Res.* 2003; **12**(3): 275–80.

22 Malla AK, Norman RMG, McLean TS, *et al.* Determinants of quality of life in first-episode psychosis. *Acta Psychiat Scand.* 2004; **109**(1): 46–54.

23 Strauss JS. The person with schizophrenia as a person: approaches to the subjective and the complex. *Brit J Psychiat.* 1994; **164**(S23): 103–7.

24 Sumsion T. The client-centred approach. In: Sumsion T, editor. *Client-Centred Practice in Occupational Therapy*. 2nd ed. Edinburgh: Churchill Livingstone Elsevier; 2006. pp. 19–28.

25 Corring D, Cook J. *Client-Centred Practice: an exchange of views*. Research Insights: Regional Mental Health Care London & St. Thomas. London, ON: RMHC; 2008.

26 Mishler EG. *Research Interviewing: context and narrative*. Cambridge, MA: Harvard University Press; 1986.

27 Stewart M, Brown JB, Weston WW, *et al.*, op. cit. p. 83.

28 Nagle, S. *I'm Doing as Much as I Can: pathways to occupational choice*. University of Western Ontario: London, ON; 1997.

29 Rose D, Thornicroft G, Slade M. Who decides what evidence is? Developing a multiple perspectives paradigm in mental health. *Acta Psychiat Scand.* 2006; **113**(Suppl. 429): 109–14.

30 Ibid.

31 Phelan M, Slade M, Thornicroft G, *et al.* The Camberwell Assessment of Need (CAN): the validity and reliability of an instrument to assess the needs of people with severe mental illness. *Brit J Psychiat.* 1995; **167**(5): 589–95.

32 Butzlaff R, Hooley J. Expressed emotion and psychiatric relapse: a meta-analysis. *Arch Gen Psychiat.* 1999; **55**(6): 547–52.

33 Rush AJ Jr, First MB, Blacker D, editors. *Handbook of Psychiatric Measures*. 2nd ed. Washington, DC: American Psychiatric Publishing; 2008.

34 Ibid.

35 Hogarty, Flesher, Ulrich, *et al.*, op. cit.

36 Medalia A, Revheim N, Casey M. Remediation of problem-solving skills in schizophrenia: evidence of a persistent effect. *Schizophr Res.* 2002; **57**(2–3): 165–71.

37 Gorske TT, Smith SR. *Collaborative Therapeutic Neuropsychological Assessment*. New York: Springer; 2009.

38 Haddock G, Shaw J. Understanding and working with aggression, violence, and psychosis. In: Mueser KT, Jeste DV, editors. *Clinical Handbook of Schizophrenia*. New York, NY: Guilford; 2008. pp. 398–410.

39 Heisel MJ. Suicide. In: Mueser KT, Jeste DV, editors. *Clinical Handbook of Schizophrenia*. New York, NY: Guilford; 2008. pp. 491–504.

40 Oquendo MA, Giner L, Harkavy FJ, *et al.* Suicide risk measures. 2nd ed. In: Rush AJ Jr, First MB, Blacker D, editors. *Handbook of Psychiatric Measures*. Washington, DC: American Psychiatric Publishing; 2008. pp. 237–48.

41 Suris A, Coccaro EF. Aggression measures. In: Rush AJ Jr, First MB, Blacker D, editors. *Handbook of Psychiatric Measures*. 2nd ed. Washington, DC: American Psychiatric Publishing; 2008. pp. 731–44.

42 Fiscella K, Meldrum S, Franks P, *et al.*, op. cit.

43 Ibid.

44 Corring DJ. *Client-Centred Care Means I am a Valued Human Being* [unpublished master's dissertation]. London, ON: University of Western Ontario; 1996.

45 Fiscella K, Meldrum S, Franks P, *et al.*, op. cit.

46 Corring D, Cook J. Use of qualitative methods to explore the quality of life construct from a consumer perspective. *Psychiat Serv.* 2007; **58**: 240–4.

47 Dumont JM, Ridgway P, Onken SJ, *et al. Recovery Oriented Systems Indicator Measure (ROSI). Measuring the Promise: a compendium if recovery measures, Volume II.* Cambridge, MA: The Evaluation Center at the Human Services Research Institute; 2005. pp. 3–6.

48 O'Connell M, Tondora J, Croog G, *et al.* From rhetoric to routine: assessing perceptions of recovery-oriented practice in a state mental health and addiction system. *Psychiatr Rehabil J.* 2005; **28**(4): 378–86.

49 Prochaska JO, DiClemente CC, Norcross JC. In search of how people change. *Am Psychol.* 1992; **47**(9): 1102–4.

50 Teague GB, Caporino NE. Patient perceptions of care measures. In: Rush AJ Jr, First MB, Blacker D, editors. *Handbook of Psychiatric Measures*. 2nd ed. Washington, DC: American Psychiatric Publishing; 2008. pp. 163–91.

51 Mezzich JE, Salloum IM, Cloninger CR, *et al.* Person-centered integrative diagnosis: conceptual bases and structural model. *Can J Psychiatry.* 2010; **55**: 701–8.

52 Rush, First, Blacker D, op. cit.

6.2 Person-Centered Approaches to Psychopharmacology for People with Serious Mental Illness

Abraham Rudnick and Joel Lamoure

INTRODUCTION

Psychotropic medications are now widely considered a key component of mental health care for many people with SMI, such as those with schizophrenia and bipolar disorder. Approaches to psychotropic medication prescribing vary from authoritarian to collaborative (when possible); the latter may be viewed as part of PCC. These approaches may be related to a medical model or to a biopsychosocial model, respectively. This section will examine issues in relation to person-centered approaches to psychotropic medications for people with SMI, focusing on adherence, competence/capacity, ethnic and metabolic factors, and adverse effects, as well as psychosocial and biophysical alternatives and adjuncts in brief. We will exclude from our discussion self-prescribing, as it is a possibility that has not materialized in mental health care to date (unlike self-provision of psychotherapy such as cognitive behavioral therapy (CBT) by audiotapes or by Internet). We will also exclude from our discussion alternative/complementary/herbal medications, recognizing that is an emerging field in mental health care, e.g. it is part of the newly developed notion of personal medicine, which refers to non-conventional as well as conventional strategies that a person chooses to use in order to cope with his or her mental health related challenges.[1] Non-pharmacological alternative and adjunct interventions will also be discussed, albeit briefly. It will be assumed that most prescribers are physicians, although we recognize that some prescribers of psychotropic medications are now other health care providers, such as psychologists and advance practice nurses in North America.[2] We will first briefly present some definitions, philosophy, history and classification of psychotropic medications.

Definitions, Philosophy, History and Classification of Psychotropic Medication

Psychotropic medications are widely considered a central part of treatment for individuals with psychiatric disorders. Treatment can be defined as any health care intervention that aims to reduce or alleviate symptoms directly, if not induce full and sustainable remission (which has not been common for SMI to date). Thus, treatment is in contrast to other types of health care interventions, such as rehabilitation, which can be defined as any health care intervention that aims to reduce functional disability or role disruption directly; psychiatric treatment and PSR are considered complementary and may impact on each other's aims.[3] The science of psychotropic medications, termed psychopharmacology, may be more or less person-centered, depending in part on its philosophical assumptions. Thus, reductionist assumptions that reduce psychopathology and psychotropic medications to (only) neurochemical phenomena move away from person-centered approaches, whereas systemic (holistic) assumptions that consider psychopathology and psychotropic medications in the context of neural and other relevant biological and social systems and factors (including personal preferences of service users), move towards person-centered approaches.[4,5,6] The technology of psychotropic medication prescribing, somewhat confusingly also termed psychopharmacology, may be more or less person-centered too, depending on its practice and marketing. For instance, critical psychopharmacology is recently emerging, advocating for involvement of people with mental illnesses, including individuals with SMI, in decision-making related to psychotropic medications – from (scientific) bench to markets and practice.[7,8,9] Such involvement will not be discussed in this chapter (in spite of its centrality to PCC, as another chapter – on communication – does so), other than to mention that it involves a partnership and environment in which honesty, choice and individual responsibility can thrive.[10]

For example, an individual with major depressive disorder comes to the psychiatrist seeking help. It is prudent that the psychiatrist collaborate with that service user in an honest manner in order to find the most appropriate antidepressant that matches the medical needs of the service user as well as meets the individual goals of the service user. This includes what the service user's personal goals of therapy are as well as carefully considering what side effect profile is acceptable to the service user. This physician-service user collaboration also encourages service user autonomy and individual responsibility. By collaborating with the service user in a shared decision-making process, a strong therapeutic alliance will be formed, which in turn will enhance the likelihood of service user adherence to recommended best practice and positive clinical outcomes. Thus, person-centered approaches to exploring psychopharmacology have the potential for significant impacts on current and future clinical outcomes.

Modern psychopharmacology began in the late 1940s and early 1950s, with the discovery of the mood stabilizing effect of lithium, the antipsychotic effect of chlorpromazine, and the antidepressant effect of impiramine. Interestingly, psychotropic effects of these medications were mostly discovered by serendipity.[11,12] In the 1990s, new mood stabilizers, antipsychotics and antidepressants were developed and marketed, although there have not been major breakthroughs, other than clozapine – which was actually developed in the 1970s but remarketed in North America in the 1990s – for refractory schizophrenia.[13,14] Current classifications of psychotropic medications for SMI mostly focus on their main symptomatic effects, i.e. as mood stabilizers for manic episodes, antipsychotics for psychotic episodes, and antidepressants for major depressive disorders.[15,16] Some of these medications are prescribed for other indications, such as antipsychotics for manic episodes, and other psychotropics are sometimes prescribed for individuals with SMI, e.g. anti-anxiety medications such as benzodiazepines for comorbid anxiety symptoms. In the following sections, we will refer to all psychotropic medications that are commonly prescribed for people with SMI, with a focus on schizophrenia for the purpose of illustration.

Adherence to Medications

One of the most commonly discussed issues in relation to psychopharmacology for people with SMI is adherence to psychotropic medications, previously termed compliance and more recently termed concordance (we will use the term adherence as it is more well-known than concordance, although we recognize that the term concordance is taken by some to imply more respect for persons than the term adherence). The importance of adherence is illustrated by the fact that, among service users with schizophrenia, approximately 40% stop their antipsychotic medication within one year and up to 75% or so stop them by the second year.[17] In a study of adherence over a four-year period, about 38% of individuals with schizophrenia had challenges with adherence in any given year, i.e. they did not take all or part of their medication, while 60% of individuals had challenges with adherence (similarly defined) at some point over the four years.[18] Among individuals with long-term schizophrenia, adherence to antipsychotic medications is relatively low (up to 40%), which is lower than adherence to medications of individuals who have other mental disorders such as depression or of individuals suffering from physical illnesses.[19] This lack of adherence of many individuals with schizophrenia has been associated with high rates of relapse, repeated hospitalizations and longer hospital stays, resulting in disruption to individuals' lives and in societal costs.[20] Also, non-adherence to antipsychotics is a predictor of violence committed by individuals with schizophrenia.[21]

Lack of adherence to psychotropic medications, such as antipsychotics, can be explained by four sets of factors: 1. Person-related factors; 2. Disorder-related factors; 3. Treatment-related factors; and 4. Environment-related factors.[22] Person-related factors include relevant personal knowledge, health beliefs and preferences, among others; disorder-related factors include cognitive impairments, such as working memory impairment and lack of illness awareness/insight (particularly lack of awareness of need for treatment), among others; treatment-related factors include adverse effects such as weight gain, inconvenient medication regimes such as frequent dosing, and poor therapeutic relationships, among others; and environment-related factors include lack of funding, poverty, lack of access to services, stigma or discrimination and lack of family support, among others. Interventions that address all these sets of factors in a flexible manner are not yet established, but some evidence-based and promising interventions that improve some of these factors are available. Some approaches address cognitive impairments, e.g. by means of behavioral tailoring or pairing that cues the person who has memory impairments to take the medication on time[23] – a typical example is that of locating night medications near an object that is routinely used at night, such as a toothbrush, where water is also available so that oral medication ingestion can immediately follow the visual cue; admittedly, although this strategy may be convenient, caution should be noted about bathroom medicine cabinets for storage of medications, as high humidity in bathrooms may affect medication stability (hence locating a reminder note – to take the medications – near the toothbrush may be safer than locating the medications there). Other approaches are the use of motivational interviewing to address and enhance motivation for adherence by developing discrepancy between the person's goals and his or her lack of adherence, among other strategies.[24] And family support to improve adherence can be enhanced by family psychoeducation that increases family knowledge of the disorder and its care, as well as family problem-solving skills, such as in relation to a person with SMI who lacks insight.[25] Enhancing adherence may require going beyond the above classification, both because these four different domains and factors within them interact, and because using this classification rigidly may not be motivating to the person with the SMI and thus may not be person-centered.

A complex medication regimen with multiple medications and administration times may lead to poor adherence. Monotherapy can increase adherence by ensuring a more simple medication regimen and reducing adverse effects and drug-drug interactions; it is easier to monitor, and may be more cost-effective. Moreover, if the dose of a medication needs to be adjusted due to the development of adverse effects, an attempt should usually be made to first reduce the dose rather than add a second medication to treat adverse effects. This will provide a more simple medication regimen and hence may improve adherence.[26,27,28] The use of long-acting (mostly injectable) medication formulations may also improve adherence because they are administered infrequently (once every few weeks). Individuals who may especially benefit from a long-acting formulation include those who relapse repeatedly due to non-adherence, and those who prefer a long-acting injectable medication.[29,30,31]

The service user's concurrent medical conditions must be considered in getting the right medication to the right person at the right time for the right condition.[32] Careful screening of the person's medication profile and identification of potential drug-drug interactions that may result in increased antipsychotic levels and consequently adverse effects is yet another approach that prescribers should use to help promote adherence.[33] In addition to screening the medication profiles for potential drug-drug interactions, the pharmacist should proactively monitor service users who appear to be over-using prescription medications with a potential for abuse, e.g. benzodiazepines and narcotics. Alerting the prescriber as needed is critical for the service user to receive the needed help and care, because comorbid medication abuse is a major risk factor for non-adherence.[34,35]

There are various educational strategies that may be employed to promote adherence, such as training in IMR, which is a person-centered, recovery-oriented psychoeducation and coping enhancement approach that has been endorsed federally in the U.S.[36] Education with respect to the SMI and its biological basis may improve adherence by decreasing the stigmatized perception of the disease.[37] Still, two recent reviews of the literature have concluded that the use of an education intervention alone to promote adherence is less successful than an approach that combines education, problem-solving, behavioral tailoring, and motivational interviewing/

enhancement.[38,39] Specifically, psychoeducation stresses the importance of: taking medications consistently and on a daily basis for them to be effective; continuing medications even if symptoms subside, in order to prevent relapse; and consulting a pharmacist or other health care provider before taking over-the-counter medications and/or herbal products, in order to avoid drug interactions.[40] Education should be provided about potential adverse effects. For instance, weight gain due to psychotropic medications is one of the most common reasons for non-adherence. Providers can help service users create proactive strategies to help manage their weight and prevent weight gain. Minimizing adverse effects and optimizing the risk-benefit balance of psychotropic medications is a mainstay of prescribing practice. A person-centered approach to adverse effects attempts to explore and strike this balance according to the preferences of the person with the SMI.

A person-centered approach to psychopharmacology for people with SMI involves not only decision-making and prescribing but also dispensing of psychotropic medications. This is particularly helpful for persons with cognitive impairments, who benefit from dispensing methods such as blister packs or dosettes, which organize the medications in containers per dosing schedule. Medication deliveries to the person's home, as commonly done by ACT teams, also supports disorganized persons in their medication adherence.[41] In addition, self-monitoring calendars, reminder telephone calls, computer alarms, or having someone else administer the medication may also enhance adherence in service users with cognitive impairments.[42,43] Another strategy that may be employed to augment adherence is that of drug use control (DUC), where limited amounts of medication are dispensed at more frequent intervals. One issue with DUC is overcoming challenges of third-party coverage and practical support, such as transportation. The key for success is to create an individualized plan that meets the person's needs and addresses situational challenges.

It is essential for adherence to build a supportive therapeutic alliance over time with all members of the care team. This will foster a more trusting and open relationship, in which the service user is willing to be honest about adherence and to actively problem solve with the provider. As a therapeutic relationship is being established, the provider will have the opportunity to understand the person's goals and desired outcomes, as well as to understand potential barriers to adherence. Changes to medication regimes, e.g. a switch to a pharmacologically identical generic brand in order to reduce cost, must be made collaboratively, as these changes may disrupt trust of services users in prescribers and other providers and hence may disrupt adherence, due to reasons such as lack of knowledge about generic medications or persecutory ideas in relation to medications. Providers may improve adherence by discussing family and/or social support programs that are available in the community that may be able to address the other factors that help to promote adherence.[44]

Competence/Capacity to Consent to Treatment

Another important issue in relation to psychopharmacology for people with SMI is the question of competence or capacity to decide on psychiatric treatment. People with SMI are more likely than the general population to be impaired in their capacity to decide on their treatment, specifically their psychotropic medications, due to lack of insight or other factors such as cognitive impairment, as mentioned above; still, many individuals with SMI are considered capable for such decisions, and such capacity (or lack of it) should be determined for each person separately.[45] It should also be recognized that disagreement of an individual who has SMI with a provider about mental health care does not necessarily imply lack of capacity of that individual, as it can be related to capable personal choice.[46] Also, there are variants of capacity that should not be considered abnormal.[47] If a person is determined as incapable of deciding on his or her own psychiatric treatment, most jurisdictions require a substitute decision-maker to decide on his or her treatment. Such substitute decision-makers can be appointed by the court, by the treating physician or by a lawyer, depending on the local legislation and legal approach used.

If a person is determined as incapable of deciding on his or her own psychiatric treatment, the substitute decision-maker is usually required to make treatment decisions that align with that person's preferences when he or she was capable, if known (in which case the decisions are person-driven; if those preferences are not known, the substitute decision-maker can still be person-centered by considering the apparent needs of the person, hence being person-focused). An alternative is to establish an advance directive when the person with the SMI is capable, so that if he or she becomes incapable, the advance directive will be followed.[48] If a person is determined as incapable, a person-centered approach attempts to explore his or her assent (which is defined as incapable agreement), and when possible, to enhance the individual's capacity so that he or she becomes capable; in simple cases, this can be done by providing background information such as by psychoeducation, and in more challenging cases, this may be done by more in-depth interventions that can reduce psychosis or cognitive impairment (or their impact on the person's decision-making), such as CBT or cognitive remediation.[49]

Ethnic and Metabolic Factors

Individualizing psychotropic medication prescription as part of PCC may require consideration of many factors – biological, psychological, sociocultural and economic. This is clearly illustrated in ethno-psychopharmacology, where both race and culture are taken into consideration as part of tailoring psychotropic medications to the particular person for which they are prescribed.[50] For instance, health beliefs differ between Caucasians and Asians, with the latter having more negative attitudes to medications.[51] Pharmacodynamics (the effects of the medication on the body) and pharmacokinetics (the effects of the body on the medication) differ between Caucasians and Asians, with the latter requiring lower doses of antipsychotics such as haloperidol.[52] Interactions occur with complementary medications such as herbal remedies that are more commonly taken by Asians than Caucasians,[53] which may be explained in part by genetic polymorphisms that occur primarily within the CYP-2 group of cytochrome P450 isoenzymes in the liver.[54] The

P450 system in the liver is generally important for psychotropic effects and interactions with other medications and with smoking, as blood levels of medications may vary significantly with such interactions, requiring monitoring and adjustment of doses.[55,56] Food and use of substances such as cigarettes and alcohol may also play a role in the impact of medication, due to impact on absorption and metabolism. This is seen with antipsychotics such as quetiapine and ziprasidone, where higher-fat diets may increase the amount of medication absorbed in the intestines, which can lead to fluctuations in blood levels of these antipsychotics.[57] In addition and related to such ethnic factors, sociocultural factors play a role in individuals' beliefs, values and related actions in relation to psychotropic medication; for cultural aspects of PCC, see Section 4.2, *Trans-Cultural Issues in Person-Centered Care for People with Serious Mental Illness.* Also, family related factors play a similar role, partly because culture and family are interrelated, and partly because family can provide support (or lack of it) in relation to medication; for family aspects of PCC, see Section 4.1, *Collaborating with Families of People with Serious Mental Illness.*

Adverse Effects of Medications

A person-centered approach to adverse effects of psychotropic medications considers the pros and cons of the medications with service users by listening to their concerns, discussing them, and supporting them in aligning medication use with their personal goals. In this approach, the service user determines the significance of adverse effects and their balance with benefits of the medications (with evidence-based information offered by relevant providers such as physicians and nurses). For instance, typical or first generation antipsychotics (FGAs) such as haloperidol and even lower potency FGAs such as perphenazine may cause more movement disorders (particularly dystonia, akathisia, parkinsonism, and dyskinesia) but less metabolic syndrome complications (such as obesity, hypertension, hyperlipidemia and diabetes mellitus) than some atypical or second-generation antipsychotics (SGAs) such as olanzapine and clozapine.[58] A service user with schizophrenia who has a sensitive body image and a strong family history of diabetes mellitus may decide to take an FGA rather than an SGA, and thus knowingly take the risk of developing a movement disorder, which may sometimes be irreversible (as is commonly the case with tardive dyskinesia); alternatively, one of the best current antipsychotics for that particular service user may be ziprasidone (provided it is effective for his or her psychotic symptoms), which is an SGA that does not induce much if any weight gain nor hyperlipidemia nor glucose dysregulation, and therefore the risk of diabetes mellitus is not significantly increased with it.[59]

Example

The following is an illustration of the significant impact that adverse effects may have on adherence and clinical outcomes:

Marcus is an 18-year-old male, newly diagnosed with bipolar disorder with psychotic features (consisting of auditory/visual hallucinations). As a result of his psychiatric symptoms and new diagnosis, Marcus is started on olanzapine 30 mg at bedtime. After three months of treatment at this dose, a review of his blood work reveals that his triglyceride: total cholesterol ratio is elevated at 6.1. He has also developed an elevated level of glycosylated hemoglobin (HbA1c), which is currently 10.9%. Moreover, his psychiatrist notes that his weight has increased by 15 kg over the past three months. Given these markers, this service user is already experiencing significant metabolic adverse effects at the age of 18. If Marcus continues down this medication path, he will be at significant risk of developing cardiovascular sequelae early in his life. Given the relative importance of physical health at his age, Marcus is also at significant risk of non-adherence to his medication due to treatment-related factors, e.g. the obvious physical changes (particularly weight gain) that it has induced over the past three months.

Consequently, this is an illustrative situation where a psychiatrist can collaboratively work with the service user in an SDM process to find the most appropriate medication in the short- and long-term. Knowing that weight gain will be a significant concern for this service user now and in the future, both with respect to adherence and health, the physician and the service user can examine weight-neutral antipsychotic options together. Moreover, by listening to the concerns of the service user, discussing them, and aligning medication choices with personal goals, the physician can help to encourage adherence and promote positive outcomes of the service user, while building a strong therapeutic alliance with him.

A Psychosocial Alternative/Adjunct to Antipsychotic Medication

CBT is now used to alleviate or reduce persistent psychotic symptoms (or their disruptive impact), such as delusions or hallucinations that persist as part of refractory schizophrenia, i.e. schizophrenia that does not respond sufficiently to antipsychotic medication.[60,61] As such, CBT is mostly used in conjunction with antipsychotic medication. A person-centered approach may consider using CBT for persistent psychosis without using antipsychotic medication or with using lower than usual medication doses, e.g. if the medication at a standard dose is causing more harm than benefit by inducing adverse effects and/or by not reducing the psychotic symptoms much. Future research on such an approach could be helpful, particularly in relation to individuals with refractory schizophrenia, perhaps using randomized controlled trials of CBT with and without antipsychotics (with placebo as a medication control) for individuals with refractory schizophrenia.

Biophysical Interventions

Biophysical evidence-based or promising interventions for individuals with SMI include electric and magnetic brain stimulation therapies (BSTs), particularly ECT, vagus nerve stimulation (VNS) and repetitive transcranial magnetic stimulation (rTMS). ECT is considered helpful for alleviating severe, refractory or psychotic depression, as well as life-threatening mania and catatonia; VNS (by pacemaker) is considered helpful for reducing refractory depression; and rTMS is considered helpful for alleviating mild to moderate depression and for reducing persistent auditory hallucinations in schizophrenia.[62] As part of a person-centered approach, they should be offered when they are indicated and available (and they should be made available when they are not in place, as part of health care advocacy). Their adverse effects, which are partly different but usually no worse (and commonly milder) than those of psychotropic medications, include temporary memory impairment with ECT, possible surgical risks with VNS, and rare seizures with rTMS, among a few others. An individual who has schizophrenia with persistent and disruptive auditory hallucinations can choose to try rTMS (most probably with one antipsychotic) instead of antipsychotic polypharmacy, if he or she wants to avoid more adverse effects of medications. Providing care according to such a choice is not only person-centered, but also not less (if not more) evidence-based, considering that antipsychotic polypharmacy is not evidence-based for refractory schizophrenia.[63,64] Importantly, there is emerging evidence that such choice, and SDM, does not compromise and may even enhance outcomes of health care, both in general and in relation to mental health.[65,66] More research is required on this matter, particularly in relation to people with SMI who may be especially challenged in such choice and decision-making due to personal and environmental barriers, as addressed in many other sections in this book, such as the section on PCA, the section on psychiatric and cognitive rehabilitation, and more.

CONCLUSION

Person-centered approaches to psychopharmacology and biophysical interventions for people with SMI include many factors and considerations. SDM, substitute decision-making while exploring assent with incapable service users, as well as individualized medication prescribing and dispensing constitute important aspects of such person-centered approaches. Research is needed to further explore and provide more evidence-based interventions that align with such person-centered approaches.

REFERENCES

1 Deegan PE. The importance of personal medicine: a qualitative study of resilience in people with psychiatric disabilities. *Scand J Public Health*. 2005; **66**: 29–35.
2 Forchuk C, Kohr R. Prescriptive authority for nurses: the Canadian perspective. *Perspect Psychiatr C*. 2009; **45**(1): 3–8.

3 Anthony W, Cohen M, Farkas M, *et al. Psychiatric Rehabilitation.* 2nd ed. Boston, MA: Center for Psychiatric Rehabilitation; 2002.

4 Rudnick A. Towards a rationalization of biological psychiatry: a study in psychobiological epistemology. *J Med Philos.* 1990; **15**(1): 75–96.

5 Rudnick A. The molecular turn in psychiatry: a philosophical analysis. *J Med Philos.* 2002; **27**(3): 287–96.

6 Stein DJ. *Philosophy of Psychopharmacology: smart pills, happy pills, and pepp pills.* Cambridge: Cambridge University Press; 2008.

7 Deegan PE, Rapp C, Holter M, *et al.* Best practices: a program to support shared decision-making in an outpatient psychiatric medication clinic. *Psychiatr Serv.* 2008; **59**(6): 603–5.

8 Porter D. The critical theory of psychopharmacology: the work of David Healy and beyond. In: Phillips J, editor. *Philosophical Perspectives on Technology and Psychiatry.* Oxford: Oxford University Press; 2009. pp. 115–34.

9 Rudnick A. Psychiatric rehabilitation and the notion of technology in psychiatry. In: Phillips J, editor. *Philosophical Perspectives on Technology and Psychiatry.* Oxford: Oxford University Press; 2009. pp. 203–13.

10 Deegan PE, Drake RE. Shared decision-making and medication management in the recovery process: from compliance to alliance. *Psychiatr Serv.* 2006; **57**(11): 1636–9.

11 Ayd JF, Blackwell B, editors. *Discoveries in Biological Psychiatry.* Philadelphia, PA: Lippincot; 1970.

12 Healy D. *The Creation of Psychopharmacology.* Cambridge, MA: Harvard University Press; 2002.

13 Lieberman JA, Stroup TS, McEvoy JP, *et al.* Effectiveness of antipsychotic drugs in patients with chronic schizophrenia. *New Engl J Med.* 2005; **353**(12): 1209–23.

14 Sajatovic M, Madhusoodanan S, Fuller MA. Clozapine. In: Mueser KT, Jeste DV, editors. *Clinical Handbook of Schizophrenia.* New York, NY: Guildford; 2008. pp. 178–85.

15 Healy D. *Psychiatric Drugs Explained.* 4th ed. Edinburgh: Elsevier; 2005.

16 Stein DJ, Lerer B, Stahl S, editors. *Evidence-Based Psychopharmacology.* Cambridge: Cambridge University Press; 2005.

17 Lieberman, Stroup, McEvoy, *et al.*, op. cit.

18 Pohar R. Adherence to second-generation antipsychotics. *Pharmacy Practice.* 2007 Oct; (Continuous Education Suppl.): 1–8.

19 Cramer JA, Rosenheck R. Enhancing medication compliance for people with serious mental illness. *J Nerv Ment Dis.* 1999; **187**(1): 53–5.

20 Weiden PJ, Olfson M. Cost of relapse in schizophrenia. *Schizophr Bull.* 1995; **21**(3): 419–29.

21 Swartz MS, Swanson JW, Hiday VA, *et al.* Violence and severe mental illness: the effects of substance abuse and nonadherence to medication. *Am J Psychiatry.* 2008; **155**(2): 226–31.

22 Fenton WS, Blyler CR, Heinssen RK. Determinants of medication compliance in schizophrenia: empirical and clinical findings. *Schizophr Bull.* 1997; **23**(4): 637–51.

23 Velligan DI, Bow-Thomas CC, Huntzinger C, *et al.* Randomized controlled trial of the use of compensatory strategies to enhance adaptive functioning in outpatients with schizophrenia. *Am J Psychiatry.* 2000; **157**(8): 1317–23.

24 McCracken SG, Corrigan PW. Motivational interviewing for medication adherence in individuals with schizophrenia. In: Arkowitz H, Westra HA, Miller WE, *et al.*, editors. *Motivational Interviewing in the Treatment of Psychological Problems.* New York, NY: Guilford; 2008. pp. 249–76.

25 McFarlane W, Dixon L, Lukens E, *et al.* Family psychoeducation and schizophrenia: a review of the literature. *J Marital Fam Ther.* 2003; **29**(2): 223–45.

26 Pohar, op. cit.

27 Burton SC. Strategies for improving adherence to second-generation antipsychotics in patients with schizophrenia by increasing ease of use. *J Psychiatr Pract.* 2005; **11**(6): 369–78.

28 Nose M, Barbui C, Gray R, *et al.* Clinical interventions for treatment non-adherence in psychosis: meta-analysis. *Brit J Psychiat.* 2008; **183**: 197–206.

29 Lieberman, Stroup, McEvoy, *et al.*, op. cit.

30 Pohar, op. cit.

31 Burton, op. cit.

32 Lamoure J. Schizophrenia: getting the right drug to the right patient. *Pharmacy Practice.* 2007; **23**(4): 48–64.

33 Pohar, op. cit.

34 Ibid.

35 Meyer JM. Strategies for the long-term treatment of schizophrenia: real-world lessons from the CATIE trial. *J Clin Psychiat.* 2007; **68**(Suppl. 1): 28–33.

36 Mueser KT, Corrigan PW, Hilton DW, *et al.* Illness management and recovery for severe mental illness: a review of the research. *Psychiatr Serv.* 2002; **53**(10): 1272–84.

37 Poulin MJ, Cortese L, Williams R, *et al.* Atypical antipsychotics in psychiatric practice: practical implications for clinical monitoring. *Can J Psychiat.* 2005; **50**(9): 555–62.

38 Dolder CR, Lacro JP, Leckband S, *et al.* Interventions to improve antipsychotic medication adherence: review of recent literature. *J Clin Psychopharm.* 2003; **23**(4): 389–99.

39 Zygmunt A, Olfson M, Boyer CA, *et al.* Interventions to improve medication adherence in schizophrenia. *Am J Psychiatry.* 2002; **159**(10): 1653–64.

40 Pohar, op. cit.

41 Bond GR, Drake RE, Mueser KT, *et al.* Assertive community treatment for people with severe mental illness: critical ingredients and impact on patients. *Dis Manage Health Outcomes.* 2001; **9**: 141–59.

42 Dodds F, Rebair-Brown A, *et al.* A systematic review of randomized controlled trials that attempt to identify interventions that improve patient compliance with prescribed antipsychotic medications. *Clin Eff Nurs.* 2000; **4**: 47–53.

43 Perkins DO. Predictors of noncompliance in patients with schizophrenia. *J Clin Psychiatry.* 2002; **63**(12): 1121–8.

44 Pohar, op. cit.

45 Grisso T, Appelbaum PS. *Assessing Competence to Consent to Treatment: a guide for physicians and other health professionals.* New York, NY: Oxford University Press; 1998.

46 Roe D, Lereya J, Fennig S. Comparing patients and staff members' attitudes: does patients' competence to disagree mean they are not competent? *J Nerv Ment Dis.* 2001; **189**(5): 307–10.

47 Rudnick A, Roe D. Normal variants of competence to consent to treatment. *HEC Forum.* 2004; **16**: 129–37.

48 Henderson C, Swanson JW, Szmukler G, *et al.* A typology of advance statements in mental health care. *Psychiatr Serv.* 2008; **59**(1): 63–71.

49 Stroup S, Appelbaum P, Swartz M, *et al.* Decision-making capacity for research participation among individuals in the CATIE schizophrenia trial. *Schizophr Res.* 2005; **80**(1): 1–8.

50 Ng CH, Lin K-M, Singh B, editors. *Ethno-psychopharmacology: advances in current practice.* Cambridge: Cambridge University Press; 2008.

51 Ng CH, Klimidis S. Cultural factors and the use of psychotropic medications. In: Ng CH, Lin KM, Singh B, Chiu E, editors. *Ethno-Psychopharmacology: advances in current practice.* Cambridge: Cambridge University Press; 2008. pp. 123–34.

52 Lambert T, Norman TR. Ethnic differences in psychotropic drug response and pharmacokinetics. In: Ng CH, Lin KM, Singh B, *et al.* Ibid. pp. 38–61.

53 Yu X. Complementary medicines in mental disorders. In: Ng CH, Lin K-M, Singh B, *et al.* Ibid. pp. 118–22.

54 Stahl SM, Grady MM, Munter N. *Essential Psychopharmacology: the prescribers guide.* Cambridge: Cambridge University Press; 2005.

55 Ibid.

56 Lyon ER. A Review of the effects of nicotine on schizophrenia and antipsychotic medications. *Psychiatr Serv.* 1999; **50**(10): 1346–50.

57 Lamoure J, Bush H. Atypical antipsychotics as poison in overdose. *Canadian Journal of CME.* 2005; **17**: 71–3.

58 Haddad PM, Dursun S, Deakin B, editors. *Adverse Syndromes and Psychiatric Drugs: a clinical guide.* Oxford: Oxford University Press; 2004.

59 Kingsbury SJ, Fayek M, Trufasiu D, *et al.* The apparent effects of ziprasidone on plasma lipids and glucose. *J Clin Psychiatry.* 2001; **62**(5): 347–9.

60 Kingdon DG, Turkington D. *Cognitive Therapy of Schizophrenia.* New York, NY: Guildford; 2005.

61 Peuskens J. The evolving definition of treatment resistance. *J Clin Psychiatry.* 1999; **60**(Suppl. 12): 4–8.

62 Higgins ES, George MS. *Brain Stimulation Therapies for Clinicians.* Washington, DC: American Psychiatric Publishing; 2009.

63 Miller AL, Craig CS. Combination antipsychotics: pros, cons and questions. *Schizophr Bull.* 2002; **28**(1): 105–9.

64 Honer WG, Thornton AE, Chen EY, *et al.* Clozapine alone versus clozapine and risperidone with refractory schizophrenia. *New Engl J Med.* 2006; **354**(5): 472–82.

65 Joosten EA, DeFuentes-Merillas L, *et al.* Systematic review of the effects of shared decision-making on patient satisfaction, treatment adherence and health status. *Psychother Psychosom.* 2008; **77**(4): 219–26.

66 Duncan E, Best C, Hagen S. Shared decision making interventions for people with mental health conditions. *Cochrane Database Syst Rev.* 2010; **20**(1): CD007297.

6.3 Person-Centered Individual Psychotherapy for Adults with Serious Mental Illness

Paul H. Lysaker, Nicole L. Beattie and Amy M. Strasburger

INTRODUCTION

As detailed clearly in the introduction to this book, PCC is currently a conceptual cornerstone of mental health services for adults with SMI. According to this model, treatment must seek to understand and address the strengths and needs of the whole person. As is the focus of this volume, exactly what this entails across a range of treatment approaches has yet to be fully detailed and studied. In this section we will explore one way of conceptualizing a person-centered approach to individual psychotherapy for persons with SMI. To that end we will describe one set of conditions sometimes found in SMI, specifically a subjective experience of a diminished sense of self, which a person-centered psychotherapy might be uniquely prepared to address. We next describe some of the possible requirements of that psychotherapy, focusing first on three principles related to the development of the therapeutic relationship and then three principles in terms of goal setting. This will be illustrated with an example and finally we will discuss possible ways to assess outcome.

Of note, it is not our intent in this section to suggest that there is only one way to approach these issues or to suggest a treatment that is superior to others, e.g. other cognitive behavioral approaches.[1] Indeed, we refer the reader to relevant sections in this book, such as Section 6.4, *Cognitive and Psychiatric Rehabilitation: person-centered ingredients for success*. We do though intend to suggest a person-centered psychotherapy that is available to any recovering person including those who experience disabling symptoms or deficits. We are not proposing a therapy that applies or is viable only during periods of greater levels of wellness and health. We hope to outline one set of principles that could be used to assist anyone with SMI, regardless of his or her condition, in the hopes of spurring dialogue, debate and research.

Possible Conditions for a Person-Centered Individual Psychotherapy for Serious Mental Illness

Recovery from mental illness is now widely thought to occur in both objective and subjective domains.[2] Along with things such as symptom remission and return to work, recovery is thought to also sometimes involve a recovery of a fuller sense of self. This may be an especially important issue for recovery based treatments to address, given that many forms of mental illness are often characterized as involving at some point during their course profound diminishments in the subjective experience of oneself as able to make meaning of daily experience and an individual's larger place in the world.[3,4,5] Here we are not referring to merely disorganized or confusing verbalization about facts, affects, thoughts and any of their contexts, but to the subjective experience in SMI of one's core identity as diminished relative to how that identity was previously experienced. To clarify matters, we are not referring to issues related to self-doubt, disappointment with oneself or the experience of oneself as changing in undesirable ways. What is reported instead is an experience of oneself as radically losing or lacking depth and richness.[6] Intimately tied to periods of dysfunction and anguish, this may include feeling oneself as having lost a basic sense of personhood or having become an object that is controlled by others.[7,8] These diminishments may also involve the sense that one cannot organize and account for the events that unfold in one's life in a manner that others can accept and empathize with.[9,10] They can also involve the experience of an inability to represent oneself as someone who possesses basic human dignity and is meaningfully connected to others.[11,12,13]

We would suggest that person-centered psychotherapy might facilitate recovery for some persons with SMI when they struggle with these issues. As noted in Rudnick and Roe's Section 1.1, *Foundations and Ethics of Person-Centered Approaches to Individuals with Serious Mental Illness*, the tradition of person-centered treatment in general is closely linked to efforts to explore "both the disease and illness experience" and the "whole person." Beyond that, the psychotherapy for many forms of SMI has been noted to be concerned with issues of narrative or ways people construct stories to make sense of their lives, emotions and challenges.[14,15] Psychotherapy in general has also been widely recognized as a process that can assist persons facing many predicaments to enrich narrative understanding of themselves and their life.[16]

Thus we suggest one role for person-centered psychotherapy might be to help persons with SMI recover a fuller and richer sense of self. In small frame, the focus of such a psychotherapy might be to help persons recapture a subjective experience of themselves as possessing dignity and competence as well as the ability to make sense of pain and confusion. In the larger frame, such psychotherapy could be thought of as helping persons to regain authorship over their lives. But what would concrete requirements of this be?

The Therapeutic Relationship in Person-Centered Psychotherapy for Serious Mental Illness

One natural place to start our discussion of person-centered psychotherapy for SMI is with the development of the therapeutic relationship. Not only is this the foundation for any work that will follow, but the development of a therapeutic relationship with persons with SMI is a notoriously delicate process to negotiate and may challenge even experienced providers. Much has been made about how persons with SMI may find intimacy overwhelming as well as how stigma may incline mentally ill persons to reject the possibility they are ill and distrust mental health providers.[17,18]

We would suggest that there are three related issues that have to be addressed in a person-centered psychotherapy as the possibility of a therapeutic relationship emerges. First, many with SMI may be wary of that relationship and may be distant initially. They may, for instance, find interpersonal relationships confusing or, anticipating rejection, be unwilling to engage initially in the relationship. They may fear that their families will be blamed for their illness or that they will be stigmatized if it is discovered that they are mentally ill. In response to this, painstaking efforts may need to be undertaken to understand the service users and how they experience the potential relationship with their providers. A frank discussion may need to be invited and supported in which service users can freely voice doubts or fears they hold without fears of repercussions, and this is an invitation service users should be allowed to regard with distrust as well.

A second issue that follows this pertains to how to respond to ambivalence or distance. In particular, one common set of errors can occur when a provider assumes the best way to establish rapport with such service users is to offer considerable support, education and empathy. If the service user seems withdrawn or untrusting, it might be intuitively appealing to offer friendly support and information until a trusting relationship is formed. Providing immediate empathy might be thought of by providers as welcoming. This stance, however, risks patronization and the reinforcement of stigma. We suggest that a person-centered approach may need to emphasize that service user distrust should be accepted empathically. This does not mean to empathize with the service users' general dilemmas but with their specific distrust of the provider. In this instance the issue is the object of empathy. We are suggesting that the provider can empathize with how difficult it is to trust the provider but not necessarily with the things that may later be disclosed once trust has been established.

Ambivalence may need to be accepted as a realistic and understandable response to stigma and not a sign of service user weakness. As a relatively simple illustration of this, a service user confessed to the first author that he felt guilty because he was uncomfortable in therapy and feared the first author would punish him. When the first author accepted these feelings and rejected the possibility the service user should feel guilty, the service user went on to explain that the only way he could imagine being comfortable in therapy was to first "thrash" the provider "in a friendly boxing match." In other words beneath what was presented as guilt were strong feelings of anger at the provider. From there it was explored how his anger at the provider was natural given his deep sense of mistreatment in the past by mental health providers. He was consequently not rushed into a trusting relationship, offered support or education he did not ask for, but allowed to be in charge of his own feelings about the meaning of therapy sessions.

Consistent with this, a third issue concerns the importance of establishing the therapeutic relationships in a non-hierarchical manner. We suggest one way to think about this is for providers to see themselves as "consultants" and not as "experts."

We use this distinction to suggest a more desirable role for providers wherein they feel free to take their time to learn about the service user's needs and perspective, and to reject the possibility that any uncertainty is a sign of incompetence. This has the possibility of suggesting to distant service users that there is an interest in getting to know them and help them, but not with any preformed solution or knowledge that the provider has about them. The service user's sense of their own identity is accepted as-is, and providers must be slow to offer alternative ideas relating to sense of self. Taking on the role of a consultant instead of an expert is also consistent with the imperative that providers relate to persons with mental illness in a non-stigmatizing manner. Continuing the illustration from above, the provider, in the manner of a consultant, accepted ongoing criticism of him by the service user but also felt free to challenge the service user in matters where he appeared to be denying he had feelings about tragic events or in which his behavior appeared to be sabotaging opportunities for success in a range of settings, without worrying these challenges would be destructive. Some service users may want the provider to be an expert. Our own view of this may be controversial. We would suggest that while there is nothing wrong with providing information or openly sharing opinions, a request to be an expert risks making the provider the principle agent of meaning-making, and consequently we fully avoid playing that role. We respond to these requests by sharing just this view and invite conversations regarding the meaning of the request for the provider to be an expert.

Goal Setting in a Person-Centered Psychotherapy for People with Serious Mental Illness

In addition to the formation of the therapeutic relationship, it is essential that in any person-centered individual therapy the provider and service user set mutually agreed upon goals for treatment. Although this can be a straightforward process, we can think of three issues that may need to be addressed. First, there may be times when finding a goal may be confusing; service users consumed with a particular delusion may offer a goal that could not be mutually agreed upon, for example, "Can you make me become God?" Alternatively, service users with negative symptoms may say they have no goals, for example: "I don't know about that – that's up to you, doctor." Service users with severe cognitive symptoms may offer thoughts that seem unconnected to one another. Still others may deny that they have a mental illness or offer overly simplistic, e.g. to become physically attractive, or unrealistic goals, e.g. to become a TV anchor person.

Here the provider must see that the development of goals may take time and careful thought. In the spirit of being a consultant the provider should not forcibly supply his or her own goals in the face of confusion. For instance, it is tempting to respond to a delusional goal with the suggestion that reducing delusions should be a goal. Others may want to respond to a service user unaware of his or her illness by suggesting awareness of illness should be a goal. If the service user hallucinates, the provider might jump to thinking that reducing hallucinations should be the goal.

Of course these may be goals, but the issue is that they must be supplied by the service user. To avoid these pitfalls, providers must tolerate the anxiety that naturally arises when service user and provider are unsure of the treatment's purpose. When meeting with a service user who thinks that therapy is useless and wants to leave, but attends only to conform to expectations of a commitment, the provider may need to develop a comfort level with being in the position of a consultant rather than an expert who assists the service user in the process of understanding and giving a name to the individual's thoughts, feelings and behaviors.

Once a provider has become comfortable with not supplying a goal when the process is confusing, a second issue is that the provider must listen to the authentic message of the service user as a whole person, noticing the content of the message as well as how the service user says it, and to seek consensually valid meaning, which could be the agreed upon focus of treatment. In the example of the service user who wants to be God, providers might consider that to be God could mean relief from feelings of guilt and inadequacy. Similarly, the provider might consider the possibility that the service user who says he or she has no mental illness may have been trying to communicate that he or she feels unfairly ostracized by others and is unsure how to fit in. Maybe the service user feels his or her life story is over or that it is unworthy of being told. In each of these examples then, the provider should be expected to find a wealth of possible goals, e.g. managing guilt, making sense of rejection or revisiting service user's experience that he or no longer is a subject worthy of a narrative. Goals in this way emerge and evolve as the provider gets to know the whole person, again in keeping with the key tenets of PCC.

From a different angle, one which may be more complicated, there is also the need for the provider to not accept that everything could be an equally valid goal of therapy. If the provider can assume the position of a consultant, he or she should see that he or she has permission to have his or her own opinions about what makes sense. Consider, for example, the service user who says: "I know I'm a schizophrenic with a chemical imbalance, so I take my medication every day." Some providers might see this as successful learning and fail to consider that this statement also harbors the possibility that the service user has defined himself or herself by his illness and is counting on external forces exclusively to solve problems. As providers work with service users, many of who will have internalized stigma, they must be ready to inquire about what their perceptions of being ill mean and then to challenge self-stigma as it arises.

Importantly, our view in this example is that the provider's role is not to merely see a need to educate the service user to think of himself or herself as a person with schizophrenia, but to encourage him or her to make his or her own sense of his or her life as a whole person. It may be tempting to tell discouraged persons with mental illness that they are heroes. Indeed many rehabilitation providers might endorse this as a good practice. Our view though deviates from this practice. To tell service users they are heroes might be a part of the provider's story, but as such it is not the service user's story. Adopting another's story as one's own, no matter how positive, may result in the experience again of being an object controlled by others, or of needing the praise of a more powerful other in order to be able to have a positive self-definition.

A third issue with regard to goal-setting is the risk that once concrete goals have been established, providers may lose sight of the whole person and see the process of recovery as the taking of a series of small, unambiguous steps. A goal, for example, may be set to increase socialization by joining a horseback riding club. In helping the service user pursue that goal, the provider may need to continue to recognize the need to know the service user as a whole person and to evolve an ever deeper shared understanding of what recovery means. It is important that the meeting of a concrete goal, while an accomplishment, should not eclipse the process of relating and continuous reassessment. For instance, in joining the club, what if the service user is shocked by his success and attributes it to the excellence of the provider, accepting quietly the stigmatizing belief that mental illness means incompetence? What if the service user discovers that he or she does not like his or her club mates or misses solitude in the evening but does not want to withdraw in fear of disappointing the provider? Our point then is regardless of whether the goal is attained or not, the process of assisting the service user to see him or herself as a whole person must remain ongoing.

Person-Centered Therapy for Serious Mental Illness and the Assessment of Outcomes

A final set of issues we will address pertains to outcomes. How does the provider know change is occurring? Definitions of recovery are at present still evolving. and there is no consensus regarding how one should assess progress.[19] Regardless, it is irresponsible to not try and objectively determine how matters are unfolding. Providers may inquire routinely in an unstructured manner if interventions are helpful but then to inquire in depth about what was helpful and/or what was not helpful. Beyond general inquiries, providers can also assess outcome using any of a number of formal questionnaires designed to assess related constructs such as hope, self-esteem and stigma. Administering instruments such as these at fixed intervals has the benefit of tracking small degrees of change over time, something which may be important to do given the nonlinear course of recovery. As illustrated in intensive case studies, growth from week to week may be miniscule, such that the provider can have the impression that nothing has changed, leading to discouragement.[20]

Regarding the assessment of global changes in sense of self, one scale that may be used to quantitatively evaluate outcomes in this domain is the Scale to Assess Narrative Development (STAND).[21,22] The STAND assesses the extent to which persons have developed a coherent story of themselves and their psychiatric challenges. The STAND can be rated by providers at the end of a session and, as above, compiled over time to produce a record of progress that may be too slow or uneven for the eye to track from week to week. It includes Likert scales to assess four outcomes for recovering persons: *Illness Conception*, or the extent to which psychiatric or psychological challenges are plausibly elucidated; *Alienation*, or the extent to which persons experience themselves as linked to at least one fulfilling intimate tie; *Agency*, or the extent to which the self is portrayed as actively affecting one's life course; and *Social Worth*, or the extent to which the self is portrayed as intrinsically valuable in one's community. The STAND may offer a way to quantify movement along this most personal and subjective continuum of recovery, and as such can be used to both identify need, e.g. lack of agency, as well as to quantitatively track change. Of note, this tool may also help providers avoid focusing on concrete goals, during either periods of loss or gain, to the extent that the whole person is lost from view.

Example

This is an illustration of the principles laid out about as demonstrated in a single session of psychotherapy:

Handel is a single man in his 20s who has struggled with symptoms of psychosis since his early teenage years. He has struggled with the abuse of drugs and alcohol and had several incarcerations for aggressive behavior while intoxicated. He has had two suicide attempts in the past and has a brother who also has been diagnosed with a severe mental illness. He has had multiple experiences in which he has rejected different treatment providers. For the session illustrated here, he arrives 20 minutes early and during the week prior had canceled, saying he was ill. He and the provider have been meeting weekly for two years at this point. Recent gains include his first episode of continuous community tenure of six months.

The interaction begins in the waiting room. The two men say hello and there is a warm handshake. They walk silently into the provider's office, and once the door is closed Handel sits in silence until the provider asks Handel where he "wants to start." Handel calls attention to the fact that he is wearing a tie today, something that feels uncomfortable. There is a general discussion of how Handel is doing several things which are in line with treating himself and his body with "more respect" and that "does not feel like me." When asked if this is something to explore Handel says, "No, it was only a thought on my mind." He talks next about his mother, who has appeared in a newspaper article about gardening. But after a little of inquiry Handel says it was just another thought. He says he is not sure what he wants of the provider today.

After a few minutes to think, Handel says his major issue is work and he has gone another week without looking for a job. He states this is something he wants to talk about. He is not sure what to say, and the provider asks if Handel is looking for help figuring out how to put in job applications. Handel says "yes," and the provider offers some thoughts about concrete solutions for this issue. This brings a look of displeasure to Handel's face. When that is noticed, Handel says he really didn't want any advice and actually when the provider suggests solutions he ends up resenting them and feeling bad about himself. It is agreed the advice was not helpful.

What emerges next is a reflection by Handel that he has not looked for work since he expected to fail if he did find another job. He notes that foremost he wishes to avoid humiliation in life, and he also remarks that his identity is one of a failure. There is some discussion about how this view of himself has emerged over his whole life story. Pain and indecision in the present is understood in a storied and narrative context. The provider asks if Handel wants to form a different picture of his life and Handel says he does but he is just "too uncomfortable" at the moment to consider thinking differently about himself. There are examples of ways in which Handel is currently not acting like a failure and even a joke about how Handel should be careful not to ruin his image as a failure with all these recent gains. Handel comes back to how his way of living is to avoid as much as he can "as often as possible." The provider asks if Handel was avoiding when he called in sick and whether he was not sick. Handel confesses this is, in fact, what happened. When asked if he considered it rude of the provider to think and ask this, Handel says, "no – it is a relief." When asked by the provider if next time Handel may not just say in the future that he wanted to avoid the session rather than lie, Handel offered an emphatic "no." He went on say, "If I confessed that to you I couldn't fool myself and I would make myself come in." This is followed by a period of laughter over the issue by both parties. The provider asks Handel if it was worth his time coming today and he says it was, that it made him more "comfortable with myself and being open with someone else." There is a warm handshake at the end and an agreement to meet again next week at the same (usual) time.

When compared to previous sessions in general, a STAND rating of the current session would show improvements in the areas of the enhancement of sense of Agency and Social Worth.

CONCLUSION

In summary, we have suggested that person-centered psychotherapy may be appropriate in assisting persons with SMI to make larger narrative sense of their strengths and weaknesses, particularly during periods of illness in which they experience a diminishment of their sense of self. To begin to describe the requirements of such a psychotherapy, we have offered three general principles in reference to the formation of the therapeutic alliance. Specially, we suggested that it may be challenging to form such a relationship and that the provider must accept distance or ambivalence on the part of the service user as possible and reasonable given levels of illness and previous experiences with stigma. The provider must also allow a non-hierarchical relationship to develop at a pace dictated by the service user, one which moves past stigmatizing dynamics and allows for a mutual focus on the service user as someone who is making his or her own meaning of his or her life. Second, we suggested that goal setting is essential to such a therapy but that therapy should not become fixed in the setting and achievement of goals. Providers may need to sustain a dialogue with the service user that develops a meaningful sense of the service user's life and perspective of his or her recovery. Finally, the measurement of outcomes can be useful to providers both as a means of understanding where the service user is in recovery and also for gaining a perspective of non-linear growth over time.

Importantly, the speculations laid out here are a beginning. As noted above, we have not intended to suggest a better treatment than any other, only to begin a dialogue about the principles of person-centered psychotherapy for persons with SMI that could address both the illness experience and the whole person. Future case study and controlled research is necessary to define and test the usefulness of these methods as the field develops. Current projects underway by the authors' group include in-depth analyses of the interpersonal process occurring between providers and service users that help service users to tolerate the painful feelings that emerge when confronting loss. We are also exploring how those same interpersonal processes facilitate the development of more awareness of service users' own thoughts and feelings and their ability to accurately detect the thoughts and feelings of others around them. Finally we are attempting to operationalize the practices outlined above and plan to explore whether sessions that conform to these qualities have superior outcomes relative to ones that do not.

REFERENCES

1 Tarrier N, Wykes T. Is there evidence that cognitive behaviour therapy is an effective treatment for schizophrenia? A cautious or cautionary tale? *Behav Res Ther.* 2004; **42**(12): 1377–401.
2 Lysaker PH, Buck KD. Is recovery from schizophrenia possible: an overview of concepts, evidence and clinical implications. *Prim Psychiatry.* 2008; **15**(6): 60–6.
3 Horowitz R. Memory and meaning in the psychotherapy of the long term mentally ill. *Clin Soc Work J.* 2006; **34**: 175–85.
4 Silverstein SM, Bellack AS. A scientific agenda for the concept of recovery as it applies to schizophrenia. *Clin Psychol Rev.* 2008; **28**(7): 1108–24.
5 Staghellini G. *Disembodied Spirits and Deanimated Bodies.* Oxford: Oxford University Press; 2004.
6 Lysaker PH, Lysaker JT. *Schizophrenia and the Ffate of the Self.* Oxford: Oxford University Press; 2008.
7 Roe D. Recovering from severe mental illness: mutual influences of self and illness. *J Psychosoc Nurs Ment Health Serv.* 2005; **43**: 35–40.
8 Rudge T, Morse K. Re-awakening?: a discourse analysis of the recovery from schizophrenia after medication change. *Aust N Z J Ment Health Nurs.* 2001; **10**(2): 66–76.

9 Gallagher S. Self narrative in schizophrenia. In: Kirshner T, David A, editors. *The Self in Neuroscience and Neuropsychiatry*. Cambridge: Cambridge University Press; 2003. pp. 336–53.

10 Holma J, Aaltonen J. Narrative understanding and acute psychosis. *Contemporary Family Therapy*. 1998; **20**: 253–63.

11 Lysaker, Lysaker, op. cit.

12 Laithwaite H, Gumley A. Sense of self, adaptation and recovery in patients with psychosis in a forensic NHS setting. *Clin Psychol Psychother*. 2007; **14**: 302–16.

13 Roe D, Ben-Yaskai AB. Exploring the relationship between the person and the disorder among individuals hospitalized for psychosis. *Psychiatry*. 1999; **62**: 372–80.

14 Dimaggio G, Semerari A, Carcione A, *et al*. *Psychotherapy of Personality Disorders: metacognition, states of mind and interpersonal cycles*. London: Brunner Routledge; 2007.

15 Fenton WS. Evolving perspectives on individual psychotherapy for schizophrenia. *Schizophr Bull*. 2000; **26**(1): 47–72.

16 Neimeyer RA, Raskin JD. *Constructions of Disorder: meaning-making frameworks for psychotherapy*. Washington, DC: APA Press; 2000.

17 Weiden P, Havens L. Psychotherapeutic management techniques in the treatment of outpatients with schizophrenia. *Hosp Community Psychiatry*. 1994; **45**: 549–55.

18 Lysaker PH, Roe D, Yanos PT. Toward understanding the insight paradox: internalized stigma moderates the association between insight and social functioning, hope and self-esteem among people with schizophrenia spectrum disorders. *Schizophr Bull*. 2007; **33**: 192–9.

19 Silverstein, Bellack, op. cit.

20 Lysaker PH, Davis LD, Eckert GJ, *et al*. Changes in narrative structure and content in schizophrenia in long term individual psychotherapy: a single case study. *Clin Psychol Psychother*. 2005; **12**: 406–16.

21 Lysaker, Buck, op. cit.

22 Lysaker PH, Taylor A, Miller A, *et al*. The scale to assess narrative development: associations with other measures of self and readiness for recovery in schizophrenia spectrum disorders. *J Nerv Ment Dis*. 2006; **194**(3): 223–5.

6.4 Cognitive and Psychiatric Rehabilitation: person-centered ingredients for success

Joel O. Goldberg

INTRODUCTION

> ### Example
>
> An individual with serious mental illness who attended our CBT for psychosis group reported that he often heard "voices" that told him to "stay home" and not attend his vocational program.[1] When asked how it was that he managed to come to the CBT group, he indicated that a valued service provider (who recognized his paranoid fears of bus travel) had arranged for special car transportation, overcoming what for him seemed to be an insurmountable attendance barrier. Through the course of the therapy, he participated actively in discussions. He witnessed how others with serious mental illness increased their self-insight regarding symptoms, and he inquired how they had been able to discover "positive self-talk" methods to cope with auditory hallucinations.[2] His learning was enhanced through watching a note-taking assistant who wrote key points on a flip chart, which was used to help group members absorb the information. He modeled his own compensatory strategies after theirs, using a "letting go" strategy of saying to himself, "I'm going to leave the voices at the bus stop" and a "volitional" strategy of telling himself, "I'm not going to allow the voices to run my life". He continues to take medication, from which he feels he derives benefit, but it is his discovery of cognitive self-instruction coping methods that have enabled him to travel comfortably on buses and to actually attend meaningful activities in the community.

This brief vignette provides an example of three key person-centered ingredients to cognitive and psychiatric rehabilitation that will be highlighted in this section. The first ingredient is that of readiness and unawareness of illness. In the example, it was an empathic service provider whose influence was crucial in identifying and overcoming barriers to engage in rehabilitation, tipping the balance of fears and indecision over attendance. The second ingredient is that of identification of cognitive impairments and application of cognitive strategies to enhance learning. In the vignette, the environment support of a flip chart provided a kind of "closed caption" text display device to help focus and guide attention. The third ingredient is that of peer support. In this example, it was peer group members who shared their personal discoveries of cognitive coping methods that contributed to this individual's increased illness awareness and led to his success in functional improvements, and which inspired his more hopeful recovery orientation. Note that this section is complementary to many other sections in this book, such as Section 6.1, *Person-Centered Assessment of People with Serious Mental Illness,* and Section 6.3, *Person-Centered Individual Psychotherapy for Adults with Serious Mental Illness,* which the reader is referred to.

Readiness and Unawareness of Illness

While an important initial focus of psychopharmacological interventions has been concerned with consent for treatment initiation and concordance with service providers about taking medication,[3] the parallel concern in the realm of PSR has been the issue of readiness,[4] since this is a key prerequisite for engagement in the process of recovery. Traditional approaches have at times emphasized power-oriented strategies, in which the service providers try to be convincing and persuasive, but then there is unfortunately a potential to go too far and become coercive in their efforts. Service providers who lack a person-centered perspective are prone to adopting either confrontation or "withdrawal of services" strategies and to just "let him or her hit rock bottom" until the service users finally concede and acquiesce, or else they become frustrated and drop out. Too often it is the service users who get blamed for failures to engage in treatment, they are said to be somehow at fault or in denial or else, and this is crucial for this discussion, as they are said to lack insight. Now, in fact, research evidence does confirm that individuals who are diagnosed with schizophrenia are more likely to be unaware of their illness, compared with individuals diagnosed with mood disorders.[5]

Indeed, what might seem ironic on the surface is that there are examples of individuals with SMI who are acutely aware and even sensitive to psychosis in others while at the same time show a marked failure of self-monitoring, a failure to recognize those same kinds of symptoms, such as paranoia, in themselves. This phenomenon is also evident in referral patterns in which persons with depression are poignantly self-aware that they are disturbed by sleep problems or forgetfulness or troubled moods and so refer themselves for help. In stark contrast, some individuals with SMI fail to refer themselves for help and may suffer from long periods of untreated psychosis,[6] in part due to their genuine lack of illness awareness, and so they need to rely on others, and in particular, their families, to assist in accessing required treatment.

Given this context, what is missing for those service providers who label service users in an almost accusatory way of lacking insight is a more nuanced understanding of how issues related to unawareness of illness impact on individuals' readiness for rehabilitation. Amador and colleagues[7] have argued that illness unawareness cannot be assumed to reflect antagonism towards help-givers but rather service providers may be failing to recognize and understand problems related to the neuropsychological aspects of illness unawareness. Illness insight is a crucial factor that needs to be considered and even formally examined, whether it is through brief methods or through use of more comprehensive assessment tools that have been developed to assess unawareness of mental disorder in a variety of domains of illness experience.[8,9] Another illness insight measure has been developed specifically to evaluate unawareness of cognitive impairments.[10] Once the nature of unawareness of illness has been identified, it is possible to work with persons who feel "I am not sick, I don't need help"[11] using empathic techniques to help achieve better self-understandings; in fact, this text is a useful resource for families who are struggling to understand failed illness awareness in their relative. Illness management approaches have been demonstrated to be effective in improving knowledge about illness and increased recovery-orientation, as have peer mentor approaches.[12,13] As well, CBT methods have been shown to have impact in improving insight.[14,15] Increased awareness of illness can be an important and often essential prerequisite for supporting persons with SMI to participate in rehabilitation and become oriented towards recovery.

In a related vein, assessing readiness for rehabilitation has been studied for decades and yet it has been a somewhat controversial topic particularly in the employment domain.[16] Traditional assessments of readiness, much like the traditional assessments of insight that simply label the person as being in denial, much too frequently determine that an individual shows a "failure to be ready," which then results essentially in the person being denied access to employment opportunities because he or she has been deemed to be uninterested in vocational training.[17] The Individual Placement and Supports model provides an alternative by first accessing job placements for individuals, then supporting them on-site to maintain their employment, which, in a sense, bypasses the "barrier" aspects of not showing "readiness" to engage in lengthy pre-employment training.[18] Nevertheless, there still remains clinical utility in considering person-centered approaches to readiness interventions that are geared not towards restricting people from accessing resources but rather towards helping people move forward in identifying and articulating desired personal goals.[19] The personal development process of "growing" readiness for rehabilitation has been carefully mapped out.[20] The view is to help individuals gain increased self-understanding by proceeding through a stepwise process of determining their need for change (through assessing levels of dissatisfaction), commitment to change (belief that change is possible), self-awareness (pertinent to skills, interests, values and preferences), environmental awareness (pertinent to opportunities and levels of demands), and willingness to establish a working alliance. Planned motivational activities play a part in moving towards readiness. Such an approach, which helps to articulate personal needs, is seen as a prerequisite to person-centered (as opposed to practitioner-defined) goals.

Finally, motivational interviewing techniques have been adapted for people with SMI.[21,22] The method considers a stage-based approach to change in which a person moves from pre-contemplation to contemplation and preparation before finally being truly ready to take action and make a change.[23] Some research has shown that clinicians fail to consider the stages of readiness and therefore overlook opportunities for change.[24] Motivational interviews use empathy to emphasize a "discovery" (not confrontational) orientation, help people deal with barriers to change, and support self-efficacy. Unfortunately, clinical experience has found that some individuals have trouble managing the cognitive demands of listing costs and benefits, which are some of the motivational interview techniques, while others show significant anhedonia and anergia (so-called "negative" symptoms found among some people with schizophrenia); thus they fail to articulate sources of motivation. In this regard, there is some evidence that it is these negative symptoms (such as apathy), more than self-efficacy, which are the biggest obstacle to functional improvements and which need to be addressed in rehabilitation efforts.[25]

Cognitive Impairments and Coping Enhancements

Traditional approaches have tended to focus on delusions and other psychotic symptoms as key "targets" for interventions, but actually it is cognitive impairments and associated negative symptoms that are crucial to recognize and address when working in a rehabilitation context with people to help them overcome barriers towards functional recovery.[26] Even when these persistent deficits are acknowledged, some scientific "broken brain" conceptualizations convey a rather pessimistic view of recovery potential.[27,28] Instead, what is critical is to identify core cognitive barriers and acknowledge their importance in rehabilitation planning.[29] Unfortunately, some clinicians have been prone to falsely labeling service users as "difficult" or "unmotivated" when in fact it is the service providers who fail to recognize these crucial neuropsychological deficits. For example, frontal systems "planning" deficits can cause impaired capacity to set goals (the negative symptom of "apathy"), but there are practitioners who mistake these "executive function" impairments for "laziness." Attention deficits have been linked to what has been pejoratively labeled as "lack of motivation," but in fact the problem may be due to failure to show the inclination to maintain focus over time. Further, attention impairments, which can affect a person's capacity to absorb information, are often quite difficult to detect and therefore can lead to the person being misjudged as "treatment resistant." Person-centered approaches can address these critical barriers to recovery through the enhancement of behavioral strategies and through the developmental of environmental coping supports. Behavioral approaches can serve to empower persons with SMI and increase opportunities and functional independence.[30]

A number of research studies, mainly using surveys and qualitative methods have identified coping methods that persons with persistent mental illness have discovered as being helpful methods, beyond medication management, to manage their serious psychotic symptoms, such as delusions and hallucinations.[31,32] Other important work has examined coping methods that persons with schizophrenia and their families had discovered on their own to be effective in managing symptoms such as apathy and inattention.[33] Such findings are consistent not only with a person-centered approach but also encourage a more hopeful recovery orientation and suggest the potential for expanded coping opportunities with further development, especially when considering applications through the development of cognitive compensatory approaches. A systematic focus on the development of environmental supports to assist persons with their adjustment has been developed using a method termed *cognitive adaptation training*.[34] This rehabilitation intervention employs assistive devices such as signs, checklists, alarms and calendars in order help to sequence and cue adaptive behavior. A critical element in the use of these environmental supports is that they be individually tailored, which is consistent with a person-centered approach. Indeed, previous work with individuals who have known brain-related memory impairments has shown that the use of a diary or "memory book" is a useful compensatory strategy,[35] but the assistive memory aid (including the commonly used techniques of weekly schedule reminders) cannot simply be handed to the person. Instead, therapeutic collaboration is required to teach and implement its use.

Consideration of information processing deficits that are evident in many individuals with SMI requires the use of teaching aids and learning accommodations. Specifically, learning capacity has been found, perhaps not surprisingly,[36] to be a key predictor of success in skills-training efforts, but what this implies is that teaching methods must incorporate strategies designed to enhance attention, memory and learning for those who show impairments. The length of classes may need to be shorter to accommodate limited capacity, while visual aids and handouts may be required to accompany verbal instruction. Attention-shaping strategies, such as social skills training, can be incorporated into groups.[37,38] The content of skills training follows a common process, beginning with instruction, demonstration, role play, corrective feedback and finally generalization.[39] However, it is the generalization component, namely, having the learner use the skills outside the classroom, which is most challenging, especially when service users are faced with frontal brain systems-based mental perseveration that cause failures to transfer learning.[40] Skills interventions require careful use of homework and "field trips" to overcome barriers to change in the "real world." Understanding the person-centered ingredients that work in various skills training curricula will help to enhance success in implementing specific rehabilitation programs.

There have been some attempts to use cognitive training to actually remediate cognitive impairments, but the early efforts seemed to meet with only mixed success based on only a few controlled outcome studies.[41] Nevertheless, research into cognitive remediation has continued and suggests that improvement is indeed possible but depends on important person and treatment factors,[42] namely, the approach must be person-centered, not simply applied as rote, routinized teaching. Another review, this one involving a more recent comprehensive meta-analysis,[43] suggested that cognitive remediation can produce moderate improvements especially when combined with PSR efforts. Cognitive training typically involves the use and repeated practice of mental exercises in order to enrich cognitive experience.[44] Some training has focused on practicing problem-solving skills through the use of stimulating computer-based games.[45] Other approaches employ "paper-and-pencil" tasks, but this training is individualized to begin with simple demands and then is progressively shaped to increasing difficulty levels using errorless learning and scaffolding teaching strategies.[46] A more comprehensive approach, developed by Hogarty and colleagues[47] has been termed *cognitive enhancement therapy*, which combines the use of computer-based exercises to improve attention, memory and problem-solving with a focus on social cognition including the use of peer partners in the training itself.

Peer Support and Role Model Learning

Example

Mark is a tutor who works part-time in the computer room at a psychiatric rehabilitation clinic. Diagnosed with paranoid schizophrenia years ago, his psychotic symptoms stabilized through treatment, but he was bored and dissatisfied. With encouragement from his case manager, he began attending one on one computer tutorial sessions at the clinic taught by a community college trained volunteer. Over time, he learned basic skills in word processing, surfing the Internet and use of email. Not a man of many words, Mark liked the sense of mastery in making things happen at the touch of his hand and the click of his mouse. He likes that he feels more focused and that his mind doesn't wander.

His case manager arranged for him to a get a computer for his apartment, providing an older model that had been donated to the agency. In fact, he became so engaged in spending time on the computers, he put his name forward when a part-time job opening was advertised at the clinic for a computer peer support tutor. He was hired and found himself an almost instant success; his schedule is full in showing others the skills that he has learned. He provides teaching using well-prepared curriculum modules for each computer skill, saying that the work "relaxes me"; he finds that he is less bored and that he really enjoys interactions with others. He has sought out further training experiences for himself, obtaining peer support worker certification through formal training at a local program and enrolling in an online course in computer repairs. He has become aware through his tutoring work that many of his peers often struggle to manage on their own, that for some, no matter how often he shows them how to open a browser or check their email, they are still unable to do it on their home computers, reflecting a failure in transfer of skills. But he is there for them and they value their experiences with him;[48] their self-esteem is bolstered, and they describe feeling a sense of being included – not isolated – from others.

Conveying an attitude that "recovery" is possible has not evolved from scientists whose outlook has traditionally emphasized the chronic course and persistent aspects of schizophrenia.[49] Instead, the message of hope that is so important for inspiration in PSR often comes from peers. Such optimism is not without substance, for indeed the negativism that darkened traditional perspectives has been challenged by evidence from longitudinal research that has demonstrated that up to half of service users do in fact have more favorable outcomes, such as enhanced quality of life.[50] Such findings have not been lost on public policy advocates who have worked to develop a more recovery-oriented system that highlights personal empowerment as well as featuring peer supports as a critical element of service delivery. Unfortunately, the integration of peers into rehabilitation programs has tended to be overlooked or disparaged by some providers and so its value needs to be highlighted.[51]

The use of peer providers holds much promise as a key ingredient to enhance rehabilitation success,[52] though to date there are few formal controlled studies which have been conducted to help identify the nature of the contributions and the circumstances that provide greatest benefit. In fact, as addressed and elaborated in this book, there are different kinds of peer-delivered interventions including actual peer service providers, mutual support groups, and the utilization of peer workers in adjunctive treatment support roles. Person-centered approaches incorporate peer supports because of the value placed on lived experiences that are shared; the peer has actually been there while the provider, not matter how strong their expertise, has not. What will be described here is what is speculated to be a crucial aspect of peer support, namely that of role-model learning.

Role-model learning has been found to be quite powerful and influential, based on decades of research conducted by Bandura[53] and colleagues. Opportunities for this kind of learning can be made available when there is the presence of a peer who has been successful in overcoming personal adversity and who thus provides a visible, personal and convincing demonstration of efficacy. Some recent empirical findings based on an investigation of peer service providers who shared their personal experiences with illness indicated that peer providers are not only able to validate the service user's experiences more convincingly than a traditional service provider, at least in the short-run, but they are also able to challenge erroneous beliefs in efficacious ways; they can relate because they have "been there."[54] As role models, peers are able to convey that personal recovery is indeed possible, which is a message of hope that is simply not the same when such messages attempt to be delivered by non-peer service providers. Unfortunately, traditional approaches have generally neglected such potential beneficial impact of having peer supports involved in treatment services.

In contrast, person-centered approaches employ peers in a variety of PSR contexts such as social skills groups, where the practical use of role modeling is quite explicit. Specifically, individuals who have already graduated from previous social skills training can be hired as role-play instructors, who provide teaching enriched by their personal experiences and can tell stories of what has been most challenging to them and what has contributed to their success. In fact, there are many opportunities for peer workers in every kind of rehabilitation program, for example, cooking instructors in kitchen collectives, teaching assistants in smoking management programs and leaders in mutual self-support groups, including those specifically aimed at enhancing an attitude of hope and recovery.[55] Furthermore, the effective inclusion of peer workers in rehabilitation programs may have important influences on social cognition and is an important and growing area of study.[56] Taken together, it has come to be recognized that psychosocial interventions are showing promise beyond symptom stabilization as a way of helping service users achieve adaptive functional recovery.[57]

CONCLUSION

Person-centered rehabilitation practice can be enhanced through the recognition of various cognitive impairments that affect many individuals with schizophrenia and other SMIs, including those which may cause unawareness of illness that affect readiness to engage and those attention and motivational deficits that disrupt learning and so may require accommodations. In turn, both empirical work and clinical experience suggest that cognitive remediation practices, in order to be successful, need to incorporate a person-centered approach when individually tailoring skills-training interventions. Peer supports have been underutilized in traditional health care settings and only minimally examined in empirical work, yet clinical experience suggests that they provide crucial opportunities for role-model learning and sharing of coping strategy discoveries in moving forward towards recovery.

REFERENCES

1 Goldberg JO, Wheeler H, Lubinsky T, *et al.* Cognitive coping tool kit for psychosis: development of a group-based curriculum. *Cognitiv Behav Pract.* 2007; **14**: 98–106.
2 McNally SE, Goldberg JO. Natural cognitive coping strategies in schizophrenia. *Br J Med Psychol.* 1997; **70**(Pt. 2): 159–67.
3 Canadian Psychiatric Association. Clinical practice guidelines. Treatment of schizophrenia. *Can J Psychiatry.* 2005; **50**(13 Suppl. 1): 7S–57S.
4 Ferdinandi AD, Yoottanasumpun V, Pollack S, *et al.* Predicting rehabilitation outcome among patients with schizophrenia. *Psychiatr Serv.* 1998; **49**(7): 907–9.
5 Pini S, Cassano GB, Dell'Osso L, *et al.* Insight into illness in schizophrenia, schizoaffective disorder, and mood disorders with psychotic features. *Am J Psychiatry.* 2001; **158**(1): 122–5.
6 Norman RM, Malla AK. Duration of untreated psychosis: a critical examination of the concept and its importance. *Psychol Med.* 2001; **31**(3): 381–400.
7 Rickelman BL. Anosognosia in individuals with schizophrenia: toward recovery of insight. *Issues Ment Health Nurs.* 2004; **25**(3): 227–42.
8 Lacro JP, Dunn LB, Dolder CR, *et al.* Prevalence and risk factors for medication nonadherence in patients with schizophrenia: a comprehensive review of recent literature. *J Clin Psychiatry.* 2002; **63**(10): 892–909.
9 Amador XF, Flaum M, Andreasen NC, *et al.* Awareness of illness in schizophrenia and schizoaffective and mood disorders. *Arch Gen Psychiatry.* 1994; **51**(10): 826–36.

10 Medalia A, Thysen J. Insight into neurocognitive dysfunction in schizophrenia. *Schizophr Bull.* 2008; **34**(6): 1221–30.

11 Amador X, Johanson AL. *I Am Not Sick I Don't Need Help!: how to help someone with mental illness accept treatment.* Peconic, NY: Vida Press; 2000.

12 Mueser KT, Meyer PS, Penn DL, *et al.* The illness management and recovery program: rationale, development, and preliminary findings. *Schizophr Bull.* 2006; **32**(Suppl. 1): S32–43.

13 Turkington D, Kingdon D, Utner T. Effectiveness of a brief cognitive-behavioural therapy intervention in the treatment of schizophrenia. *Br J Psychiatry.* 2002; **180**: 523–27.

14 David AS. Insight and Psychosis. *Br J Psychiatry.* 1990; **156**: 798–808.

15 Zito W, Greig TC, Wexler BE, *et al.* Predictors of on-site vocational support for people with schizophrenia in supported employment. *Schizophr Res.* 2007; **94**(1–3): 81–8.

16 Lucksted A, McNulty K, Brayboy L, *et al.* Initial evaluation of the peer to peer program. *Psychiatr Serv.* 2009; **60**(2): 250–3.

17 Roberts MM, Pratt CW. Putative evidence of employment readiness. *Psychiatr Rehabil J.* 2007; **30**(3): 175–81.

18 Bond GR. Supported employment: evidence for an evidence-based practice. *Psychiatr Rehabil J.* 2004; **27**(4): 345–59.

19 Farkas M, Sullivan Soydan A, Gagne C. Introduction to rehabilitation readiness. Boston, MA: Center for Psychiatric Rehabilitation; 2000.

20 Cohen MR, Anthony WA, Farkas MD. Assessing and developing readiness for psychiatric rehabilitation. *Psychiatr Serv.* 1997; **48**(5): 644–6.

21 Miller WR, Rollnick S, editors. *Motivational Interviewing: preparing people for change.* New York, NY: Guilford Press; 2002.

22 Rusch N, Corrigan PW. Motivational interviewing to improve insight and treatment adherence in schizophrenia. *Psychiatr Rehabil J.* 2002; **26**(1): 23–32.

23 Prochaska JO, DiClemente CC, Norcross J. In search of how people change. *Am Psychol.* 1992; **47**(9): 1102–14.

24 Archie SM, Goldberg JO, Akhtar-Danesh N, *et al.* Psychotic disorders, eating habits, and physical activity: who is ready for lifestyle changes? *Psychiatr Serv.* 2007; **58**(2): 233–9.

25 Pratt SI, Mueser KT, Smith TE, *et al.* Self-efficacy and psychosocial functioning in schizophrenia: a mediational analysis. *Schizophr Res.* 2005; **78**(2–3): 187–97.

26 Goldberg JO, Cook PE. Cognitive rehabilitation for negative symptoms. In: Corrigan PW, Yudofsky SC, editors. *Cognitive Rehabilitation for Neuropsychiatric Disorders.* Washington, DC: American Psychiatric Press; 1996. pp. 349–70.

27 Andreason NC. *The Broken Brain: the biological revolution in psychiatry.* New York, NY: Harper & Row; 1984.

28 Lieberman JA, Drake RE, Sederer LI, *et al.* Science and recovery in schizophrenia. *Psychiatr Serv.* 2008; **59**(5): 487–96.

29 Silverstein SM, Hitzel H, Schenkel L. Identifying and addressing cognitive barriers to rehabilitation readiness. *Psychiatr Serv.* 1998; **49**(1): 34–6.

30 Corrigan PW. Behaviour therapy empowers persons with severe mental illness. *Behav Modif.* 1997; **21**(1): 45–61.

31 Lee PWH, Lieh-Mak F, Yu KK, *et al.* Coping strategies of schizophrenic patients and their relationship to outcome. *Br J Psychiatry.* 1993; **163**: 177–82.

32 McNally SE, Goldberg JO. Natural cognitive coping strategies in schizophrenia. *Br J Med Psychol.* 1997; **70**(Pt. 2): 159–67.

33 Mueser KT, Valentiner DP, Agresta J. Coping with negative symptoms of schizophrenia: patient and family perspectives. *Schizophr Bull.* 1997; **23**(2): 329–39.

34 Velligan DI, Mueller J, Wang M. Use of environmental supports among patients with schizophrenia. *Psychiatr Serv.* 2006; **57**(2): 219–24.

35 Schmitter-Edgecombe M, Fahy JF, Whelan JP, *et al.* Memory remediation after severe closed head injury: notebook training versus supportive therapy. *J Cons Clin Psychol.* 1995; **63**(3): 484–9.

36 Fiszdon JM, McClough JF, Silverstein SM, *et al.* Learning potential as a predictor of readiness for psychosocial rehabilitation in schizophrenia. *Psychiatry Res.* 2006; **143**(2–3): 159–66.

37 Silverstein SM, Spaulding WD, Menditto AA, *et al.* Attention shaping: a reward-based learning method to enhance skills training outcomes in schizophrenia. *Schizophr Bull.* 2009; **35**(1): 222–32.

38 Kopelowicz A, Liberman RP, Zarate R. Recent advances in social skills training for schizophrenia. *Schizophr Bull.* 2006; **32** (Suppl 1.): S12–S23.

39 Liberman RP, Mueser KT, Wallace CJ, *et al.* Training skills in the psychiatrically disabled: learning coping and competence. *Schizophr Bull.* 1986; **12**(4): 631–47.

40 Martino D, Bucay D, Butman J, *et al.* Neuropsychological frontal impairments and negative symptoms in schizophrenia. *Psychiatry Research.* 2007; **152**(2–3): 121–8.

41 Hayes RL, McGrath JJ. Cognitive rehabilitation for people with schizophrenia and related conditions. *Cochrane Database Syst Rev.* 2000; (3): CD000968.

42 Medalia A, Richardson R. What predicts a good response to cognitive remediation interventions? *Schizophr Bull.* 2005; **31**(4): 942–53.

43 McGurk SR, Twamley EW, Sitzer DI, *et al.* A meta-analysis of cognitive remediation in schizophrenia. *Am J Psychiatry.* 2007; **164**(12): 1791–1802.

44 Lindenmayer JP, McGurk SR, Mueser KT, *et al.* A randomized controlled trial of cognitive remediation among inpatients with persistent mental illness. *Psychiatr Serv.* 2008; **59**(3): 241–7.

45 Medalia A, Revheim N, Casey M. Remediation of problem-solving skills in schizophrenia: evidence of a persistent effect. *Schizophr Res.* 2002; **57**(2–3): 165–71.

46 Wykes T, Reeder C, Landau S, *et al.* Cognitive remediation therapy in schizophrenia: randomised controlled trial. *Br J Psychiatry.* 2007; **190**: 421–7.

47 Hogarty GE, Greenwald DP, Eack SM. Durability and mechanism of effects of cognitive enhancement therapy. *Psychiatr Serv.* 2006; **57**(12): 1751–7.

48 Koblick M, Kidd SA, Goldberg JO, *et al.* So I wouldn't feel like I was excluded: the learning experience in computer education for persons with psychiatric disabilities. *Psychiatr Rehabil J.* 2009: **32**(4): 306–8.

49 Lieberman JA, Drake RE, Sederer LI, *et al.* Science and recovery in schizophrenia. *Psychiatr Serv.* 2008; **59**(5): 487–96.

50 Bellack AS. Scientific and consumer models of recovery in schizophrenia: concordance, contrasts, and implications. *Schizophr Bull.* 2006; **32**(3): 432–42.

51 Davidson L, Chinman M, Sells D, *et al.* Peer support among adults with serious mental illness: a report from the field. *Schizophr Bull.* 2006; **32**(3): 443–50.

52 Solomon P. Peer support/peer provided services: underlying processes, benefits and critical ingredients. *Psychiatr Rehabil J.* 2004; **27**(4): 392–401.

53 Bandura, A. *Social Learning Theory.* New York, NY: General Learning Press; 1977.

54 Sells D, Black R, Davidson L, *et al.* Beyond generic support: incidence and impact of invalidation in peer services for clients with severe mental illness. *Psychiatr Serv.* 2008; **59**(11): 1322–7.

55 Spaniol L, Koehler M, Hutchinson D. *The Recovery Workbook.* Boston, MA: Center for Psychiatric Rehabilitation; 1994.

56 Brekke JS, Hoe M, Long J, *et al.* How neurocognition and social cognition influence functional change during community-based psychosocial rehabilitation for individuals with schizophrenia. *Schizophr Bull.* 2007; **33**(5): 1247–56.

57 Kern RS, Glynn SM, Horan WO, *et al.* Psychosocial treatments to promote functional recovery in schizophrenia. *Schizophr Bull.* 2009; **35**(2): 347–61.

CHAPTER 7

Prevention and Health Promotion

This (seventh) chapter of the book addresses physical health and wellness as well as peer support of persons with SMI. It is relevant to many other chapters of this book, as physical health and wellness and peer support, formal or informal, are matters that arise in many other aspects of the lives of persons with SMI, and can challenge as well as enable PCC for persons with SMI.

Section 7.1, *Cultivating Physical Health and Wellness Utilizing a Person-Centered Approach*, argues that there is a large gap between physical and mental health services, which has led to an excess of medical morbidity and mortality among people with SMI. The section points to wellness resources and tools that can improve the physical wellness of people with SMI. Section 7.2, *Self-Help and Peer-Operated Services*, addresses types of self-help groups and peer-operated services deemed person-centered. The section discusses the growing body of literature illustrating the beneficial aspects of both self-help groups and peer-operated services for people with mental illnesses, including SMI.

7.1 Cultivating Physical Health and Wellness Utilizing a Person-Centered Approach

Betty Vreeland, Anna Marie Toto, Marie Verna and Jill Williams

INTRODUCTION

> "People used to say things to me like: if you don't lose 20 pounds or if you don't quit smoking you're going to die ten years early. Well, I didn't care if I died early. I didn't care until I met a man and we fell in love. We got married, had a child and I wanted to live to see my grandchildren."
>
> – Anonymous service user

Many service users face the harsh reality that they or their peers may die an average of 25 years earlier than people without mental illness.[1,2] This is during a time when the life expectancy of other Americans continues to lengthen. Behavioral health service providers, advocates and service users recognize that the gap between behavioral (or mental) and physical health is growing larger and that health disparities are likely to continue to worsen without immediate changes.[3,4,5,6,7] Note that we use the term behavioral health rather than mental health, as although we consider them substantively synonymous in this context, the term behavioral health is more commonly used in the public mental health system in the U.S., with which we are experienced.

Leading organizations involved in influencing public policy are prioritizing the problem of excess medical morbidity (including cardiovascular disease, obesity, diabetes, respiratory disease and infectious diseases) and mortality and have made an urgent call to action to transform the current behavioral health care system into one that can better integrate physical health,[8,9,10,11,12] such as including physical health care services within the behavioral health care system. There is considerable work ahead needed to heal the mind-body split and develop a holistic system of care. Integrated care and the path toward delivering it are not yet well-defined. We hope this section provides support and direction to those interested in working towards bridging the gap that currently exists between physical and behavioral health. In the U.S., the Substance Abuse and Mental Health Services Administration (SAMHSA)'s "10 by 10 Pledge" is an example of a national action plan to promote wellness and reduce early mortality by 10 years over the next 10-year time period.[13] Additionally, the World Federation of Mental Health highlighted the need for the integration of physical and mental health during World Mental Health Day (2004–2005) and at its 2009 conference.[14] Furthermore, service user organizations have begun to advocate for public policy and funding to address the physical needs of people with mental illness. For example, the Highland Users' Group held a series of meetings across Scotland in 2007 and compiled a comprehensive report containing first-person views about the difficulty service users deal with as they work to improve wellness.[15]

It is important to utilize PCC as new models, programs and strategies continue to evolve to address and integrate behavioral and physical health care. However, how to do this may seem challenging. Service users may feel that their resources are already taxed and have few options to turn to. Family members may wonder how they can support their loved ones' physical health needs or whether it's even possible to improve their physical health. Others may ask who's responsible to coordinate the integration of care: the behavioral health service provider or the physical health service provider? Physical health service providers may feel ill-prepared to care for people with behavioral health issues. And behavioral health service providers may feel they lack the knowledge and skills to address physical health problems.

While the practice of integrating physical health into behavioral health care may seem new, the concept of holistic health has been around for quite some time. For example, over 50 years ago the WHO defined health as *"a state of complete physical, mental, and social well-being and not merely the absence of disease or infirmity."*[16] People living with SMI have higher rates of co-occurring physical health problems including obesity, diabetes, hypertension and tobacco dependence.[17,18] These problems can lead to a reduced quality of life and premature death. This section will discuss the urgent need to address the physical health of people with SMI from a person-centered perspective and will also explore how to integrate physical health care into behavioral health practice. The following topics are included: key contributing factors to poor health (modifiable lifestyle risk factors such as tobacco use and obesity); how medications can impact health; person-centered approaches and other wellness solutions that can cultivate health and wellness; and how organizational change and advocacy can help bridge the gap between mental and physical health. Note that while the authors primarily explore the American health care experience, the information presented has international applicability. Note also that this section addresses some matters that are relevant to and addressed in part in other sections in more detail, such as collaboration of physical and behavioral health services, addressed in detail in Section 5.3, *Shared/Collaborative Care for People with Serious Mental Illness.*

Key Contributing Factors to Poor Health

"Premature death from medical conditions prevents recovery from mental illness. It's a medical fact that once you're dead of a heart attack you cannot recover from schizophrenia."

– Joe Parks, M.D.

A number of issues, some of which are discussed below, contribute to the high rate of medical problems in people with SMI. While these factors pose challenges to optimal health, the good news is, there are solutions and strategies emerging.

Modifiable Lifestyle Risk Factors

Much of the increased morbidity and mortality of people living with SMI are due to preventable conditions.[19,20] Cardiovascular disease, diabetes, respiratory diseases and infectious diseases are caused by a higher rate of modifiable risk factors including smoking, poor nutrition, obesity, lack of physical activity, substance abuse and unsafe sexual behavior.[21] Additionally, SAMHSA identifies a similar set of risk factors associated with early death: smoking, hypertension, cholesterol, diet, exercise, diabetes and accidents. SAMHSA's report states that if these conditions were managed, the resulting care would most likely "make the biggest difference in the health of consumers."[22] Heart disease has been identified as the leading cause of death in individuals with SMI, with obesity and hypertension as the most prevalent medical co-morbidities.[23] Adopting healthier behaviors such as eating nutritious foods, being physically active and avoiding tobacco use is important in preventing or controlling the devastating effects of many diseases. This is the case whether or not the individual has a co-occurring mental illness.

There is scientific evidence to support that individuals with SMI can change health risk behaviors related to tobacco, weight loss, healthy eating and increased physical activity.[24,25,26,27,28,29,30,31] Tobacco use and obesity are two of the top causes of preventable death and are therefore focused upon in this section. Specialized comprehensive programs designed to improve the physical health of service users are limited. Therefore, two manualized psychoeducational wellness programs, specifically designed to inspire and assist service users to achieve their physical health and wellness goals, are highlighted.[32,33] These resources are scientifically based, widely used, and freely available via the Internet. There are other programs such as NAMI's Hearts and Minds, WRAP and IMR that address the importance of integrating physical health and wellness into recovery and should also be utilized.[34,35,36]

All of these programs are based on the expectation that service users can learn and implement a self-directed plan for their own wellness and recovery. NAMI's Hearts and Minds is an educational program for service users, family members and other supporters delivered by people who have personal experience managing both behavioral and physical health issues. WRAP is a structured program to teach participants recovery and self-management skills and strategies for dealing with mental health difficulties. IMR is a program in which providers work collaboratively with service users, offering a variety of information, strategies and skills to help manage their recovery, with a strong emphasis on helping service users identify and achieve personally meaningful goals. Since their inception, both WRAP and IMR have added wellness components (which address physical health issues) to their materials.

Tobacco Use

Tobacco dependence is a leading cause of death, causing at least one in five deaths annually.[37] Current smokers have poorer health habits and health-related quality of life than those who have never smoked.[38] About 70% of individuals with SMI are tobacco dependent,[39] and more broadly, 44% of all the cigarettes consumed in the U.S. are by individuals with a current DSM-IV mental illness or addiction.[40] Although nicotine may have some beneficial aspects in certain mental disorders,[41,42,43,44] tobacco is not a pharmaceutical, and nicotine can be delivered more safely in gum, nasal spray, lozenge, inhaler and patch. Despite this opportunity, mental health providers infrequently assess or treat tobacco use.[45,46,47,48]

Research suggests that although there are strong associations in neurobiology and behaviors that link nicotine, smoking and mental disorders, the role of psychosocial factors, such as role modeling of peers, are important as well. Also, smokers with schizophrenia, bipolar disorder, depression, and personality disorder describe smoking as an existential "need" that helps them to cope.[49] Smoking has traditionally been used as a behavioral reward in mental health facilities and continues to be a shared social activity. In a recent paper, Lawn[50] described cigarettes as "the currency by which economic, social and political exchange took place" among hospitalized Australian individuals with mental disorders.

In addition to health problems, tobacco use can have other disruptive consequences, which may be influential factors in helping to motivate individuals with SMI to quit smoking. For example, smokers with mental illness suffer financially, spending at least one third of their income on cigarettes.[51] Smoking also influences community integration, as smokers have less income to spend on clothing and housing. As the smoking rate decreases among the general population, there is stigma in being a smoker, in addition to the stigma of having mental illness.[52,53] This can reduce success in obtaining employment, housing or interpersonal relationships.[54] Smoking also increases the metabolism of several widely used psychiatric medications, resulting in increased dosage requirements.[55,56]

Although many smokers with SMI understand that smoking is harmful and that quitting can improve health, it is estimated that only 10–25% are interested in quitting within the next month.[57,58,59,60] This highlights the need to increase an individual's motivational level before tobacco treatment can commence. In one study, brief motivational interventions with education and personalized feedback were effective in encouraging individuals with schizophrenia to seek tobacco treatment.[61] Applying Prochaska and DiClimente's Transtheoretical Model of Change when using motivational interventions can be helpful.[62] Research shows that 50–60% are in the pre-contemplation stage, 40% of smokers are in the contemplation stage, and only 10–15% of smokers are prepared for action.[63] Therefore, motivational interventions that build upon tobacco awareness, self-efficacy and the pros and cons of using tobacco are important in an individual's efforts to make healthier choices. *Learning About Healthy Living: tobacco and you,* is a manualized resource for behavioral health service providers on how to address tobacco with people with SMI. The goal of the intervention is to increase an individual's awareness about the risks of tobacco use and treatment options, as well as to enhance motivation to address tobacco and to begin by making healthier choices. The manual was tested for feasibility in a brief outcome study[64] and is available as a publicly available resource on the Internet.[65]

Weight-Related Problems

Obesity is a complex, multifactorial chronic disease that develops from the interaction between genotype and the environment, is considered a medical disease,
and has been identified as a growing global public health crisis. It is estimated that
1.6 billion adults are overweight and at least 400 million adults are obese. Obesity
can be viewed as a "complex condition, one with serious social and psychological
dimensions, that affects virtually all age and socioeconomic groups and threatens
to overwhelm developed and developing countries."[66]

The fundamental cause of obesity and overweight is an energy imbalance
between calories consumed and calories expended. Excess body weight increases
the risk for many medical problems, including type 2 diabetes, coronary heart disease, osteoarthritis, hypertension, gallbladder disease, stroke and certain forms of
cancer. The health consequences of obesity range from increased risk of premature
death to serious chronic conditions that reduce the overall quality of life.[67] Additionally, obese individuals experience stigma and discrimination.

Overweight and obesity are more prevalent in people with SMI, and obesity is
one of the most common physical health care problems in this population. Among
individuals with SMI, an unhealthy lifestyle, as well as the effects of psychotropic
medications, such as atypical antipsychotics, can contribute to the development of
this problem, among other – partly related – things, such as lack of sufficient income
for a healthy diet, lack of adequate knowledge and living skills to make use of such
a diet, and more. Additionally, "people with co-occurring mental illness and obesity may face a double whammy: stigma associated with mental illness and stigma
related to body weight."[68] The National Association of State Mental Health Program
Director (NASMHPD) issued a report titled *Obesity Reduction and Prevention Strategies
for Individuals with SMI*, which states: "the epidemic of obesity in persons with mental illness is a major cause of morbidity and early death and a significant obstacle to
wellness and recovery that requires action by policy makers, administrators, health
care providers, and consumers. Effective interventions are available."[69]

In addition to the stigma and discrimination associated with mental illness and
obesity, the health of people with SMI may be further challenged by the low expectations of others who may not believe that people with SMI can make healthier
lifestyle choices. The Healthy Living study is one example of what's possible.[70,71]
This lifestyle intervention for overweight and obese subjects with schizophrenia
who had gained weight on psychotropic medications consisted of nutrition, exercise
and behavioral interventions. Persons who received the Healthy Living intervention demonstrated a significant reduction in weight, whereas subjects who received
"treatment as usual" gained weight.[72] In addition, subjects in the intervention group
showed statistically significant improvement in minutes per week of exercise, knowledge of nutrition, exercise stage of change, weight stage of change, systolic and
diastolic blood pressure, body mass index (BMI), waist circumference, and hemoglobin A1c (a marker of fasting blood glucose).[73] The Healthy Living results were
compared to a study by Dansinger and colleagues,[74] which assessed adherence rates

and effectiveness of four popular diets (Atkins®, Zone®, Weight Watchers®, and Ornish®) in 160 overweight adults without a known mental illness. After one year, overall adherence rates ranged from 50–65%, with a mean weight loss among the four diet groups ranging from 2.1 kg to 3.3 kg. In contrast the Healthy Living subjects with schizophrenia and schizoaffective disorder at one year had a mean adherence (attendance) rate of 69% and a mean weight loss of 3.7 kg – which is clinically significant, and even more so if it continues – in study completers.[75,76] The reader is referred to the original article for more information about the clinical significance of this amount of weight change in people taking antipsychotic medications.[77] This research suggests that when some adults with schizophrenia participate in specialized wellness programs it may be possible for them to lose more weight than people without mental illness who participate in weight-loss programs. Additionally, research suggests that programs like the Solutions for Wellness (SFW) personalized and manualized programs, which are also designed to inspire and assist people with mental illness to choose healthier eating, physical activity, and other lifestyle behaviors, can also improve weight and other health outcomes in some people with mental illness.[78,79,80,81] The SFW manualized program is publicly available on the Internet.[82] Other strategies and programs that may help prevent and reverse weigh gain in service users are available and described elsewhere in further detail.[83,84,85,86]

The Added Burden of Medication

Medications are often the mainstay of behavioral health treatment, especially for psychotic disorders. Unfortunately, these medications carry the burden of side effects, which can contribute to poor physical health.[87] Many major classes of psychotropic medications, such as antidepressants, antipsychotics and mood stabilizers, cause weight gain as a side effect.[88] In addition to weight gain, however, the risks of metabolic disturbances in glucose regulation and hyperlipidemia, especially from the newer atypical antipsychotics, may contribute to metabolic syndrome that greatly increases the risk of developing cardiovascular disease and diabetes.[89]

Service providers are increasingly aware of these conditions and metabolic concerns that may cause significant distress among service users and contribute to problems with medication concordance.[90,91] Many providers feel that monitoring of blood pressure, blood glucose/lipids and measurements of weight and abdominal obesity fall within the scope of psychiatric practice.[92,93] Recent practice guidelines and expert consensus urge behavioral health service providers to play a larger role in the detection and intervention of medical conditions such as these.[94,95] A multidisciplinary team approach, including an active service user role, may help meet practice guidelines and help integrate physical health into behavioral health care.[96,97]

Poor Quality Physical Health Care

For various reasons, people with SMI often experience substandard health care, which may contribute to excess mortality.[98,99,100] Providers from both medical and behavioral health settings, service users and the health care system itself all contribute to this problem. Service users may experience challenges with health literacy and navigating the health care system. Bureaucratic barriers in the health insurance system create financial and other disincentives for service providers and service users seeking integrated solutions to health concerns. As in the case of depression or anxiety, medical bias may predispose primary care providers and service users to adopt medical explanations in preference to behavioral health diagnoses. Alternately, the stigma often associated with mental illness may predispose service providers and service users to adopt behavioral explanations when the cause is physical. Furthermore, service users may be less likely to receive evidence-based medical care. A review by Druss[101] found potential deficits in the health care of persons with mental disorders in a variety of situations including the care of hypertension, diabetes, and cardiovascular disorders as well as preventative health.

Many individuals with SMI have difficulty accessing health, dental and vision services and often rely on the use of emergency room services for their health care needs.[102] In addition to having higher rates of physical health problems, a meta-analysis revealed that 35% of people with SMI had at least one undiagnosed medical disorder.[103] Behavioral health service providers/facilities may be the primary source of contact with physical health service provider. Therefore, to improve the accessibility and quality of care, a holistic approach that forms a partnership between primary care and behavioral health is recommended. The development of person-centered health care homes, which take a team-based approach to provide care management and support individuals in their self-management goals, are evolving.[104] At the most integrated level, this model would co-locate primary health service providers in behavioral health facilities (such as community mental health agencies), where they would work together with service users to achieve optimal health.

Cultivating Health and Wellness Utilizing Person-Centered Approaches and Other Wellness Solutions

The impact of physical health on one's overall well-being is often not well understood. Physical health can affect quality of life on many levels including one's daily routine, work and educational activities, relationships, recreational activities and achieving recovery goals.

Example

This is an illustration of how a behavioral health service provider could utilize a person-centered approach while integrating physical health issues into a behavioral health service plan:

Calvin is a 28-year-old, single male who has diagnoses of bipolar disorder, nicotine dependence, hypertension and obesity. Calvin lives at home with his parents, participates in a self-help center, volunteers in his local church, attends a day treatment program two days per week, and recently obtained a part-time job working as a server in a restaurant. Calvin says he feels "good" that he has his own job. However, he voices frustration that he needs to rely on his parents to drive him to and from work, and he also says he is lonely. Calvin identifies goals of wanting to buy a car, move into his own apartment, and become involved in a long-term relationship.

Utilizing a person-centered approach will offer an opportunity to engage individuals like Calvin by respecting their current preferences as well as their existing capacity and resources.[105] An integrated approach addresses the behavioral health and physical health needs of the individual. For example, if Calvin cuts down on his tobacco use it could help him save money to buy a car and also work on his goal to live independently. Additionally, losing weight may increase his self-esteem and help him feel more confident about asking someone out on a date. If a provider explores with Calvin the physical health aspects of losing weight and tobacco use without linking Calvin's personal goals, the probability of Calvin addressing his tobacco use and weight problem would be less likely.

Integrated service planning should be specific to the needs of persons served and hence provide for person-centered service and not a "one size fits all" process. It should also include strategies, education/materials, and a menu of program options to help individuals such as Calvin achieve their goals. Effective resources that can maximize efforts in this endeavor include programs such as IMR and WRAP.[106,107] Calvin, for example, may also benefit from participating in the SFW and *Learning About Healthy Living: tobacco and you* programs. The SFW program may also help him control weight-related physical health problems such as hypertension.

Additionally, collaboration between service users, service providers and family members/significant others *can* better assess what is needed to improve one's quality of life. Calvin may choose to involve his family in service planning to discuss how he can achieve his goals such as living independently. Service planning can serve as a time to ensure that Calvin, behavioral health service providers, and physical health service providers are collaborating. For example, Calvin's psychiatrist or other member of the behavioral health team could call or send a coordination of care letter to Calvin's primary care provider. A coordination of care letter could include an update on Calvin's current psychiatric medications and ask for the following information to be sent in return: all physical health diagnoses, prescribed medications, blood pressure readings and copies of laboratory and other diagnostic tests. Service planning is also an ideal opportunity to: 1. Update Calvin's physical health status and records, which should include monitoring of health measures such as BMI, waist circumference, tobacco use and blood pressure; and 2. For behavioral health service providers to educate Calvin on the importance of monitoring his own health measures throughout the year and finding user-friendly tools (such as the *Progress Record Log* found in Solutions for Wellness) to track this information. Ultimately, this integrated process can empower Calvin to become more aware of his physical health issues, i.e. obesity, hypertension and tobacco use, while he is pursuing his recovery goals.

In the next section we discuss how a behavioral health service provider can begin a dialogue about physical health with service users.

Beginning the Collaborative Health Dialogue and Key Strategies to Sustain It

Building competency in addressing physical health begins by having a collaborative dialogue with service users about their personal health needs and goals. While a background in health is helpful it is not necessary. If a concern arises, it's important to have access to service providers who can assist. Beginning the dialogue with a simple question about wellness such as, "What does *wellness* mean to you?" can prove helpful. In a recent study designed to study the effects of a wellness intervention,[108] 67 service users were asked that same question. As part of the study, subjects were asked to fill out several questionnaires, one of which included the aforementioned question. Responses were analyzed and the most common wellness factors were identified as: mind and body or mind/body/spirit, which represented 26.1% of responses; healthy eating/exercise 20%; stable/recovery 11.5%; functioning 7.2%; and making healthy choices 1.4% (*see* Figure 7.1).

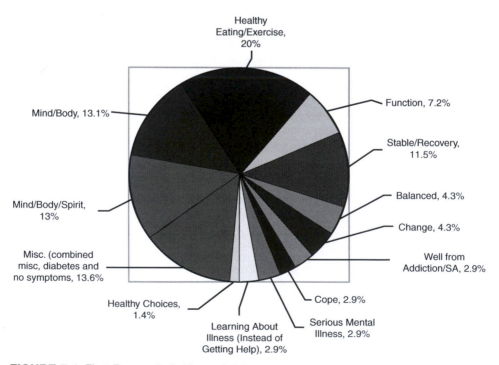

FIGURE 7.1 First-Person Definitions of "Wellness"

By asking one or more of the following health assessment questions an assessment and referral process may begin that assists individuals with achieving optimal health:

1 When was the date of your last physical exam? Do you have a primary care practitioner whom you see regularly? If not, do you know how to find a primary care practitioner?

2 Do you have any known physical health problems? If yes, what are they and how do you take care of them? Do you have any other concerns about your health?

3 Do you know the names and doses of all your medications, including over the counter medications and vitamins? (Ask for a written list).

4 When was your last dental exam?

5 When was your last eye exam?

6 Do you smoke? If yes, how many cigarettes do you smoke per day? On a scale of 1 (not interested) to 10 (very interested), how interested are you in quitting in the next six months?

7 How many minutes of regular physical activity/exercise do you get per day/per week? What type of physical activity/exercise do you do?

8 On a scale of 1 (unhealthy) to 10 (very healthy), please rate the food choices you make on a daily basis. Consider asking for a 24-hour food and beverage recall, i.e. tell me everything you ate and drank over the past 24 hours.

9 Do you have any concerns about your weight?

10 How many hours of sleep to you generally get per night? Do you feel well-rested when you wake up?

Additionally, as part of the health dialogue and a way to empower individuals to take responsibility for their own health record, consider asking service users to record and monitor their health data such as vital signs, medication information and physical activity and/or food logs. Finally, all service team members including the service user, family members/support system, and the prescriber should review available health data, discuss health concerns and begin to work toward optimizing the individual's health. Begin work on the most pressing areas of need and interest. Keep in mind that with the exception of urgent problems, this is a work in progress.

A stage-based motivational approach can assist with the integration of personal health goals.[109,110] Furthermore, a "small steps approach" has been found to be a useful practice to help prevent weight gain and is highlighted in the NASMHPD's technical report on obesity and SMI.[111,112] Such an approach can be utilized across the continuum of care and with a spectrum of health and lifestyle issues to build an individual's personal belief that good health can be achieved one *"small step"* at a time.

"I had gained a lot of weight and developed diabetes. Professionals kept telling me what to do. They told me what to eat and to start exercising. I decided to quit drinking soda. A year later I weighed over a hundred pounds less."

– Anonymous

When asked why (out of all the options available) he chose to cut out soda, he replied: *"Because I thought I could."* He also reported drinking at least two liters of soda per day. NASMHPD's technical report titled *Measurement of Health Status for People with Serious Mental Illness*, as a first step on creating capacity to measure baseline data and the impact of interventions, recommends that standard set of 10 health indicators, including BMI, blood pressure, and tobacco use, be gathered regularly to inform care.[113]

What Can Organizations Do?

It would be remiss to talk about PCC without addressing the integration of physical and mental health on an organizational level. As a way to help bridge the gap between physical and mental health, hundreds of behavioral health care organizations from across the U.S. have been trained on implementing a "complete wellness" or holistic (mind/body/spirit) approach.[114] Just as PCC meets the service user where they are, so too the organization should begin wherever their services will allow.[115] The facilities trained were asked to look at a place in their organization that was most ready to implement a "complete wellness" initiative, beginning with one small achievable step to be completed in two weeks' time. The "small steps" in numerous cases led to large-scale changes. For example, an organization that began with the "small step" of asking service users about smoking during the intake process led to the formation of three smoking cessation groups in one year's time. Another organization implemented the "small step" of a lunchtime walking group to promote physical activity which led to the creation of a gym. Another organization's "small step" of asking service users (new to their system) if they were linked to a primary care practitioner eventually led to a "primary care referral/linkage" quality improvement (QI) initiative to increase the percentage of service users linked with a primary care practitioner.

What Can Advocacy Do?

Advocacy can influence policy, regulation and funding to help integrate physical health into behavioral health care.[116] To this end, elected officials must champion laws that encourage collaboration, coordination and communication across agencies and promote the use of consistent and accessible medical records. Additional funding for longitudinal research using consistent instruments is needed to add to the growing body of evidence about the crisis of mortality and morbidity.[117] QI initiatives at the organizational level that measure physical health outcomes can help build upon this body of evidence and are encouraged.[118]

Advocacy can help address the significant changes in financing of health care needed, so that organizations providing care can provide high-quality integrated care. Public health insurance must: 1. "Provide coverage for health education and prevention services (primary prevention) that will reduce or slow the impact of disease; 2. Establish rates adequate to assure access to primary care;

3. Cover smoking cessation and weight reduction treatments; and 4. Use community case management to improve engagement with and access to preventive and primary care".[119] As health care reform for the general public progresses, advocates should ensure that those with SMI are included in dialogues about the importance of a "medical home."[120] A "medical home" model for people for SMI is being explored and has been referred to as a "person-centered health care home."[121] At the core of the clinical approach of the patient-centered medical home is team-based care that provides coordination of physical health care and promotes independence and self-care.[122] This emphasis on self-care resonates with the behavioral health system movement fostering recovery and resilience and its focus on integrating primary care and behavioral health provides evidence-based approaches that may address the health disparity seen in people with SMI.[123]

Finally, advocacy is needed to improve health literacy about how to integrate physical health into behavioral health care at the public mental health system level. This would help raise awareness of the importance of integrating physical and mental health and provide education at the community level. This education should include health literacy for service providers, service users and family members, as well as mental health literacy for primary care providers and those who traditionally provide only physical health care.

CONCLUSION

There is a huge gap between physical and behavioral health. This has led to an excess of medical morbidity and mortality among service users. Many things, including poor quality and usage of health care, modifiable lifestyle factors, low socioeconomic status, psychotropic medication and other issues discussed in this section can contribute to this health disparity. A holistic (mind/body/spirit) framework and PCC approaches and programming can help cultivate optimal health and well-being. Connecting health and wellness goals to recovery goals can motivate individuals to improve their health. Wellness resources and tools exist that can also assist in this process. The person-centered health care home is being explored as an integrated care model. Organizational change and advocacy are essential to help bridge the gap between physical and behavioral health that currently exists. While there are many challenges in integrating physical health into behavioral health, we hope this section has provided the reader with a few *"small steps"* about how to get started and a belief that it is possible.

REFERENCES

1 Colton CW, Manderscheid RW. Congruencies in increased mortality rates, years of potential life lost, and cause of death among public mental health clients in eight states. *Preventing Chronic Disease.* 2006; **3**(2): 1–14. Available at: www.cdc.gov/pcd/issues/2006/apr/05_0180.htm (accessed 16 May 2011).

2 National Association of State Mental Health Program Directors (NASMHPD) Medical Directors Council. *Morbidity and Mortality in People with Serious Mental Illness.* 2006. Available at: www.nasmhpd.org (accessed 16 May 2011).

3 Ibid.

4 Bazelon Center for Mental Health Law. *Get It Together: how to integrate physical and mental health care for people with serious mental disorders.* 2004. Available at: www.bazelon.org (accessed 16 May 2011).

5 Everett A, Mahler J, Biblin J, *et al.* Substance Abuse and Mental Health Services Administration (SAMHSA), Center for Mental Health Services (CMHS) Wellness Summit. *Improving the Health of Mental Health Consumers: effective policies and practices* [paper]. 2007. Available at: www.oregon.gov/DHS/mentalhealth/wellness/policies-and-practices.pdf?ga=t (accessed 16 May 2011).

6 NASMHPD) Medical Directors Council. *Integrating Behavioral Health and Primary Care Services: opportunities and challenges for state mental health authorities.* 2005. Available at: www.nasmhpd.org (accessed 16 May 2011).

7 National Council for Community Behavioral Healthcare. *Behavioral Health/Primary/Primary Care Integration and the Person Centered Healthcare Home.* 2009. Available at: www.thenationalcouncil.org (accessed 16 May 2011).

8 NASMHPD Medical Directors Council, 2006, op. cit.

9 Bazelon Center for Mental Health Law, op. cit.

10 Everett, op. cit.

11 NASMHPD Medical Directors Council, 2005, op. cit.

12 National Council for Community Behavioral Healthcare, op. cit.

13 Substance Abuse and Mental Health Services Administration (SAMHSA), Center for Mental Health Services (CMHS). *Wellness Summit and 10x10 Pledge.* 2007. Available at: www.promoteacceptance.samhsa.gov (accessed 16 May 2011).

14 www.wfmh.org/01WMHDayArchives.htm

15 Highland Users' Group: mental health and physical health. 2008. Available at: www.hug.uk.net (accessed 16 May 2011).

16 World Health Organization: Preamble to the Constitution of the World Health Organization as adopted by the International Health Conference. New York; 1946 June. Entered into force 7 April 1948. Available at: www.who.int/governance/eb/who_constitution_en.pdf (accessed 26 May 2011).

17 NASMHPD Medical Directors Council, 2006, op. cit.

18 Bazelon Center for Mental Health Law, op. cit.

19 NASMHPD Medical Directors Council, 2006, op. cit.

20 Everett, op. cit.

21 NASMHPD Medical Directors Council, 2006, op. cit.

22 Everett, op. cit.

23 Miller BJ, Paschall CB, Svendsen DP. Mortality and medical comorbidity among patients with serious mental illness. *Psychiatr Serv.* 2006; **57**(10): 1482–7.

24 Meyer JM. Effects of atypical antipsychotics on weight and serum lipid levels. *J Clin Psychiatry.* 2001; **62** (Suppl. 27): 27–34. Discussion 40–1.

25 Williams JM, Foulds J. Successful tobacco dependence treatment in schizophrenia. *Am J Psychiatry.* 2007; **164**(2): 222–7.

26 Baker A, Richmond R, Haile M, *et al.* A randomized controlled trial of a smoking cessation intervention among people with a psychotic disorder. *Am J Psychiatry.* 2006; **163**(11): 1934.

27 George TP, Ziedonis DM, Feingold A, *et al*. Nicotine transdermal patch and atypical antipsychotic drugs for smoking cessation in schizophrenia. *Am J Psychiatry*. 2000; **157**(11): 1835–42.

28 Vreeland B, Minsky S, Menza M, *et al*. A program for managing atypical antipsychotic-associated weight gain. *Psychiatric Serv*. 2003; **54**(8): 1155–7.

29 Menza M, Vreeland B, Minsky S, *et al*. Managing atypical antipsychotic-associated weight gain: 12 month data on a multimodal weight control program. *J Clin Psychiatry*. 2004; **65**(4): 471–7.

30 Pelletier JR, Nguyen M, Bradley K, *et al*. A study of a structured exercise program with members of an ICCD Certified Clubhouse: program design, benefits, and implications for feasibility. *Psychiatric Rehab J*. 2005; **29**(2): 89–96.

31 Senn TE, Carey MP. HIV testing among individuals with a severe mental illness: review, suggestions for research, and clinical implications. *Psychol Med*. 2008; **8**: 1–9.

32 Williams J, Ziedonis D, Speelman N, *et al*. Learning about Healthy Living: tobacco and you. State of New Jersey, Division of Mental Health Services. Revised June 2005. Available at: http://ubhc.umdnj.edu/nav/LearningAboutHealthyLiving.pdf (accessed 16 May 2011).

33 Vreeland B, Toto AM, Sakowitz M. Solutions for Wellness. 3rd ed. Indianapolis, IN: Eli Lilly & Co.; 2008. Available at: www.treatmentteam.com/tools_to_help/help_with_your_patients.jsp (accessed 16 May 2011).

34 National Alliance on Mental Illness (NAMI). NAMI Hearts & Minds. 2003. Available at: www.nami.org/heartsandminds (accessed 16 May 2011).

35 Substance Abuse and Mental Health Services Administration (SAMHSA), Center for Mental Health Services (CMHS). *Illness Management & Recovery Toolkit*. Rockville, MD. Available at: www.mentalhealth.samhsa.gov/cmhs/communitysupport/toolkits/illness (accessed 16 May 2011).

36 Copeland ME. *Wellness Recovery Action Plan*. 2nd ed. U.S.A.: Peach Press; 2000.

37 Hyland A, Vena C, Bauer J, *et al*. Cigarette smoking-attributable morbidity – United States, 2000. *Morbidity and Mortality Weekly Report*. 2003; **52**(35): 842–4.

38 Strine TW, Okoro CA, Chapman DP, *et al*. Health-related quality of life and health risk behaviors among smokers. *Am J Prev Med*. 2005; **28**(2): 182–7.

39 Williams JM, Ziedonis DM. Addressing tobacco among individuals with a mental illness or an addiction. *Addictive Beh*. 2004; **29**(6): 1059–270.

40 Lasser K, Wesley BJ, Woolhandler S, *et al*. Smoking and mental illness: a population-based prevalence study. *JAMA*. 2000; **284**(20): 2606–10.

41 Adler LE, Hoffer LD, Wiser A, *et al*. Normalization of auditory physiology by cigarette smoking in schizophrenic patients. *Am J Psychiatry*. 1993; **150**(12): 1856–61.

42 Conners CK, Levin ED, Sparrow E, *et al*. Nicotine and attention in adult ADHD. *Psychopharmacol Bull*. 1996; **32**(1): 67–73.

43 Sacco KA, Termine A, Seyal A, *et al*. Effects of cigarette smoking on spatial working memory and attentional deficits in schizophrenia: involvement of nicotinic receptor mechanisms. *Arch Gen Psychiatry*. 2005; **62**(6): 649–59.

44 George TP, Vessicchio JC, Termine A, *et al*. Effects of smoking abstinence on visuospatial working memory function in schizophrenia. *Neuropsychopharmacology*. 2002; **26**(1): 75–85.

45 Phillips KM, Brandon TH. Do psychologists adhere to the clinical practice guidelines for tobacco cessation? A survey of practitioners. *Prof Psychology: research and practice*. 2004; **35**: 281–5.

46 Peterson AL, Hryshko-Mullen AS, Cortez Y. Assessment and diagnosis of nicotine dependence in mental health settings. *American Journal of Addictions*. 2003; **12**(3): 192–7.

47 Montoya I.D, Herbeck DM, Svikis DS, *et al*. Identification and treatment of patients with nicotine problems in routine clinical psychiatry practice. *Am J Addictions*. 2005; **14**(5): 441–54.

48 Thorndike AN, Stafford RS, Rigotti NA. U.S. physicians' treatment of smoking in outpatients with psychiatric diagnoses. *Nicotine Tob Res*. 2001; **3**(1): 85–91.

49 Lawn SJ, Pols RG, Barber JG. Smoking and quitting: a qualitative study with community-living psychiatric clients. *Soc Sci Med*. 2002; **54**(1): 93–104.

50 Lawn SJ. Systemic barriers to quitting smoking among institutionalised public mental health service populations: a comparison of two Australian sites. *Int J Social Psychiatry*. 2004; **50**(3): 204–15.

51 Steinberg ML, Williams JM, Ziedonis DM. Financial implications of cigarette smoking among individuals with schizophrenia. *Tobacco Control*. 2004; **13**(2): 206.

52 Corrigan PW. *Marlboro Man and the Stigma of Smoking*. In: Gilman SL, Xun Z, editors. *Smoke: a global history of smoking*. London: Reaction Books; 2004.

53 Williams JM, Ziedonis DM, Vreeland B, *et al*. A Wellness Approach to Addressing Tobacco in Mental Health Settings: learning about healthy living. *Am J Psychiatr Rehabil*. 2009; **12**(4): 352–69.

54 Ibid.

55 de Leon J, Diaz FJ. A meta-analysis of worldwide studies demonstrates an association between schizophrenia and tobacco smoking behaviors. *Schizophrenia Research*. 2005; **76**(2–3): 135–57.

56 Desai HD, Seabolt J, Jann MW. Smoking in patients receiving psychotropic medications: a pharmacokinetic perspective. *CNS Drugs*. 2001; **5**(6): 469–94.

57 Ziedonis DM, Trudeau K. Motivation to quit using substances among individuals with schizophrenia: implications for a motivation-based treatment model. *Schizophenia Bull*. 1997; **23**(2): 229–38.

58 Carosella A, Ossip-Klein DJ, Owens, CA. Smoking attitudes, beliefs, and readiness to change among acute and long term care inpatients with psychiatric diagnoses. *Addict Behav*. 1999; **24**(3): 331–44.

59 Addington J, el-Guebaly N. Group treatment for substance abuse in schizophrenia. *Can J Psychiatry*. 1998; **43**(8): 843–5.

60 Hall RG, DuHamel M, McClanahan R, *et al*. Level of functioning, severity of illness, and smoking status among chronic psychiatric patients. *J Nervous Mental Disease*. 1995; **183**: 468–71.

61 Steinberg, op. cit.

62 Miller WR, Rollnick S. *Motivational Interviewing: preparing people for change*. 2nd ed. New York, NY: Guilford Press; 2002.

63 Prochaska JO, DiClemente C, Norcross JC. In search of how people change: applications to addictive behaviors. *Am Psychol*. 1992; **47**(9): 1102–14.

64 Williams, Ziedonis, Vreeland, *et al.*, op. cit.

65 Williams, Ziedonis, Speelman, *et al.*, op. cit.

66 World Health Organization. *Controlling the Global Obesity Epidemic*. Available at: www.who.int/nutrition/topics/obesity/en (accessed 16 May 2011).

67 World Health Organization. *What is Overweight and Obesity?* Available at: www.who.int/mediacentre/factsheets/fs311/en/index.html (accessed 16 May 2011).

68 National Association of State Mental Health Program Directors (NASMHPD) Medical Directors Council. *Obesity Reduction and Prevention Strategies for Individuals with Serious Mental Illness*. 2008. Available at: www.nasmhpd.org/general_files/Obesity%2010-8-08.pdf (accessed 16 May 2011).

69 Ibid.

70 Menza M, Vreeland B, Minsky S, *et al.*, op. cit.

71 Vreeland B. Treatment decisions in major mental illness: weighing the outcomes. *J Clin Psychiatry*. 2007; **68**(Suppl. 12): 5–11.

72 Menza M, Vreeland B, Minsky S, *et al.*, op. cit.

73 Ibid.

74 Dansinger ML, Gleason JA, Griffith JL, *et al.* Comparison of the Atkins, Ornish, Weight Watchers, and Zone diets for weight loss and heart disease risk reduction: a randomized trial. *JAMA*. 2005; **293**(1): 43–53.

75 Vreeland, 2007, op. cit.

76 Dansinger, Gleason, Griffith, *et al.*, op. cit.

77 Menza M, Vreeland B, Minsky S, *et al.*, op. cit.

78 NASMHPD Medical Directors Council, 2008, op. cit.

79 Hoffmann VP, Ahl J, Meyers A, *et al.* Wellness intervention for patients with serious and persistent mental illness. *J Clin Psychiatry*. 2005; **66**(12): 1576–9.

80 Littrell KH, Hilligoss NM, Kirshner CD, *et al.* The effects of an educational intervention on antipsychotic-induced weight gain. *J Nurs Scholarsh*. 2003; **35**(3): 237–41.

81 Vreeland B, Minsky S, Gara MA, *et al.* Solutions for wellness: results of a manualized psychoeducational program for adults with psychiatric disorders. *Am J Psychiatric Rehab*. 2010; **13**(1): 55–72.

82 Vreeland, Toto, Sakowitz, 2008, op. cit.

83 Citrome L, Vreeland B. Schizophrenia, obesity, and antipsychotic medications: what can we do? *Postgrad Med*. 2008; **120**(2): 18–33.

84 Citrome L, Vreeland B. Obesity and mental illness. In: Thakore J, Leonard BE, editors. *Metabolic Effects of Psychotropic Drugs*. Basel, Switzerland: Karger; 2009.

85 Allison DB, Newcomer JW, Dunn AL, *et al.* Obesity among those with mental disorders: a National Institute of Mental Illness meeting report. *Am J Prev Medicine*. 2009; **36**(4): 341–50.

86 Ness-Abramof R, Apovian CM. Drug-induced weight gain. *Drugs Today (Barc)*. 2005; **41**(8): 547–55.

87 Citrome, Vreeland, 2008, op. cit.

88 Ness-Abramof, Apovian, op. cit.

89 Newcomer JW. Antipsychotic medications: metabolic and cardiovascular risk. *J Clin Psychiatry*. 2007; **68**(Suppl. 4): 8–13.

90 Johnson FR, Ozdemir S, Manjunath R, *et al.* Factors that affect adherence to bipolar disorder treatments: a stated-preference approach. *Med Care*. 2007; **45**(6): 545–52.

91 Covell NH, Weissman EM, Schell B, *et al.* Distress with medication side effects among persons with severe mental illness. *Adm Policy Ment Health*. 2007; **34**(5): 435–42.

92 Cohn TA, Sernyak MJ. Metabolic monitoring for patients treated with antipsychotic medications. *Can J Psychiatry*. 2006; **51**(8): 492–501.

93 NASMHPD Medical Directors Council. *Measurement of Health Status for People with Serious Mental Illness*. 2008. Available at: www.nasmhpd.org (accessed 16 May 2011).

94 Ibid.

95 Goff DC, Cather C, Evins AE, *et al.* Medical morbidity and mortality in schizophrenia: guidelines for psychiatrists. *J Clin Psychiatry.* 2005; **66**(2): 183–94. Quiz 147, 273–4.

96 Vreeland B. Bridging the gap between mental and physical health – a multidisciplinary approach. *J Clin Psychiatry.* 2007; **68**(4): 26–33.

97 National Council for Community Behavioral Healthcare, op. cit.

98 Bazelon Center for Mental Health Law, op. cit.

99 NASMHPD Medical Directors Council, 2005, op. cit.

100 Druss BG. Improving medical care for persons with serious mental illness: challenges and solutions. *J Clin Psychiatry.* 2007; **86**(4): 40–4.

101 Ibid.

102 NASMHPD Medical Directors Council, 2005, op. cit.

103 Felker Bl, Yazel J, Short D. Mortality and medical comorbidity among psychiatric patients: a review. *Psychiatric Serv.* 1996; **47**(12): 1356–63.

104 National Council for Community Behavioral Healthcare, op. cit.

105 Tondora J, Picklington S, Gorges AG, *et al. Implementation of Person-Centered Care and Planning: how philosophy can inform practice* [paper]. Available at: www.psych.uic.edu/uic-nrtc/cmhs/pcp.paper.implementation.doc (accessed 16 May 2011).

106 SAMHSA, CMHS, op. cit.

107 Copeland, 2000, op. cit.

108 Vreeland, Minsky, Gara, *et al.*, op. cit.

109 Miller, Rollnick, op. cit.

110 Prochaska, DiClemente, Norcross, op. cit.

111 Hill JO, Wyatt HR. Small changes: a big idea for addressing obesity. *Obes Manage.* 2006; **2**: 227–331.

112 NASMHPD Medical Directors Council, 2008, op. cit.

113 NASMHPD Medical Directors Council. *Measurement of Health Status for People with Serious Mental Illness.* 2008. Available at: www.nasmhpd.org (accessed 16 May 2011).

114 Druss, op. cit.

115 Tondora, Picklington, Gorges, *et al.*, op. cit.

116 NASMHPD Medical Directors Council, 2006, op. cit.

117 Manderscheid R, Druss B, Freeman E. *Data to Manage the Mortality Crisis* [paper]. Substance Abuse and Mental Health Services Administration (SAMHSA), Center for Mental Health Services (CMHS) Wellness Summit. 2007.

118 NASMHPD Medical Directors Council, 2006, op. cit.

119 Ibid.

120 Everett, Mahler, Biblin, *et al.*, op. cit.

121 National Council for Community Behavioral Healthcare, op. cit.

122 Ibid.

123 Ibid.

7.2 Self-Help and Peer-Operated Services

Margaret Swarbrick

INTRODUCTION

Self-help groups and peer-operated services have come to be considered a viable resource for persons diagnosed with mental illness. In fact, there is a growing body of literature illustrating their beneficial aspects. These groups and services are relevant to PCC for various reasons, e.g. these groups and services are person-driven (as defined in Section 1.1, *Foundations and Ethics of Person-Centered Approaches to Individuals with Serious Mental Illness*), at least more than many other services. The current section will present an overview of self-help groups and three types of peer-operated services. The first part of the section will offer an overview of the range of self-help groups available to address emotional and social needs. Aspects of the self-help group model, research and types of groups will be reviewed. The second part of the section will examine three types of peer-operated services (peer- or consumer-operated, peer partnership, and service users as employees). Service providers using a person-centered approach, e.g. as characterized in this book's chapter on foundations of PCC, are encouraged to explore these important resources. Service providers should be inspired to collaborate with persons served to empower them to become involved in designing, delivering and evaluating services. Note that this section addresses matters such as stigma and its relevance to other sections of this book, such as Section 3.1, *The Lived Experience: narratives through the lens of wellness*, and Section 4.4, *Mental Health Systems and Policy in Relation to People with Serious Mental Illness* (which self-help and peer-operated services can be viewed as part of).

Self-Help Groups

Throughout the mental health system, the line between "SMI" and conditions where people spend most of their time "not disabled" is blurry. This is true for many reasons, including the episodic nature of mental illness and the trajectories of recovery, as people move beyond their illnesses to find new meaning and purpose and to pursue their hopes and dreams. This is extremely true in self-help and peer support, where the doors are open to anybody, and people at all levels of recovery can and do benefit. Most self-help groups would acknowledge Alcoholics Anonymous (AA) as the "father" of all self-help groups. AA's "How It Works" is a set of guidelines generally read aloud at every AA meeting, and it embeds the phrase: "There are those, too, who suffer from grave emotional and mental disorders, but many of them do recover if they have the capacity to be honest." That serves as another cue to various self-help groups to welcome people at all levels of emotional distress, including "grave."

Many mental health self-help groups were started by "ex-patients" with long histories of hospital stays. In most groups the empathy that people have for their peers does not seem to be diluted by an "us versus them" mentality. All self-help groups have basic structures, or "rules for interaction," which they ask all attendees to abide by. It is a rare occurrence for a group to ask a person to leave or not to return due to his or her inability to follow the basic rules.

The author of this section and her colleagues have had the experience of wanting group members to tolerate a person who did not fully follow the group rules. It was heartening to see the group members strengthen themselves by extending their tolerance to a peer having a hard time "there but for the grace of God go I," as well as to see that person benefitting from the practical knowledge and empathy around her. This writer and her colleagues have also had the experience of watching people who are longer-term state hospital patients get on a van and proceed to attend sessions at in-community peer support self-help centers. "It was tough to tell the players without a scorecard."

One key reason that self-help groups work for people at all levels of recovery is that people's issues are often comparable regardless of their extent of disability. Self-help groups concentrate on coping skills: how to reduce stress, how to get along with colleagues, how to manage treatment-related issues such as medicine side-effects, how to maximize family roles and responsibilities, how to cope with limited incomes, etc. People apply their various coping skills and personal medicine and can share their effective techniques, regardless of their extent of disability.

Self-help is based on the notion that people facing similar problems learn from and support one another when they share their experiences and strengths with an understanding and accepting community of service users.[1] Self-help groups are offered outside the conventional mental health system, and service users simply volunteer to help their peers. Self-help groups are voluntary associations of people who share a common desire to manage a mental health condition or otherwise improve one's sense of emotional well-being. Self-help groups are described in the literature using a variety of terms including *mutual self-help, mutual aid* and *mutual support group*. In this section, the term *self-help group* will be used.

Self-help groups are widely available for many different kinds of difficult life experiences including most illnesses, addictions, disabilities, bereavement situations, abuse experiences, parenting problems and other stressful life problems. Self-help groups are an important resource that can benefit persons living with serious and persistent mental illnesses (service users). Some persons living with more serious forms of the illness may not fully benefit from participation in self-help.

Self-help groups are member run, not professionally run, and are typically held outside the conventional mental health system, in informal local community settings. These types of groups are financially accessible because they do not charge fees. Self-help groups can serve as a bridge to professional treatment, since many members are aware of the different professional services available and can often attest to the value of those services. Over the last decade, online self-help or mutual support networks have developed, and many have their own online message boards, e-mail discussion groups, and/or scheduled real-time chat meetings.[2] Online self-help networks may eliminate barriers that previously kept people from participating in a community group, including the lack of any local support group or the lack of transportation.

A tremendous number and variety of member-run self-help groups have evolved since the formation of AA in 1935. The first national self-help group for persons living with mental illness was Recovery Inc., which started in 1937 by a psychiatrist, Dr. Abraham A. Low.[3] Some of the various types of self-help groups include those at a grassroots level that have been independently organized in local communities, local affiliates of national groups, e.g. Schizophrenic's Anonymous, Depression and Bipolar Support Alliance (DBSA), as well as organizations at the international level, e.g. Emotions Anonymous, GROW and Recovery Inc. Although some self-help groups may follow a similar approach in their methods, service users have the option of finding a group that is right for them. For example, Emotions Anonymous offers an approach similar to AA (a 12-step strategy), Recovery Inc. employs a self-help cognitive therapy approach, and GROW has incorporated both approaches in their strategy (*see* Table 7.1 for main types of self-help groups).

Participation in self-help groups for some seems to have a positive impact on psychological and social functioning. Practical participation in self-help groups is believed to be an effective way for people to learn to cope and deal with a variety of problems.http://en.wikipedia.org/wiki/Self-help_groups_for_mental_health - cite_note-DAVIDSON1999-4#cite_note-DAVIDSON1999-4 Self-help group participation is voluntary, which has made it difficult to conduct controlled empirical studies examining the full range of characteristics, benefits and implications associated with membership. Humphreys and Rappaport[4] discuss the problems of conducting self-help outcomes research. Rigorous research designs that include random assignment violate the spirit of open access to self-help and change the nature of the group in fundamental ways. Qualitative and naturalistic evaluation research approaches, as well as the Participatory Action Research (PAR) model, which will be discussed later in this section, may be more appropriate to better understand outcomes.

TABLE 7.1 Example of Self-Help Groups and Clearinghouses

Organization	Website
GROW	www.GROWinAmerica.org
DBSA	www.dbsalliance.org
Dual Recovery Anonymous	www.draonline.org
Emotions Anonymous	www.emotionsanonymous.org
New Jersey Self-Help Group Clearinghouse	www.medhelp.org/NJGroups
	www.selfhelpgroups.org
Recovery, Inc.	www.recovery-inc.org
Schizophrenics Anonymous	www.sanonymous.com
Walkers in Darkness	www.walkers.org

Despite the challenges, there have been some studies that provide evidence that self-help group participation is beneficial. Empirical studies examined how participation in mutual help groups for service users can lead to improved psychological and social functioning. There have been several reviews of mental health self-help group outcome studies.[5,6,7] Roberts *et al.*[8] studied members of GROW groups and found significant positive correlations between measures of psychosocial adjustment and the amount of help given, which is in keeping with the *helper-therapy principle* as described by Riessman.[9] The *helper-therapy principle* refers to the notion that those who help others help themselves in terms of an increased sense of self-worth and self-esteem.[10,11] In this way, groups turn what society considers a liability, e.g. one's experience as a person dealing with an addiction, or the experience of living with an illness, into an asset by their unique ability to provide understanding and help to others. Members who are further along in managing problems can demonstrate to one another that recovery is possible. Peers model competence and show how problems can be handled effectively. Peers provide one another needed encouragement and hope that otherwise is not available, since such role models are rarely found outside the group.[12]

A series of qualitative studies suggest that progress towards recovery is facilitated by membership in GROW groups.[13,14] Bright and associates[15] found that in relieving symptoms of depression, self-help groups led by service users were just as effective as cognitive behavioral therapy groups led by trained providers.

New data indicate that 2.3 million people who participate in self-help groups for alcohol or illicit drug use currently abstain from use of these substances. Based on a nationwide survey conducted by the SAMHSA, the report offers other data highlighting the use and benefits of these groups.[16] An annual average of 5 million persons aged 12 or older attended a self-help group in the past year because of their use of alcohol or illicit drugs. Of these, 45.3% attended a group because of their alcohol use only, 21.8% attended a group because of their illicit drug use only, while 33% attended a group because of their use of both alcohol and illicit drugs. This report adds to the substantial body of research indicating that participation in self-help groups can help support people battling substance abuse problems. Self-help groups often are used in conjunction with specialty treatment and support for individuals seeking help for sustaining their recovery.

Self-help groups serve as a preventive function by enhancing social connections that serve as a buffer to stress and by promoting people's ability to cope with stress and adversity for many of life's transitions and crises. Group members learn skills and gain support so they can better handle inevitable life stress. Self-help groups offer a connection to a social network that may address issues of loneliness and isolation. Self-help participation offers multiple ways for peers to contribute to their own and others' well-being and feel part of a community. Participants that assume leadership roles can enhance self-efficacy and self-esteem and find opportunities to utilize innate talents and skills.

Self-help groups can be an important resource for providers, and groups are a widely available cost effective resource that can serve as an important alternative or adjunct source of support. Referrals mostly come from informal sources such as word of mouth, friends and family; therefore it is important for providers to become aware of and link a service user to a self-help group when it may seem appropriate. Providers should be aware of available self-groups and clearinghouses (*see* Table 7.1 for some examples).

We will conclude the section on self-help support with a firsthand account by a man who has attended, facilitated and supervised NAMI Connection peer support groups (and groups following a similar prior model, NAMI CARE), for over a decade. Several hundred NAMI Connection peer support groups operate around the county, and the association is actively seeking to expand groups to the point where any peer in the country may locate a group any night of the week within a 30-minute drive.

Example

The following is an account shared to the author by a real service user (who provided consent for this excerpt to be used in this publication). This story will be used to illustrate the benefits that can be gained through participation in self-help groups:

"Being involved in self-help groups has been very good for me. Helping to facilitate groups has helped me overcome my natural shyness. Through group participation I learned about systems advocacy, which has helped me to become more organized, which is good for coping with my Attention Deficit Hyperactivity Disorder (ADHD). As I helped advocate for person-focused recovery services with a high level of peer control and staffing, I was constantly challenged by my lack of professional background in mental health. This led me to seek a second graduate degree, and now my career is mostly transitioned from computer programming to psychiatric rehabilitation.

The NAMI Connection model is very egalitarian, and it is a facilitator's job to do little talking and no advice-giving. We follow some structures, including a set of 'principle of support.'[17] Facilitators have a couple of days of training in group processes, and in how to use our structures effectively, and in how to keep people dealing with current issues and coping mechanisms, rather than 'wallowing in the past.' We welcome any adult with any kind of mental illness, with or without membership, with or without a diagnosis, and receiving or not receiving any kind of treatment. When groups run well, most of our time is spent discussing coping skills and their application, and most of that is about issues like school and work and money and parenting, which are not very specific to mental illness.

Our larger, twice per month group averages over a dozen people, ranging in age from 19–70. Several ethnicities are represented, as well as varying levels of recovery, from 'recent hospital graduates' to people who have been working full-time for decades. Diagnoses include depressive, bipolar, anxiety, schizo-affective, obsessive-compulsive, and attention deficit disorders.

It is always great to see how much in common group members have. Whether it's choosing a good gym, sleep management or workplace stress that causes hallucinations, we almost never have a 'one of a kind' issue. Members bring a wide variety of tools to the room, which they share readily. We have members who have experience in yoga and yoga breathing, Wellness Recovery Action Planning (WRAP), and a wide variety of other techniques they have learned on their own or from their therapists and treatment teams. We have members who bring philosophies from GROW and other 12-step groups, from Recovery International, and from other self-help structures and methods. It is also great to see group members taking on volunteer roles within our local organization."

Peer-Operated Services

Peer support is based on the belief that people who have faced, endured or overcome adversity can offer useful support, hope and encouragement to others facing similar situations.[18] Self-help groups as previously discussed are one form of peer support offered voluntarily. Another type of peer support service is the peer-operated service model (also referred to as consumer or peer run, operated or led). Peer-operated services are controlled by service users to serve their peers. In this section, three types of peer-operated services will be reviewed, including practical benefits. The final part of this section will outline some strategies regarding how service providers can empower service users to design, deliver and evaluate self-help groups and the peer-operated service models.

Peer-operated services in mental health have increased significantly over the past few decades. The peer-operated service model has been evolving throughout the world and in the U.S. is considered an essential ingredient in many people's mental health recovery.[19] The evidence base supporting the effectiveness of peer-operated services is gradually expanding.[20,21]

Peer-Operated Services

Peer-operated services are operated and controlled by service users and staffed by paid service users to serve their peers. Services are planned, managed and evaluated by service users. There is broad consensus that the Boards of Directors of these peer-operated organizations should be comprised of 51–100% self-identified service users. Some organizations also have advisory bodies that may include program members, representatives from family groups, churches, service provider organizations, banks, etc. Funded publicly or privately, they provide services that are alternative or complementary to those provided by the traditional mental health system. Peer-operated services have included employment programs, education and financial programs, education and advocacy, self-help and drop-in centers.[22,23,24,25,26] Self-help (or drop-in) centers are a type of peer-operated service where service users can connect with a peer network, gain practical assistance, and experience support in a family-like environment.[27]

The Center for Mental Health Services (CMHS) funded a multi-site research study designed to examine the extent to which consumer-operated service programs (COSP) are effective in improving outcomes of adults with serious and persistent mental illness when used as an adjunct to traditional mental health services. The COSP Initiative was a four-year project using a multi-site, random assignment, experimental design with 1,827 research participants, which aimed at generating empirical data meant to provide a more in-depth understanding of service user operated programs and services. The study investigated the extent to which service user-operated programs are effective in improving the following outcomes: empowerment, employment, housing, social inclusion and satisfaction. Rogers and associates[28] found that individuals with greater engagement in attendance at the COSP fared better in empowerment outcomes.

Peer Partnerships

Peer partnerships are service initiatives developed within the conventional system where peers offer services generally as a volunteer in one capacity or another, sometimes as an assistant within a program, program escort or role model within groups or activities. Peer partnerships can include peers who volunteer their own time to visit peers who are in state psychiatric hospitals.

The difference between peer-operated models and peer partnership is based on how much control persons in recovery have in the administration, budgeting and control of the operation. In the peer partnership model, decision-making and control is shared by peers and non-peer professionals. The executive staff and board of directors are comprised mainly of non-peer professionals; whereas on the peer-operated service model the board of directors is comprised of over 50% persons with a mental illness. Two examples of the peer partnership model include the Vet-to-Vet program[29,30] and the Recovery Network Project.[31]

Vet-to-Vet is run by veterans who have a psychiatric diagnosis.[32] The Vet-to-Vet hour-long group meetings are egalitarian, with conversations loosely organized around books written by mental health service user-service provider experts. The focus of the groups is on taking personal responsibility for mental illness, instead of relying solely on disability benefits and medication; learning to combat depressive cycles, which are marked by anger, self-destructive activity, and isolation from society; and a sense of mutual support and hope. Resnick and Rosenheck[33] compared the effectiveness of the Vet-to-Vet program, a peer education and support program, and standard care without peer support on measures of confidence, and empowerment. This study revealed that participation in the peer support and education condition (Vet-to-Vet) enhanced participant's sense of well-being.[34] This project is an excellent illustration of how a very large organizational entity, the Veterans Administration, has embraced peer support as an important component of an array of services offered to meet long-term social and support needs.

The Recovery Network Project describes how a cadre of ex-patients gained access to training opportunities and support to be able to offer a training curriculum for service users and staff at psychiatric hospitals in one state.[35] The authors share the challenges and successes of bringing wellness-oriented thinking into settings historically resistant to change.[36] This project illustrates how a peer partnership model has empowered service users to assume an important role as an educator for fellow service users and providers in a state psychiatric hospital setting.

Service Users as Providers

Peers as employees (service users as service providers) offer services within the conventional system, a non-service user-controlled entity. In this type of paid employment, a service user works within the regular mental health system in its usual programs, operated and administered primarily through an organization not considered controlled by service users. The notion that a service user can provide assistance to others with similar mental health problems is being viewed more favorably in the field of mental health. The addictions field has a long tradition of viewing service users as service providers or counselors. The service user as service provider, like an addiction counselor, offers a unique skill considered "life experience" that is believed to offer enhanced empathy, insights and foster hope.

Service users as service providers are distinct from the peer-operated or peer partnership framework outlined by Solomon[37] and Mowbray and Moxley.[38] Service users are persons who identify that they are living with a mental illness who seek *paid employment* within the regular mental health system in its usual programs, operated and administered primarily by non-service users. There are two broad types of service users as provider roles: 1. Service user or consumer designated positions; and 2. Service users who assume traditional positions. The peer specialist is generally the designated position for a service user who is considered further along in their recovery. Another example is peer advocates on an ACT team. Service users also may occupy a traditional provider position such as a case manager, staff psychologist or social worker, and just happen to be a service user. In either case, the person is paid wages for their services.

There is a small but evolving body of research indicating that service users as service providers can be as effective as service providers in professional settings. A series of research endeavors have examined the impact of these services. There were three randomized control trials[39,40,41,42,43] and a quasi-experimental studies[44,45,46] comparing outcomes of consumer provider (service users as providers) services to traditional, non-consumer provider services. All of these studies demonstrate that service users as service providers can provide services that produce at least equivalent outcomes in regards to engaging service users and helping them to maintain stability in the community.

Schmidt[47] recently demonstrated that service users with life experience but little formal training can work together successfully with service providers to offer case management services for people with an SMI. This research adds to the growing body of evidence that suggests that service users can deliver service as effectively as other service providers within conventional case management programs.[48]

Rowe and associates[49] demonstrated that early in treatment, service users as service providers may possess distinctive skills in communicating positive regard, understanding and acceptance to clients and a facility for increasing treatment participation among the most disengaged, leading to greater motivation for further treatment and use of peer-based community services. Their findings suggest that peer service providers serve a valued role in quickly forging therapeutic connections with persons typically considered to be among the most alienated from the health care service system.[50] In summary, service users are effective in service provision, at least as much as or complementary to professional service providers. Service users offer the following benefits: role modeling, hope for recovery, practical skills training and engagement and further research should examine if the factors lead to improvement in terms of outcomes on the individual served, systems level and also organizational culture.

There are challenges to integrating service users as service providers into the service delivery system. A number of authors have reported the challenges in terms of implementation, including role definition, supervision and training, impact on the organizational culture and issues related to accommodations.[51]

CONCLUSION: OPPORTUNITIES FOR COLLABORATION

This summary will outline potential roles and possible opportunities for service providers to collaborate with service users to help access, develop or even research self-help and peer-operated services. There are exciting new prospects for providers to become involved with individuals and groups to develop, implement and evaluate these services.

First, service providers should be aware of existing self-help and peer-operated services in their communities. They can contact the local or state department of mental health to identify programs receiving public funding and visit these programs. In terms of recruitment and outreach efforts, service providers can assist service users to access these resources for longer-term social support. Service providers should have the necessary information and contacts to refer service users to these resources when it seems it may be beneficial. Service providers can assist individuals or small grassroots groups in collaborating with traditional mental health programs to establish formalized referral networks.

Since there is a growing need to further research self-help and peer-operated services models, university and academic faculty can partner with individuals and groups to contribute to the body of knowledge through collaborative research endeavors. A PAR approach is an empowering form of applied research whereby the people being studied are fully engaged in the process of investigation. PAR is a method of inquiry consistent with the self-help ethos that explores practical problems and issues of concern to constituents.[52] The PAR approach involves maximum participation of stakeholders – those whose lives are affected under study – in the systematic collection and analysis of information for the purpose of taking action and making change.[53,54] Researchers can play an important role collaborating with peer groups in research to examine aspects of fidelity and efficacy.

It seems apparent that self-help groups and peer-operated services are becoming more widely available and offer a unique source of long-term support to foster mental health recovery. Mental health service providers and researchers alike should consider this emerging trend and position themselves to help develop, implement and evaluate these important practical service models.

REFERENCES

1 White B, Madara E. *Self-Help Group Sourcebook.* 7th ed. Denville, NJ: Self-Help Group Clearinghouse; 2002.
2 Ibid.
3 Low AA. *Mental Health Through Will Training.* Winnetka, IL: Willett Pub.; 1984.
4 Humphreys K, Rappaport J. Researching self-help/mutual aid groups organizations: many roads, one journey. *Applied & Preventive Psychology.* 1994; **3**: 217–31.
5 Kyrouz EM, Humphreys K, Loomis C. A review of the effectiveness of self-help mutual aid groups. In: White BJ, Madara EJ, editors. *A Review of Research on the Effectiveness of Self-Help Mutual Aid Groups.* 7th ed. Cedar Knolls, NJ: American Self-Help Clearinghouse; 2003. pp. 71–86.
6 Solomon P. Peer support/peer provided services: underlying processes, benefits, and critical ingredients. *Psychiatric Rehabilitation Journal.* 2004; **27**(4): 392–402.
7 Pistrang N, Barker C, Humphreys K. Mutual help groups for mental health problems: a review of effectiveness studies. *Am J Community Psychol.* 2008; **42**(1–2): 110–21.
8 Roberts LJ, Salem D, Rappaport J, *et al.* Giving and receiving help: interpersonal transactions in mutual-help meetings and psychosocial adjustment of members. *Am J Community Psychol.* 1999; **27**(6): 841–68.
9 Riessman F. The "helper" therapy principle. *Social Work.* 1965; **10**: 27–32.
10 Ibid.
11 Riessman F. Ten self-help principles. *Social Policy.* 1997; **27**(3): 6–12.
12 White, Madara, op. cit.
13 Corrigan P, Calabrese J, Diwan S, *et al.* Some recovery processes in mutual-help groups for persons with mental illness; I: qualitative analysis of program materials and testimonies. *Community Ment Health J.* 2002; **38**(4): 287–301.
14 Corrigan PW, Slopen N, Gracia G, *et al.* Some recovery processes in mutual-help groups for persons with mental illness; II: qualitative analysis of participant interviews. *Community Ment Health J.* 2005; **41**(6): 721–35.

15 Bright J, Baker K, Neimeyer R. Professional and paraprofessional group treatments for depression: a comparison of cognitive-behavioral and mutual support interventions. *J Consult Clin Psychol.* 1999; **67**(4): 491–501.

16 Substance Abuse and Mental Health Services Administration. *Results from the 2006 National Survey on Drug Use and Health: national findings.* Rockville, MD: Office of Applied Studies, NSDUH Series H-32, DHHS Publication No. SMA 07-4293; 2007.

17 White, Madara, op. cit.

18 Davidson L, Chinman M, Kloos B, *et al.* Peer support among individuals with severe mental illness: a review of evidence. *Clinical Psychology: science and practice.* 1999; **6**: 165–87.

19 Doughty C, Tse S. *The Effectiveness of Service User-Run or Service User-Led Mental Health Services for People with Mental Illness: a systematic review* [Mental Health Commission Report]. Wellington, New Zealand: Mental Health Commission; 2005.

20 Ibid.

21 Rogers S, Teague G, Lichenstein C, *et al.* Effects of participation in consumer-operated service programs on both personal and organizationally mediated empowerment: results of a multi-site study. *Journal of Rehabilitation Research and Development.* 2007; **4**(6): 785–98.

22 Clay S. *On Our Own Together: peer programs for people with mental illness.* Nashville, TN: Vanderbilt University Press; 2005.

23 Swarbrick M. Consumer-operated self-help centers. *Psychiatric Rehabilitation Journal.* 2007a; **31**: 76–9.

24 Swarbrick M. Consumer-operated self-help services. *Journal of Psychosocial Nursing.* 2007b; **44**(12): 26–35.

25 Swarbrick M. Consumer-operated self-help centers: the relationship between the social environment and its association with empowerment and satisfaction [doctoral dissertation]. New York, NY: New York University; 2005.

26 Swarbrick M, Duffy M. Consumer-operated organizations and programs: a role for occupational therapists. *Mental Health Special Interest Quarterly.* 2000; **23**(3): 1–4.

27 Swarbrick, 2005, op. cit.

28 Rogers, Teague, Lichenstein, *et al.*, op. cit.

29 Holter M, Mowbray C, Bellamy C, *et al.* Critical ingredients of consumer run services: results of a national survey. *Community Mental Health Journal.* 2004; **40**(1): 47–63.

30 Resnick SG, Armstrong M, Sperrazza M, *et al.* A model of consumer-provider partnership: Vet-to-Vet. *Psychiatric Rehabilitation Journal.* 2004; **28**: 185–7.

31 Resnick S, Rosenheck R. Integrating peer provided services: a quasi experimental study of recovery orientation, confidence, and empowerment. *Psychiatric Serv.* 2008; **59**(11): 1307–14.

32 Holter, Mowbray, Bellamy, *et al.*, op. cit.

33 Resnick, Armstrong, Sperrazza, *et al.*, op. cit.

34 Ibid.

35 Resnick, Rosenheck, op. cit.

36 Ibid.

37 Solomon, 2004, op. cit.

38 Mowbray C, Moxley D. A framework for organizing consumer roles as providers of psychiatric rehabilitation. In: Mowbray CT, Moxley DP, Jasper CA, *et al.*, editors. *Consumers as Providers in Psychiatric Rehabilitation.* Columbia, MD: International Association of Psychosocial Rehabilitation Services; 1997. pp. 35–44.

39 Solomon P, Draine J. The state of knowledge of the effectiveness of consumer provided services. *Psychiatric Rehabilitation Journal.* 2001; **25**: 20–7.

40 Solomon P, Draine J. One year outcomes of a randomized trial of consumer case managers. *Evaluation and Program Planning.* 1995a; **18**: 117–27.

41 Solomon P, Draine J. One year outcomes of a randomized trial of case management with seriously mentally ill clients leaving jail. *Evaluation Review.* 1995b; **19**: 256–73.

42 Solomon P, Draine J. Satisfaction with mental health treatment in a randomized trial of consumer case management. *Journal of Nervous Mental Disorders.* 1994; **182**(3): 79–184.

43 Clarke G, Herinckx H, Kinney R, *et al.* Psychiatric hospitalizations, arrests, emergency room visits, and homelessness of clients with serious and persistent mental illness: findings from a randomized trial of two ACT Programs vs. usual care. *Ment Health Serv Res.* 2000; **2**(3): 155–64.

44 Chinman MJ, Rosenheck R, Lam JA, *et al.* Comparing consumer and nonconsumer provided case management services for homeless persons with serious mental illness. *J Nerv Ment Dis.* 2000; **188**(7): 446–53.

45 Felton C, Stastny P, Shern D, *et al.* Consumers as peer specialists on intensive case management teams: impact on client outcomes. *Psychiatric Services.* 1995; **46**(10): 1037–44.

46 Klein AR, Cnaan RA, Whitecraft J. Significance of peer social support with dually diagnosed clients: findings from a pilot study. *Research on Social Work Practice.* 1998; **8**(5): 529–51.

47 Schmidt LT. Comparison of service outcomes of case management teams with and without consumer provider [dissertation]. University of Medicine and Dentistry of New Jersey: UMI Dissertation Abstracts (UMI No. 3181928); 2005.

48 Ibid.

49 Rowe M, Bellamy C, Baranoski M, *et al.* A peer-support, group intervention to reduce substance use and criminality among persons with severe mental illness. *Psychiatr Serv.* 2007; **58**(7): 955–61.

50 Ibid.

51 Chinman M, Luchsted A, Gresen R, *et al.* Early experiences of employing consumer providers in the VA. *Psychiatr Serv.* 2008; **59**(11): 1315–21.

52 Rogers ES, Palmer-Erbs V. Participatory action research: implications and evaluation in psychiatric rehabilitation. *Psychosocial Rehabilitation Journal.* 1994; **18**: 3–12.

53 Ibid.

54 Nelson G, Ochocka J, Griffith K, *et al.* "Nothing without me without me": participatory action research with self-help/mutual aid organizations for psychiatric survivors. *Am J Community Psychol.* 1998; **26**(6): 881–912.

CHAPTER 8

Constraints

This (eighth) chapter of the book presents a reasoned critique of PCC for persons with SMI. It is relevant to all other chapters of the book, as it provides an additional perspective and point to challenges of PCC. This may help improve PCC for persons with SMI by addressing such challenges explicitly and systematically.

Section 8.1, *Some Sober Reflections on Person-Centered Care*, argues that although PCC has benefits, treating and caring for individuals who have a SMI is a complex undertaking, and it is unlikely that one approach will be the best in all circumstances. This section argues for and describes some situations where a person-centered approach to people with SMI may be constrained or should be qualified.

8.1 Some Sober Reflections on Person-Centered Care

Richard O'Reilly

INTRODUCTION

The reader may be surprised to encounter this somewhat heretical section in a book devoted to PCC. As I will discuss, there are several clinical situations in the provision of mental health services where a person-centered approach is usually not taken. Failure to rigorously analyze the suitability of this approach in specific situations may lead some mental health service providers to pay lip service to person-centeredness while blithely acting in a system-centered manner. In contrast, the recognition and acknowledgement that we are deviating from a person-centered approach enables us to question whether that departure is justified. If we fail to do so it is usually obvious to others and has the effect of devaluing the concept and spawning cynicism.

Terminology

The editors of this book have asked chapter authors to use the term *service user* when describing people who are receiving mental health services. In contrast, most organizations this author works with use the term *client*. In a number of research studies, investigators asked people receiving mental health services what they would prefer to be called. Individuals attending non-hospital services, such as drop-in centers and clubhouses, generally favored the term *client*.[1,2] But individuals attending hospital programs prefer to be called *patients*.[3,4,5,6,7] So, if you work in a hospital and are genuinely *"client-centered,"* you would use the preferred term *patient* … right? Actually … no! The writer of this section works in a hospital where one of the aforementioned studies was conducted,[8] and despite the fact that the findings have been presented to the hospital staff, most service providers, and the hospital administrators, persist in referring to the people the hospital serves as *clients*. There must be some reason why we do not follow the wishes of the people we serve, but the author will leave it to the reader to speculate why that may be. In passing, please note that studies asking about the acceptability of the term *service user* reported that this term was actually less acceptable to the people receiving services than either *patient* or *client*.[9,10,11,12]

Smoking: an example

The reader probably knows that many hospitals have banned smoking on psychiatric wards. This prohibition has obvious health benefits for service users. However, banning smoking in hospitals has also generated a plethora of problems. Service users who do not have off-ward passes are often precipitously forced into nicotine withdrawal, there are frequent arguments with staff about passes, the incidence of disturbed behavior increases, physicians are pressured to prematurely grant off-ward passes to facilitate smoking and surreptitious smoking on inpatient units often causes fires. Some hospitals have been forced to follow municipal or other jurisdictional legislation on smoking in public buildings. In other hospitals, smoking bans have been adopted voluntarily, sometimes enthusiastically, by the administration.

The author of this section has had the opportunity to watch this process unfold in several hospitals. Service providers are divided in their views: some argue that hospitals must promote healthy lifestyles, while others suggest that mental health service providers should limit their attention to the psychiatric problems of the service users. Consistently ignored in this debate are the views of the service users. We know that most service users who are admitted to psychiatric units smoke cigarettes and place a high value on having smoking rooms on hospital wards.[13,14]

Nicotine replacement therapy may stop a service user from developing a full-blown nicotine withdrawal syndrome. However, service providers know that many people refuse nicotine replacement therapy and become highly agitated when forced to stay in a non-smoking unit. Moreover, we should acknowledge that nicotine replacement therapy is far from fully effective; if it were, many more people with SMI would not still be addicted to nicotine.

Whatever the views on the advantages of taking a holistic approach to the health of service users admitted to psychiatric hospitals, stopping service users from smoking is not person-centered, possibly not under any of the definitions used in Section 1.1, *Foundations and Ethics of Person-Centered Approaches to Individuals with Serious Mental Illness*.[15] Indeed, the decision whether or not to stop smoking is made for the service user, though most are capable of deciding for themselves – a decidedly paternalistic approach!

Involuntary Hospitalization and Treatment

The problems associated with banning smoking in hospital wards is greatest for those service users who have been hospitalized against their wishes. Civil commitment is a major abridgement of an individual's right to liberty, and there is a general consensus that it should be implemented in the least restrictive way possible.[16] Clinical considerations also demand that we do so in a manner that causes the least disruption to the therapeutic relationship. Not allowing service users to smoke when involuntarily confined to a ward neither meets the least restrictive principle, nor does it assist the relationship between the service user and service providers.

The inability to smoke is just one of the problems faced by service users who are involuntarily hospitalized in a psychiatric unit. These individuals are removed from their homes, must follow hospital rules, have restricted access to family and friends, are obliged to interact with strangers, may lose their pets and may be obliged to take medications they do not want. It appears that involuntary commitment over a service user's objection is the very antithesis of PCC.

Yet, civil commitment is a standard component of mental health services in all Western democracies. Most people view the use of civil commitment as justifiable in two situations: firstly, to prevent the person harming him or herself and secondly, to prevent harm to others. Many people view the prevention of self-harm as encompassing society's *parens patriae* duty to take care of citizens who lack the capacity to care for themselves.

When civil commitment is used to prevent an individual from harming him or herself it is "person-sensitive," but when used to prevent harm to others, civil commitment is clearly "society-centered."[17] As noted by Rudnick and Roe, committing an individual who is threatening to harm others may benefit the committed individual who avoids the legal consequences that would follow an assault if actually perpetrated. However, this is an incidental benefit rather than the primary rationale for the commitment.

Several studies have shown that, at the end of hospitalization or after discharge, most service users who have been hospitalized against their wishes stated that civil commitment was a good thing.[18] These findings are in accordance with Stone's "Thank You Theory,"[19] which proposes that if civil commitment is justified we would expect individuals who have been committed to be grateful following treatment. This raises the intriguing question of the identity of the person in PCC. Is it the person who refuses admission and must be compelled to enter the hospital, or is it the person who subsequently expresses gratitude for the compulsion? While this question tilts dangerously toward that quagmire of theoretical philosophy, it clearly illustrates the problem of unquestioningly taking our direction from individuals in the throes of an SMI.

While the need for civil commitment is widely acknowledged, a loose alliance of groups including right-wing libertarians, members of the mental health legal bar, some "consumer/survivor" organizations, and scientologists vigorously oppose involuntary hospitalization and any psychiatric treatment that is not voluntary. These groups argue against civil commitment from a person-centered, specifically person-driven perspective. Any interpretation of person-centeredness that demands that a service provider always acquiesce to a service user's wishes is incompatible with the "Thank You Theory," and with society's *parens patriae* duty. It is also incompatible with the equitable distribution of health services, because it would deprive a person of care and treatment when mental illness prevents the person from understanding the need for that care and treatment. By comparison, our society would not, for a moment, consider allowing individuals with non-psychotic conditions, such as intellectual disabilities or Alzheimer's disease, to refuse essential care and treatment.

The Business Model and Health Care

The mental health care system itself poses barriers to the provision of PCC. With the rising cost of health care services, hospital budgets are under significant pressure. In response to these pressures, hospital administrators are increasingly applying a business model to the provision of service. The author of this section questions how relevant a business model is in a situation where the consumer does not pay (directly) and where there is often a single service provider and thus no choice. Consumers have very little power when they do not control payment, and there is a monopoly on supply. In private health care models, where there is choice and the service user pays directly, there is more accountability. However, any advantage to individuals with SMI is usually lost due to the impairment of decision-making, which often accompanies these disorders.

The conflict between the business model and PCC is obvious. The business model demands a high level of efficiency. But efficiency is finance-centered rather than person-centered, as illustrated by the following evidence from Canada, Denmark, the UK and the U.S. Hospital utilization committees have shortened inpatient stays to the point where they are often inadequate to allow for stabilization of a service user's illness,[20] let alone to facilitate discharge planning or complex psychosocial interventions. Bed shortages lead to premature discharges and make it increasingly difficult to access hospitalization from emergency rooms when necessary.[21] Ironically, this may not save money. There is evidence that failure to provide the necessary clinical services to individuals with serious mental illness simply shifts the costs from health services to justice and correction services because these individuals have frequent contact with the police and end up in prison.[22,23]

The business model favors the use of brief, protocol-driven psychotherapies. Time-limited CBT and other modalities have been shown to be highly effective for individuals with a variety of conditions.[24,25] But one size does not fit all, and many service users require longer-term treatment and support. However, because of the high cost, administrators are reluctant to provide long-term supportive services – even for individuals with chronic illnesses.

These tensions occur throughout the mental health system and not just in services for people with SMI. Many employee assistance programs have a predetermined average number of counseling sessions, and providers are penalized if they do not remain below these averages. These benchmarks are not revealed to the service user, but put pressure on the service providers to restrict their counseling. This average can be as low as three sessions in total, which surely makes the therapy provided "time-centered" rather than "person-centered." Yet the reader will note that most employee assistance programs espouse a "person-centered" or "client-centered" approach.

The Role of Families

Finally, I will review the marginalization of families. The U.S. and Canada hold individual autonomy to be a preeminent social value. In consequence, the role of family is de-emphasized. By contrast, many other societies put a much higher value on families: placing both expectations on families and granting families certain privileges that would not be considered appropriate in North America. The clash of these values is often starkly illustrated in the delivery of mental health care.

Historically, several prominent theorists in psychiatry and psychology have accused families of causing SMIs. Think back to Fromm-Reichmann's "schizophreno-genic mother"[26] or Laing's belief that dysfunctional families cause schizophrenia.[27]

As deinstitutionalization has progressed, families have become increasingly frustrated at their inability to obtain basic treatment for an ill relative.[28] Families are often expected to accept their seriously ill relatives into their homes, to support them both emotionally and financially, and to monitor their treatment. Remarkably, even when families accept the primary burden of care, they may still not be provided with critical information, such as the nature of the medication that their relative is taking or the early signs of relapse.[29]

Anyone who has attended a single meeting of a Schizophrenia Society or the Family Council of a psychiatric hospital will have heard distressing stories of how relatives' requests for information are ignored or dismissed by providers. These reports are confirmed by systematic research.[30,31,32] It appears that many providers have developed a perverse form of "person-centered tunnel vision," which disregards the critical role that families play. Relatives are especially likely to be excluded when a service user is hostile toward the family, which is often the case when the family has sought help or asked for involuntary hospitalization. Are these not the very cases in which service providers should be actively encouraging the continued involvement of families? Undoubtedly, in many jurisdictions, privacy legislation prevents the sharing of information with the family when a service user objects. But many clinicians do not ask service users if they can communicate with relatives, let alone spend time trying to convince service users of the importance of such communication.[33]

Furthermore, clinicians seldom consider whether a service user is capable of consenting to the release or withholding of health information. Many service users do not appreciate the consequences of withholding important information from their relatives in situations where their relatives are providing financial and emotional support and monitoring for the signs and symptoms of relapse.

It is this author's belief that in many situations, we need to adopt an approach that is more family-centered. Indeed, it may be helpful at times to consider the family as our "client" as it is not only the identified service user who is distressed and dysfunctional. Family psychoeducation programs, when individualized to address the problems of the ill family member so as to align with PCC as much as possible, go a long way to meeting this goal. Of course, not every family acts in the service user's best interests. Therefore, service providers need to carefully analyze the family dynamics, but they should not start from the position of excluding family involvement.

CONCLUSION

PCC is a complex construct. The challenge for providers is not to reduce this complexity to a single person-driven dimension. As discussed above, a person-driven approach is inappropriate when SMI deprives the person of the ability to recognize his or her illness or to make rational choices about the need for care and treatment.

Some may view this position as paternalistic. This writer prefers to coin a gender-neutral term "parentalistic" and suggests that parentalism is a good thing when the alternative is abandonment of vulnerable individuals.

We should strive to provide PCC. If we cannot do this for fiscal or other reasons, this should be acknowledged honestly. Otherwise we will be seen as hypocritical. In this author's experience, the failure to acknowledge deviations from a principle quickly lead to failure to recognize these deviations.

Providers of mental health services, especially psychiatrists and psychologists, have historically viewed families as part of the problem rather than part of the solution. These views persist, albeit in a subtler form, and families are often ignored, even in situations where they will have a key role providing ongoing care for an individual. PCC must be modified in some situations to facilitate the role and the needs of families.

REFERENCES

1 Mueser KT, Glynn SM, Corrigan PW, *et al.* A survey of preferred terms for users of mental health services. *Psychiatr Serv.* 1996; **47**(7): 760–1.

2 Lloyd C, King R, Bassett H, *et al.* Patient, client or consumer? A survey of preferred terms. *Australasian Psychiatry.* 2001; **9**(4): 321–4.

3 Ibid.

4 McGuire-Snieckus R, McCabe R, *et al.* Patient, client or service user? A survey of patient preferences of dress and address of six mental health professions. *Psychiatric Bulletin.* 2003; **27**: 305–8.

5 Ritchie CW, Hayes D, Ames DJ. Service-user or client? The opinions of people attending a psychiatric clinic. *Psychiatric Bulletin.* 2000; **24**: 447–50.

6 Sharma V, Whitney D, Kazarian SS, *et al.* Preferred terms for users of mental health services among service providers and recipients. *Psychiatr Serv.* 2000; **51**(2): 203–9.

7 Simmons P, Hawley CJ, Gale TM, *et al.* Service user, patient, user or survivor: describing recipients of mental health services. *The Psychiatrist.* 2010; **34**(1): 20–3.

8 Sharma, Whitney, Kazarian, *et al.*, op. cit.

9 McGuire-Snieckus, McCabe, Priebe, op. cit.

10 Ritchie, Hayes, Ames, op. cit.

11 Sharma, Whitney, Kazarian, *et al.*, op. cit.

12 Simmons, Hawley, Gale, *et al.*, op. cit.

13 de Leon J, Tracy J, McCann E, *et al.* Schizophrenia and tobacco smoking: a replication in another U.S. psychiatric hospital. *Schizophr Res.* 2002 1; **56**(1–2): 55–65.

14 Skorpen A, Anderssen N, Oeye C, *et al.* The smoking-room as psychiatric service-users' sanctuary: a place for resistance. *J Psychiatr Ment Health Nurs.* 2008; **15**(9): 728–36.

15 Rudnick A, Roe D. *See* Section 1.1, *Foundations and Ethics of Person-Centered Approaches to Individuals with Serious Mental Illness.*

16 Lin CY. Ethical exploration of the least restrictive alternative. *Psychiatr Serv.* 2003; **54**(6): 866–70.

17 Rudnick, Roe, op. cit.

18 Katsakou C, Priebe S. Outcomes of involuntary hospital admission – a review. *Acta Psychiatr Scand.* 2006; **114**(4): 232–41.

19 Stone AA. *Mental health law: a system in transition.* Rockville, MD: National Institute of Mental Health, Center for Studies of Crime and Delinquency; 1975.

20 Munk-Jorgensen P. Has deinstitutionalization gone too far? *Eur Arch Psychiatry Clin Neurosci.* 1999; **249**(3): 136–43.

21 Capdevielle D, Ritchie K. The long and the short of it: are shorter periods of hospitalisation beneficial? *Br J Psychiatry.* 2008; **192**(3): 164–5.

22 Hoch J, Hartford K, Heslop L, *et al.* Mental illness and police interactions in a mid-sized Canadian city: what the data do and do not say. *Can J Commun Ment Health.* 2009; **28**(1): 49–66.

23 Torrey EF. *The insanity offense. how America's failure to treat the seriously mentally ill endangers its citizens.* New York, NY: W. W. Norton & Company, Inc.; 2008.

24 Leichsenring F, Leibing E. The effectiveness of psychodynamic therapy and cognitive behaviour therapy in the treatment of personality disorders: a meta analysis. *Am J Psychiatry.* 2003; **160**(7): 1223–32.

25 Hunot V, Churchill R, Lima de Silva M, *et al.* Psychological therapies for generalised anxiety disorder. *Cochrane Database Syst Rev.* 2007; (1): CD001848.

26 Fromm-Reichmann F. Notes on the development of treatment of schizophrenics by psychoanalytic psychotherapy. *Psychiatry.* 1948; **11**(3): 263–73.

27 Laing RD, Esterson A. *Sanity, madness and the family.* London: Penguin Books; 1964.

28 Jensen L. Mental health care experiences: listening to families. *J Am Psychiatr Nurses Assoc.* 2004; **10**(1): 33–41.

29 Petrila JP, Sadoff RL. Confidentiality and the family as caregiver. *Hosp Community Psychiatry.* 1992; **43**(2): 136–9.

30 Kim HW, Salyers MP. Attitudes and perceived barriers to working with families of persons with severe mental illness: mental health professionals' perspectives. *Community Ment Health J.* 2008; **44**(5): 337–45.

31 Levine I, Ligenza L. In their own voices: families in crisis: a focus group study of families of persons with serious mental illness. *J Psychiatr Pract.* 2002; **8**(6): 344–53.

32 Marshall T, Solomon P. Releasing information to families of persons with severe mental illness: a survey of NAMI members. *Psychiatr Serv.* 2000; **51**(8): 1006–11.

33 Ibid.

CHAPTER 9

Academic Activities

This (ninth) chapter of the book addresses research and its translation to practice, as well as education, in relation to PCC for persons with SMI. These academic aspects are important to address, as without them PCC cannot be practiced in an ever more evidence-based manner and by future generations of providers. This chapter is informed by issues raised in other chapters, as research, knowledge translation and education are informed by theory and practice, as discussed in Chapters 1–8.

Section 9.1, *Implications of Person-Centered Care for Evidence-Based Practices*, addresses EBP's, interventions with consistent scientific evidence of their effectiveness, and emerging practices in relation to PCC for SMI, including potential tensions between EBP and PCC. The section also considers the role of CBPR in further development of evidence-based PCC practices. Section 9.2, *Educating Service Providers and Researchers in Person-Centered Principles Related to Serious Mental Illness*, discusses the education of practitioners and researchers in the competencies necessary to provide PCC to adults with SMI. This discussion is guided by principles of psychiatric rehabilitation.

9.1 Implications of Person-Centered Care for Evidence-Based Practices

Sandra Wilkniss and Patrick Corrigan

INTRODUCTION

It is widely acknowledged by mental health authorities, providers, researchers, consumer/survivors and families that recovery and EBPs are among the most important service improvement initiatives in modern psychiatry.[1,2,3,4,5] They are essential to bridging the "quality chasm" in health care in the U.S.[6] Many feel EBPs and recovery complement and inform each other,[7,8] while others point to conflicts and suggest caution.[9,10] Still, potential sources of tension between these paradigms are: 1. Disagreement about who defines mental health objectives (the mental health provider, consumer, or a collaboration between the two); and 2. On what basis (scientific merit or value judgment). In this section, the authors frame the discussion of PCC and EBPs with the notion that it is precisely through efforts to identify and integrate EBPs and a recovery-oriented approach that high quality, person-centered mental health care can be achieved.[11,12,13] Thoughtful integration of the two initiatives forces transformation on all levels of the mental health system, i.e. policy, organizational, professional, client, towards a focus on individualized, personally defined goals and outcomes of the service user – transformation essential to PCC.[14,15,16] Of course, this is in theory. Many challenges still remain in actual practice today.

Elsewhere in this book, Section 6.4, *Cognitive and Psychiatric Rehabilitation: person-centered ingredients for success*, reviews how PCC impacts psychiatry and psychiatric rehabilitation. In this section, we focus on EBPs that correspond with rehabilitation strategies to provide a meaningful context for our points. More central to this section, however, is consideration of how PCC is key to: effective use of EBPs in the service of recovery, identification of promising practices, and how PCC informs processes essential to identifying the evidence in EBPs. Hence, the section begins with current thought about EBPs, summary of their fundamental benefits and limitations with respect to PCC, and discussion of PCC within evidence-based and emerging practice development and delivery. Finally, integral to the PCC concept, future endeavors to gather, evaluate and utilize the evidence requires CBPR, which stems from PCC. The remainder of the section considers the role of CBPR in further development of evidence-based PCC practices.

The State of Current Practice

In the past half-century, a confluence of events has led to the current revolution in mental health care.[17,18] First, the last several decades saw new data proving that recovery from SMI, even in the strictest sense (prolonged remission of symptoms and restoration of functioning to adequate levels), is not an unusual outcome.[19,20,21,22] Second, the consumer movement championing recovery in the broader sense (the personal journey) hit its stride during the same time period and served as a rallying point for consumers and families.[23] Third, on the provider side, the rehabilitation approach gained momentum with satisfaction, quality of life, and positive effects on "real-world" outcomes, rather than mere symptom remission, as the goal. Due to these simultaneous developments, national mental health priorities have been transformed. The New Freedom Commission Report[24] and the Surgeon General's Mental Health Report[25] set the national agenda for mental health care that is taking root in federal, state and local level policy initiatives and practice guidelines. Among the priorities are: 1. Recovery as the guiding vision for intervention; and 2. Rapid dissemination and routine adoption of EBPs in the service of recovery. Although the focus here is on EBPs, the authors acknowledge upfront that the recovery focus (with PCC at its heart) continually influences development, evaluation and research on EBPs. The authors provide details of this throughout the section, both in discussion of individual EBPs and in review of processes to identify, implement and study them.

Evidence-Based Practices: The SAMHSA Toolkits

EBPs are interventions with consistent scientific evidence of their effectiveness. Effectiveness is typically measured in terms of symptom reduction, functional outcomes and quality of life.[26] There are a number of practices considered effective and evidence-based for individuals with SMI. The precise list varies by source and criteria used to define evidence-based.[27,28] According to findings of the National Evidence Based Practices Project,[29] EBPs meeting the strictest criteria include pharmacotherapy with specific parameters (medical algorithms), illness self-management training, ACT, family psychoeducation, SE, and integrated treatment for co-occurring SUDs. Strict criterion, or highest standard of evidence, is superior performance of the intervention in several randomized, controlled trials comparing it with either an alternative intervention or treatment as usual (and usually summarized in a meta-analysis of multiple studies). Other types of evidence include quasi-experimental designs comparing groups with nonrandomized assignment, and open clinical trials (with no comparison group). The latter are not considered the highest standard of evidence but may be the best available evidence to date, and thus constitute "promising" or "emerging" practices as defined in the national EBP implementation project.[30] They typically involve examination by an expert panel rather than decision rules based on statistics (as in the case of randomized controlled trials), thus introducing an element of subjectivity or value judgment. The practices considered here are those most commonly referred to as evidence-based for persons with SMI by community mental health service providers. They include ACT, SE, IMR, family psychoeducation, integrated dual disorders treatment, and medication algorithms (toolkits for these can be found at www.samhsa.gov).

Person-Centered Care and Evidence-Based Practices

How does PCC influence EBPs? And how do EBPs advance PCC? We address these questions by revisiting fundamental principles of PCC as they complement the intent, structure and processes of EBPs. We assume, in this discussion, that the provider's intent is to achieve high fidelity implementation of the EBP(s). Considering others who do not value fidelity would require a lengthy discussion of workforce development issues, consumer empowerment within an agency, QI procedures and values, etc., all beyond the scope of this section.

EBPs are, by definition, practices determined to be effective based on outcomes averaged across a group or groups of individuals rather than outcomes for a particular individual. More specifically, the most rigorous research design contributing to an evidence base is the randomized controlled trial. Analysis of outcome data from this type of study relies first and foremost on comparison of group-level data, i.e. aggregated data for all participants assigned to a group. So, data from the treatment group(s) is compared with those from the control group(s) and determination of a treatment's effectiveness is grossly based on the group statistics. For this reason, EBPs and PCC may be viewed by some as incompatible.[31] Indeed, this taps into an age-old controversy around the value of universals versus particulars, or nomothetic versus idiographic methods in both assessment and treatment.[32] This is a critical debate and should remain alive in practical implementation.

The authors of this section and others argue that participation in EBPs is "both and" rather than "either or," and in theory it then should be compatible with PCC.[33,34] That is, findings that an intervention is effective based on group outcomes (replicated time and again to be considered evidence-based) are a useful starting point and should be considered in treatment planning along with individual choice and individual characteristics. For example, the IPS model of SE has been shown to effectively improve employment outcomes compared with treatment as usual. Successfully engaging a client in SE allows – indeed requires – a comprehensive understanding of that individual's personal goals for work, disclosure preference, unique needs for supports on the job, and so on. Thus, the larger evidence base stemming from group comparisons point towards best practice *and* individual choice and preference at the heart of a successful treatment partnership.

Informed personal choice by an individual is the catalyst for successful engagement in said intervention; both in choice to initiate and at critical decision nodes throughout. Sackett[35] states that EBP also involves "the more thoughtful identification and compassionate use of individual patients' predicaments, rights, and preferences in making clinical decisions." This approach is also endorsed in primary (general) health care,[36,37] further pointing out that consumers of services will not always make choices that are evidence-based but, rather, a combination of medical fact and personal values. Thus, as with any health care practice, the overarching philosophy and values of both the discipline offering the practice and the individual participating must be the foundation for any intervention. Mental health services are rooted in humanistic values, ethical principles and legal standards,[38] which should continue to apply in provision of EBPs. It is here where personal values come into play and EBPs are the tools by which someone may choose to achieve personal goals. It becomes an issue of practice rather than a fundamental flaw of EBPs in general. For example, partnership in the IMR intervention is rooted in a manualized intervention with suggested topics of discussion and therapeutic techniques but relies heavily on understanding the client's personal goals and suspension of the therapists' values in service of those goals. Further IMR encourages adoption of a supportive stance informed by ERPs such as CBT, motivational interviewing and behavioral tailoring, which may help affect change toward those goals.

Community-Based Participatory Research

CBPR is a fruitful approach for involving stakeholders of all kinds in the investigation process, an approach that parallels PCC ideas.[39,40] CBPR is a term of art, very prominent in the broader social science literature. It is not meant to distinguish community versus institutional care but to highlight the importance of the "community" (ethnic groups, people who are homosexual, people who are physically disabled) in which a study is to occur. Stakeholder is a *diverse* concept including demographics of advocates, e.g. in terms of ethnicity and gender, advocacy role (consumer or family member), and provider role (rehabilitation psychologists, psychiatrists or social workers). CBPR teams need to purposefully recruit these various stakeholders to promote research that parallels grass roots interest. Two principles illustrate the significance of CBPR: perspective and politic.[41] First, the diverse backgrounds and varied perspectives inherent in CBPR infuse theoretical understanding and corresponding research design with this diversity. Second, many advocates flex their political power by consuming research findings, integrating them into policy, and using their authority and networks to realize important change.

By virtue of diversity, dissimilar stakeholder groups vary in comprehension of an EBP and in research experiences used to test this model. For example, research suggests that interests and goals of people with Western European roots tend to be individualistic when compared to East Asian cultures, where individuals with mental illness are understood in terms of a collective, usually the person's family. As a result, goals defining the rehabilitation plan of Westerners are viewed first and foremost in terms of the individual's consideration of the costs and benefits of specific goals. East Asians, such as many Chinese, will include the active participation of authority figures that represent the needs and desires of the broader culture. These authorities are often family elders, though they may include service providers, especially physicians. In contrast, efforts to promote personal empowerment define much of the current energy of services in Western Europe and North America, where user-operated services such as mutual help programs or drop-in centers and individual users provide actual interventions to peers.

In terms of politics, "stakeholders as advocates" is the group that will consume research findings in order to act on them policy-wise. Stakeholders are likely to have a sense of key issues in the state mental health authority and use new information about CBPR to affect legislative activity (passage of budget and other mental health bills that promote a recovery-oriented system of care) and administrative efforts (the actual and day-to-day directives that make the vision of a recovery-based system a reality). Some CBPR team members may have a history of interest and authority with politicians who are likely to be responsive to constituent efforts.

We have briefly discussed the generic term "diverse stakeholder" above. Variability of the idea in terms of disorder is especially interesting. Definitions of service user may vary, for example, across type of psychiatric disability. Are the issues for people with depression the same as those with schizophrenia; and what about those with an SUD who are reactively depressed? Distinct service communities already exist in understanding and treating SUDs versus psychiatric illnesses; epidemiologic researchers, for example, have shown that people with disorders across both communities are at least half the sample of adults with mental illness or those with a SUD. As discussed earlier, evidence-based services for those with dual disorders are integrative. Rather than separate spheres of mental health and substance abuse treatment, providers from both communities need to come together and mix approaches into a sensible and solid approach for the individual.

The idea of user may also vary in terms of functional role. People with mental illness have been labeled user (the person using mental health services), ex-patient (in part, suggesting no longer needing treatment and, in part, seeking to distance one's self from the mental health system), and survivor (people who have not only overcome their illness, but endured the treatment too).[42] Inclusion of people from different roles will influence the quality of CBPR efforts. Other stakeholders may need to be included in a CBPR group. Family members of people with SMI often have different priorities than their relatives with the disability. Service providers assume important roles in implementing innovative approaches.

What exactly do we mean when we say stakeholders of different backgrounds are real partners in evaluating stigma change programs? Specific responsibilities and duties of CBPR teams include active consideration and proposal of: hypotheses; methodological design including operational decisions, e.g. hiring consumer to administer measures and manage data; and roles in the statistical process. Users and other stakeholders are meant to be equal partners in these tasks. At least one, frequently a service user, is picked as co-principal investigator and directs all aspects of the project with the other co-principal investigator who has a strong research background. Some people wonder whether this is political correctness or a truly innovative approach to assessing stigma change. True, many service user co-principal investigators do not have the sophistication to enter into the discussion of measuring stigma, though some programs include a training program to provide practical information about methods and the decisions needed to yield the best outcomes. Moreover, research decisions are not limited to design; fundamental to evaluation is hypothesis generation, recognizing the priorities and possibilities that define real-world stigma change.

CONCLUSION

PCC and EBPs are in many ways complementary and are mutually informative. Indeed, evidence-based medicine (which has now taken hold in mental health care/psychiatric rehabilitation) grew out of the movement to offer individualized, compassionate, informed care based on the best evidence available.[43] Still, PCC and EBPs diverge in some important ways, and it is at these points that the work should continue. Two important directions include developing a rich knowledge base about multiple areas of diversity, e.g. ethno-racial or faith community, and their interaction with the "best evidence" for interventions; and building on multistakeholder learning communities to ensure that evidence is collected, evaluated and acted upon in the most PCC-informed manner.

REFERENCES

1 Substance Abuse and Mental Health Services Administration. *A Guide to Evidence-Based Practices on the Web.* Washington, DC: U.S. Department of Health and Human Services; 2010.

2 Anthony WA. Recovery from mental illness: the guiding vision of the mental health service system in the 1990s. *Psychosocial Rehabilitation Journal.* 1993; **16**(4): 11–23.

3 Farkas M, Gagne C, Anthony WA, *et al.* Implementing recovery oriented evidence based programs: identifying the critical dimensions. *Community Ment Health J.* 2005; **41**(2): 141–58.

4 Fisher D. A new vision of recovery: people can fully recover from mental illness, it is not a life-long process. *National Empowerment Center Newsletter.* 1998: 12–13.

5 Torrey WC, Rapp CA, Tosh LV, *et al.* Recovery principles and evidence-based practice: essential ingredients of service improvement. *Community Ment Health J.* 2005; **41**(1): 91–100.

6 Institute of Medicine. *Crossing the Quality Chasm: a new health system for the 21st century.* National Academies Press. Available at: www.nap.edu/books/0309072808/html (accessed 17 May 2011).

7 Torrey, Rapp, Tosh, *et al.*, op. cit.

8 Frese FJ, Stanley J, Kress K, *et al.* Integrating evidence-based practices and the recovery model. *Psychiatr Serv.* 2001; **52**(11): 1462–8.

9 Anthony WA. The need for recovery-compatible evidence-based practices. *Mental Health Weekly.* 2001; **11**(42): 5.

10 Caras S. *It's Time for a New Paradigm.* Available at: www.peoplewho.org/readingroom/caras.newparadigm.htm (accessed 17 May 2011).

11 Frese, Stanley, Kress, *et al.*, op. cit.

12 Drake RE, Goldman HH, Leff HS, *et al.* Implementing evidence-based practices in routine medical health service settings. *Psychiatr Serv.* 2001; **52**(2): 179–82.

13 Wilkniss SM, Zipple A. Evidence-based practices and recovery at thresholds: transformation of a community psychiatric rehabilitation center. *Am J Psych Rehab.* 2009; **12**(2): 161–71.

14 Tondora J, Pocklington S, Gorges AG, *et al.* Implementation of person-centered care and planning: how philosophy can inform practice. *Psychiatr Serv.* 2008; **59**(11): 1242–5.

15 Osher T, Osher D. The paradigm shift to true collaboration with families. *Journal of Child and Family Studies*. 2001; **10**(3): 47–60.

16 Osher T, Osher D, Blau G. *Shifting Gears Towards Family-Driven Care*. Washington, DC: Technical Assistance Partnership for Child and Family Mental Health; 2005.

17 Bellack AS. Scientific and consumer models of recovery in schizophrenia: concordance, contrasts and implications. *Schiz Bull*. 2006; **32**(3): 432–42.

18 Silverstein SM, Spaulding WD, Menditto A. *Advances in Psychotherapy: evidence-based practices, volume 5: schizophrenia*. New York: Hogrefe & Huber; 2006.

19 Harding CM, Brooks GW, Ashikaga T. The Vermont longitudinal study of persons with severe mental illness, II: long-term outcome of subjects who retrospectively met DSM-III criteria for schizophrenia. *Am J Psychiatry*. 1987; **144**(6): 727–35.

20 Harrow M, Grossman L, Jobe TH, *et al*. Do patients with schizophrenia ever show periods of recovery? A 15-year multi-follow-up study. *Schizophr Bull*. 2005; **31**(3): 723–34.

21 Liberman RP, Kopelowicz A. Recovery from schizophrenia: a concept in search of research. *Psychiatr Serv*. 2005; **56**(6): 735–42.

22 Davidson L, McGlashan TH. The varied outcomes of schizophrenia. *Can J Psychiatry*. 1997; **42**(1): 34–43.

23 Frese FJ. Advocacy, recovery, and the challenges of consumerism for schizophrenia. *Psychiatr Clin North Am*. 1998; **21**(1): 233–49.

24 The President's New Freedom Commission on Mental Health. Achieving the Promise: transforming mental health care in America [final report]. 2003. Available at: http://store.samhsa.gov/product/SMA03-3831 (accessed 17 May 2011).

25 US Department of Health and Human Services. Mental Health: a report of the Surgeon General. Rockville, MD: US Department of Health and Human Services, Substance Abuse and Mental Health Services Administration, Center for Mental Health Services; 1999.

26 Drake, Goldman, Leff, *et al*., op. cit.

27 Lehman AF Steinwachs DM. Survey co-investigators of the PORT project: translating research into practice: the Schizophrenia Patient Outcomes Research Team (PORT) treatment recommendations. *Schizophr Bull*. 1998; **24**(1): 1–10.

28 Drake, Goldman, Leff, *et al*., op. cit.

29 Ibid.

30 Ibid.

31 Mullen EJ, Streiner DL. The evidence for and against evidence-based practice. *Brief Treatment and Crisis Intervention*. 2004; **4**(2):111–21.

32 Lamiell JT. "Nomothetic" and "idiographic": contrasting Windelband's understanding with contemporary usage. *Theory & Psychology*. 1998; **8**(1): 23–38.

33 Drake, Goldman, Leff, *et al*., op. cit.

34 Sackett DL, Rosenberg WM, Gray JA, *et al*. Evidence based medicine: what it is and what it isn't. *BMJ*. 1996; **312**(7023): 71–2.

35 Ibid.

36 Frese, Stanley, Kress, *et al*., op. cit.

37 Stewart M, Brown JB, Weston WW, *et al*. Patient-Centered Medicine: transforming the clinical method. 2nd ed. Oxford: Radcliffe Publishing; 2003.

38 Drake, Goldman, Leff, *et al*., op. cit.

39 Minkler M, Wallerstein N, editors. *Community-Based Participatory Research for Health*. San Francisco, CA: Josey-Bass; 2003.

40 Rogers ES, Palmer-Erbs V. Participatory action research: implications for research and evaluation in psychiatric rehabilitation. *Psychosocial Rehabilitation Journal.* 1994; **18**(2): 3–12.

41 Minkler, Wallerstein, op. cit.

42 Covell N, McCorkle BH, Weissman E, *et al.* What's in a name? Terms preferred by service recipients. *Adm Policy Ment Health.* 2007; **34**(5): 443–7.

43 Sackett, Rosenberg, Gray, *et al.*, op. cit.

9.2 Educating Service Providers and Researchers in Person-Centered Principles Related to Serious Mental Illness

Carlos Wilson Pratt and Kenneth Gill

INTRODUCTION

This section discusses the education of providers and researchers in the competencies necessary to provide PCC to adults with SMI. The guiding theoretical principles of PCC for these individuals have been elaborated by the field of PSR. Three relevant areas are: 1. The development of basic helping skills including active listening; 2. The acquisition of the skills needed to conduct person-centered treatment, service and rehabilitation planning; and 3. Delivery of specific person-centered practices for persons with SMI such as SDM and illness self-management. In terms of developing person-centered researchers, there will be attention to a variety of methods of engaging persons in the research process including focus groups, advisory committees and PAR.

In addition to these important content areas, this section will address education methods beyond traditional readings and lecture. These will include an explanation of skill development approaches to practice and develop skills, as well as guided practicum and work-based learning approaches to their applications with persons with SMI.

The Values Underlying Person-Centered Planning and Services

An understanding of the values and principles of PSR is critical for effective person-centered planning and services. The clubhouse movement, for example, from its inception embodied a person-centered approach that was exemplified by the full inclusion of members at all levels of clubhouse operations.[1] The expert consensus strategy used by Cnaan and colleagues to identify PSR principles highlighted several person-centered principles.[2] These principles included self-determination, and the full participation of service recipients in their treatment and rehabilitation including goal setting and the empowerment to choose interventions. Also, assessments of individualized strengths and weaknesses as well as strategies necessary for an effective person-centered approach were identified. Similarly, another synthesis of PSR principles based upon expert opinion emphasized the individualization of all services, maximum service user involvement, respect for individual preferences, a strengths focus and a partnership between the service provider and the service user.[3] *See* Table 9.1 for a listing of the goals, values and principles of PSR.

The strong relationship between PSR and person-centered planning in the U.S. is recognized at the national level. For example, the National Council on Disability recommends person-centered approaches as a possible remedy for the low levels

TABLE 9.1 The Goals, Values and Guiding Principles of PSR

GOALS

1 Recovery

2 Community integration

3 Quality of life

VALUES

1 Self-determination

2 Dignity and worth of every individual

3 Optimism

4 Capacity of every individual to learn and grow

5 Cultural sensitivity

GUIDING PRINCIPLES

1 Individualization of all services

2 Maximum service user involvement, preference and choice

3 Normalized and community-based services

4 Strengths focus

5 Situational assessments

6 Treatment/rehabilitation integration, holistic approach

7 Ongoing, accessible, coordinated services

8 Vocational focus

9 Skills training

10 Environmental modifications and supports

11 Partnership with the family

12 Evaluative, assessment, outcome-oriented focus

From: Pratt, Gill, Barrett, et al.[4]

of utilization of rehabilitation services by ethnically diverse individuals.[5] Similarly, Hasnain and Sotnik[6] outline a promising person-centered vocational rehabilitation planning approach to services for culturally diverse individuals with disabilities. The SAMHSA's National Consensus Statement on Mental Health Recovery identified "individualized and person-centered" (services) as one of the 10 fundamental components of recovery.[7] SAMHSA defines recovery as "a journey of healing and transformation enabling a person with a mental health problem to live a meaningful life in a community of his or her choice while striving to achieve his or her full potential."[8]

Evidence-Based Practices

Aspects of a person-centered approach have also been recognized as an important element in the provision of EBPs in PSR. EBPs contribute to community integration and potentially "support the maximization of consumer choice and self-determination."[9] EBPs and promising practices such as supported housing are based on the premise of individually chosen goals, and sometimes individually chosen interventions and supports. In the same text, the importance of service users' choices regarding outcomes is repeatedly stressed, as are the facilitation of empowerment and choice.[10]

Several of the staff competencies necessary to provide effective EBPs require a person-centered approach. For example, the technique of motivational interviewing, which starts from an understanding of the individual's preferences, goals and aspirations, is integral to Integrated Dual Diagnosis Treatment as it relates to substance misuse and mental health challenges.[11] The Stage of Change assessment, which helps to identify the best approaches to help elicit positive change depending on an individual's readiness for change, requires a person-centered approach. In fact, assessing an individual's readiness for change is an essentially person-centered task to determine where someone is at in his or her life.

Teaching a Person-Centered Approach

PSR students are required to adopt the attitudes and demonstrate the knowledge and skills necessary to provide person-centered services. Courses in PSR can be offered as either a distinct major or within other disciplines such as social work, psychology, rehabilitation counseling, nursing or psychiatry. An introductory course should include a review of the goals, values and principles of PSR and their practical implications. Fortunately, texts are available for both introductory and advanced students to familiarize them with the values and principles of PSR. These include *Psychiatric Rehabilitation* by Pratt and his colleagues.[12] Another recent PSR text for advanced students, *Principles and Practice of Psychiatric Rehabilitation: an empirical approach*,[13] by Corrigan and his colleagues, stresses the importance of attention to service users' personal goals and preferences for effective services. To supplement these texts, there are at least two peer-reviewed journals expressly devoted to PSR: *American Journal of Psychiatric Rehabilitation, Psychiatric Rehabilitation Journal and International Journal of Psychosocial Rehabilitation.*

Exposure to persons with SMI can begin during an introductory class with invited speakers who self-identify as service recipients and discuss their condition and experiences with services. On occasion, students in such a class will self-identify as service recipients and share their own experiences with their classmates. This exposure process is important for reducing stigma and reducing the tendency to see persons with SMI as "other" or perceiving a dichotomy of "us" (the healthy) and "them" (those with SMI). The process is especially effective when fellow students disclose. A recently developed DVD produced by persons in recovery delivers the straightforward messages that treatment and rehabilitation do promote recovery and that people with SMI can work real jobs, live on their own, and attend school.[14]

Exposure to persons with SMI is augmented by visits to community service providers. These visits might typically consist of one or two students visiting a facility after they have some didactic knowledge of the services being provided and are able to make both objective and subjective critical judgments about what they observe. For example, students might be expected to ask questions about the treatment philosophy of the service they visit and then compare what they were told with what they observe at the site. As a neutral observer, the student may get a glimpse of the services and environments from the service recipients' perspective. Later, extensive clinical practicums in such settings may be used to facilitate learning PSR skills in a hands-on or learn-by-doing fashion.

The Central Role of Communication Skills

Classes in communication skills need to stress listening coupled with reflective responding. Reflective responding is an excellent way to convey empathy and signal the other person that he or she is being heard. An effective skills training process consists of didactic instruction, in-class demonstration, in-class practice, and homework practice with audio tapes. Class objectives include the students learning the ability to demonstrate values, beliefs and attitudes consistent with the PSR field through their listening, paraphrasing and responding. Students should also be required to demonstrate communication skills "conducive to effective person-centered counseling and interviewing."[15] A useful text with a workbook includes Carkhuff's *The Art of Helping in the 21st Century*,[16] which stresses a person-centered approach to services and the helping relationship. Other important areas of study and skill development are in the areas of direct skills teaching both individually and in groups.

As an example, a student on an internship at a housing program reported that staff members scoffed when she said that as part of an assignment she wanted to use reflective responding with one of the residents; she had been assigned a five-year resident known for being uncommunicative. Using reflective responding after only a few short sessions she was able to convey the resident's history to the site supervisor, filling in a great deal of information that none of the staff had previously known.

Learning the Skills of Person-Centered Services

Historically, the assessments and treatment plans of persons with SMI focused primarily on symptoms and deficits. Borrowing from the field of occupational therapy, functional assessments specific to environments relevant to individually chosen goals were introduced to PSR by William Anthony and his colleagues. Environments include the chosen or desired setting of the individual and can be living, learning or working environments. Rapp and his colleagues went further in a person-centered direction in the area of assessment, introducing the strengths-based assessment as part of his strengths-based model.[17] Strengths-based assessments emphasize a holistic view of the individual, emphasizing strengths and preferences as opposed to problems, symptoms or a deficit orientation. These strengths may be particularly applicable in specific "niches" or settings, in which the person can apply his or her assets and thrive. An individual's strengths might include a hopeful outlook, a motivation to recover, specific skills or a helpful support network among other things. A niche might be a particular type of work setting, volunteer opportunity, home environment, educational setting or social opportunity.

Person-centered services, as opposed to program-based services, are not only individualized, but also seek to promote natural supports. Person-centered practices focus on goal setting, which is not primarily about the reduction of illness-related features, but focuses instead on the pursuit of a desirable future, sometimes referred to as "personal futures planning." Values clarification can help establish a desirable goal to pursue.[18] Followed up by functional assessments related to the environments of the chosen goal and an assessment of strengths and interests, a wellness and recovery-oriented treatment plan can be developed.[19,20] For example, for an individual whose goal is a job in retail sales, the assessment of values, strengths, interests and deficits relative to a retail environment would be assessed to develop a recovery-oriented treatment plan.

A curriculum designed to impart a person-centered approach should include two specialized intervention-related components: IMR and SDM.

Illness Management and Recovery

IMR is an EBP that is dependent on the effective utilization of person-centered principles for success. IMR is designed to assist individuals with SMI in learning about their illness, managing symptoms, preventing relapse, making progress toward their recovery goals and improving their quality of life. Effective IMR requires specialized training on the part of service providers. The manualized program contains 11 modules, including recovery strategies, mental illness related information, social support building, relapse prevention and coping skills training. IMR utilizes three types of strategies in its implementation: motivational strategies, educational strategies and cognitive-behavioral strategies. Motivational strategies help to instill interest, confidence and optimism in IMR program participants as they begin to set goals that will foster recovery. Educational strategies utilize interactive, feedback-oriented, multi-dimensional approaches to learning the information or skills necessary for pursing recovery and cognitive behavioral strategies use modeling, role-playing, shaping, cognitive restructuring and behavioral tailoring to help individuals acquire, practice and use pertinent skills as they progress toward recovery. An IMR toolkit designed to support service providers in the training, implementation and ongoing assessment of the EBP can be found at: http://store.samhsa.gov/product/SMA09-4463.[22]

Shared Decision-Making

Person-centered services imply that the individual receiving services is making informed choices and receiving support for those choices. Health and mental health care practitioners cannot know a person's set of values or know what decisions are in a person's best interest without input from the individual.[23] Traditionally, many persons with SMI have not had their values or preferences taken into consideration and thus have had neither the chance to engage in informed decision-making or the knowledge or skills necessary to do so. Effective service providers have the responsibility of: 1. Being informed about current basic practices in their field; 2. Having the skills to implement those best practices; or 3. Knowing who can be accessed to deliver these practices. Service providers owe this to the persons they serve, and it is their responsibility to share the best available advice. But the job does not end there. Service providers should develop the skills of SDM to engage service users in a process of informed choice after the consideration of all viable options. SDM is a process by which service users and service providers consider treatment options, outcomes and preferences in order to reach a health care decision based on mutual agreement.[24] In this manner, individuals will come to *own* their choices. The Ottawa Decision Making Guides provide an interesting tool to help individuals make choices through an SDM process.[25] They can also be used as a teaching tool for students to learn these skills.

Effective SDM empowers service users, which in turn can create conflicting situations for service providers. Besides assessing skills, abilities and experience, assisting an individual interested in employment implies learning about available vocational services. For example, a student intern employed SDM, assisting an individual seeking employment as an accountant at her internship site. The agency in question provided vocational services structured around a successful affirmative business that supplied baked goods for a local sports venue. The intern worked with this individual to explain the vocational services available in the area, what the services were like and their likelihood of helping to achieve regular employment. Accounting was one of the skills needed by the baked goods business, so the individual was offered a job there. Nevertheless, after learning about the available services the individual chose to attend an SE program offered by another agency. Her rationale was that she wanted regular integrated employment rather than employment in an affirmative business, even if the level of compensation was the same. SE was the best available service to achieve her goal. An SDM process gave her the information she needed to reach this decision. Of course, the student intern's agency was unhappy to lose the accounting services they needed.

Clinical Practicum

Once exposed to these techniques, the ultimate learning experience is to provide person-centered practices under supervision during clinical practicum placements. Clinical placements should last at least three to four months, affording enough time so that assessments, plans and interventions can be implemented and assessed. These should be well-documented by the students according to the most rigorous standards.

A useful general text is *The Successful Internship: transformation and empowerment in experiential learning* by Sweitzer and King.[26] These experiences work best when accompanied by a seminar that structures the applied learning. These seminars are an excellent setting for discussing the work in the field and also a chance to impart the skills of PCAs, goal setting, treatment plans and progress notes. Faculty can set an example and give feedback using person-first language. They can also work with students who are given the assignment of completing assessments, treatment plans and progress or clinical note documentation. This entails interaction with real service participants, assessing their strengths and limitations, and helping them choose and clarify their own goals. One effective strategy for practicing person-centered planning with persons with SMI is learning and then applying the WRAP pioneered by Mary Ellen Copeland[27] as a model for treatment planning. Such a plan typically includes a relapse prevention component and a plan for advance directives for managing crises. In many cases the clinical practicum or internship will also entail the application of interventions included in such plans.

Students should be required to engage in at least two forms of documentation: service provider notes for inclusion in the treatment record (also known as progress notes or chart notes) and personal logs. The format for clinician's notes or progress notes required in most settings should be learned by actual practice in the writing of them. In addition, students should learn how to incorporate relevant person-centered data and still meet traditional documentation guidelines. The instructor must provide guidelines and examples, as well as detailed written feedback on actual notes written. The product should be suitable for inclusion in service user records. A second and very different form of documentation is the student log. These logs are a diary-like document maintained by the student about his or her activities in the practicum setting. Unlike formal chart notes, students are encouraged to include personal reactions, observations and opinions. These logs often can be the basis of fruitful discussions between the faculty member and student especially regarding relevant attitudes and professional conduct. Written feedback and weekly discussion is suggested.

Designation of an experienced field supervisor is also important, as is orienting that individual to the goals and tasks of the academic program. This orientation to the field supervisor's role may take place individually or in groups, but in either case it should be well structured explicitly defining the role and expectations of the supervisor as well as the student. Regular communication between the classroom-based faculty members and the field supervisor is critical to the process. A method for mutually evaluating student progress is essential, especially since field supervisors tend to be volunteers and are typically averse to providing negative feedback, except in the most extreme cases.

Clinical practicums can be strengthened by the application of the principles of *developmental action learning* as spelled out by Raelin.[28] This strategy involves the application of workplace projects that help individuals acquire the practical skills necessary for success in the settings in which they apply them. Practicum experiences should be carefully designed by faculty familiar with the specific demands of the clinical setting and in collaboration with those who: 1. Are working in those settings; 2. Supervise staff who work there; or 3. Are service recipients. This sort of collaborative process will ensure that students engage in assignments that are directly relevant to the needs of the service recipients while meeting the demands of the workplace.

Teaching Research Competencies

The applied nature of PSR research is conducive to a person-centered approach. Such an approach is epitomized by PAR. A PAR approach requires that service recipients and/or students participate in all aspects of research on or evaluations of their own services, curricula, etc. In short, the participants of the study participate in the planning, execution and interpretation of the study. Nelson, Ochocka, Griffin et al.[29] among others, trace the emergence of PAR to two seminal sources: Paulo Freire,[30] who championed liberation of the oppressed through education, and Kurt Lewin,[31] who championed direct advocacy for system change. The inherent message of PAR is that the research process is open to everyone. In fact, given the myriad of tasks required to carry out a meaningful research or evaluation study, there are potential PAR roles for even the unskilled neophyte. PAR provides a model research approach for all levels of the curriculum and ensures that all participants are taken into consideration.

The importance of the research for the growing PSR knowledge base should be emphasized at every level of the curriculum. Consider, for example, learning about the long-term course of schizophrenia. At the associate's or bachelor of science level, students should review the findings of the Vermont Study.[32] At the graduate level students would read and critique the study and compare its findings with other longitudinal studies. In order to benefit from the current literature, undergraduate students should be exposed to introductory statistics and experimental design. In advanced PSR curricula students would have available an applied research elective in PSR mentored by a faculty supervisor with an active research program. Graduate students may also be engaged in one or two semesters of applied research practicum experiences involving outcomes research, program evaluation or controlled clinical trials.

Successful student research and evaluation projects require considerable planning and guidance combined with close faculty supervision. Students frequently propose projects that address questions that are far too large, require too many resources and would take too much time. The faculty task is to bring these parameters into line with a one- or two-semester project without demotivating the student. This can often be accomplished by changing a hypothesis or research question rather than changing an entire project. For example, a student working in an inpatient setting questioned whether participation in daily ward meetings was related to more effective discharges. While the question had merit, it is actually very complex and given the time and resources available it was unlikely that any interpretable answer might be forthcoming. By changing the focus to an assessment of the ward meetings themselves, utilizing a survey and observation, the project became viable and produced results that had some utility for improving the meetings in the future.

The applied nature of PSR research affords the student the ability to have a clear idea of the purpose and potential impact of their research efforts. Students often find that understanding the direct application of research to practice is very motivating.

CONCLUSION

Clearly, persons with SMI deserve the highest quality services organized around their individual needs and desires. Too often in the past, services for these individuals have been driven by an excessive reliance on the medical model even during non-acute phases of the illnesses. Also, emphasizing efficiency over effectiveness, many services were designed to meet the general needs of program participants rather than the individual needs of service users. Such services are rarely responsive to individual needs. The discipline of PSR offers both the theoretical and practical framework for the PCC of individuals with SMI. PCC shapes the nature of all interactions with people who have SMI and should include the nature of the assessments, goal-setting, treatment plans and interventions. The competencies of PCC can be learned through: 1. Exposure to the principles, values and practices of PSR;[33,34] 2. The practice of relevant communication and intervention skills in classroom settings, including SDM; and 3. Further skill development and application in supervised a clinical practicum with service users. In addition, the acquisition of research competencies can be enhanced through person-centered thinking and can be reflected in both PAR and other research methods.

REFERENCES

1 Propst RN. Standards for the clubhouse programs: why and how they were developed. *Psychiatr Rehabil J.* 1992; **16**(2): 25–30.
2 Cnaan RA, Blankertz L, Messinger KW, *et al.* Experts' assessment of psychosocial rehabilitation principles. *Psychiatr Rehabil J.* 1990; **13**(3): 59–73.
3 Pratt CW, Gill KJ, Barrett NM, *et al. Psychiatric Rehabilitation.* 2nd ed. San Diego, CA: Academic Press; 2007.
4 Ibid.
5 National Council on Disability. *Lift every voice: modernizing disability policies and programs to serve a diverse nation.* 1999. Available at: www.ncd.gov/publications/1999/Dec11999 (accessed 27 May 2011).
6 Hasnain R, Sotnik P. Person-centered planning: a gateway to improving vocational rehabilitation services for culturally diverse individuals with disabilities. *J Rehabil.* 2003; **69**(3): 10–16.
7 U.S. Department Of Health and Human Services. Substance Abuse and Mental Health Services Administration, Center for Mental Health Services. *Consensus Statement on Mental Health Recovery.* 2004. Available at: www.samhsa.gov (accessed 17 May 2011).
8 Ibid.
9 Drake RE. The principles of evidence-based mental health treatment. In: Drake RE, Merrens MR, Lynde DW, editors. *Evidence-Based Mental Health Practice: a textbook.* New York, NY: W. W. Norton; 2005. p. 57.

10 Rapp C, Goscha RJ. What are the common features of evidence based- practices? In: Drake RE, Merrens MR, Lynde DW, editors, op. cit. pp. 189–216.

11 Miller WR, Rollnick S. *Motivational Interviewing: preparing people for change.* 2nd ed. New York, NY: Guilford Press; 2002.

12 Pratt CW, Gill KJ, Barrett NM, *et al.*, op. cit.

13 Corrigan PW, Mueser KT, Bond GR, *et al. Principles and Practice of Psychiatric Rehabilitation: an empirical approach.* New York, NY: Guilford Press; 2008.

14 Spagnolo A, et al. *Reducing Stigma by Meeting and Learning from People with Mental Illness.* Scotch Plains, NJ: UMDNJ Department of Psychiatric Rehabilitation; 2006.

15 Basto PM. *Course Syllabus: communication skills for interviewing and counseling.* UMDNJ/ Middlesex County College, Joint Psychosocial Rehabilitation and Treatment Program; 2006. p. 1.

16 Carkhuff RR. *The Art of Helping in the 21st Century.* 8th ed. Amherst, MA: Human Resource Development Press; 2000.

17 Rapp C. *The Strengths Model.* New York, NY: Oxford University Press; 1998.

18 Center for Psychiatric Rehabilitation. *Reference Handbooks: setting an overall rehabilitation goal.* Boston, MA: Center for Psychiatric Rehabilitation; 1991.

19 Ibid.

20 Anthony W, Cohen M, Farkas M, *et al. Psychiatric Rehabilitation.* 2nd ed. Boston, MA: Boston University Center for Psychiatric Rehabilitation; 2002.

21 Gingerich S, Mueser K. Illness management and recovery In: Drake RE, Merrens MR, Lynde DW, editors, op. cit. pp. 395–424.

22 Substance Abuse and Mental Health Services Administration. *Illness Management and Recovery Toolkit.* 2003. Available at: www.mentalhealth.samhsa.gov (accessed 17 May 2011).

23 Ibid.

24 Substance Abuse and Mental Health Services Administration. *Shared Decision Making.* Available at: www.samhsa.gov/consumersurvivor/shared.asp (accessed 17 May 2011).

25 University of Ottawa. *Ottawa Personal Decision Guide for Tough Health and Personal Decisions.* 2006. Available at: http://decisionaid.ohri.ca/docs/das/OPDG_2pg.pdf (accessed 17 May 2011).

26 Sweitzer HF, King MA. *The Successful Internship: transformation and empowerment in experiential learning.* Belmont, CA: Brooks Cole-Thomson Learning; 2004.

27 Copeland ME. *Wellness Recovery Action Plan.* West Dummerston, VT: Peach Press; 2002.

28 Raelin JA, Raelin J. Developmental action learning: toward collaborative change. *Action Learning: research and practice.* 2006; **3**(1): 45–67.

29 Nelson G, Ochocka J, Griffin K, *et al.* "Nothing About Me, Without Me": participatory action research with self-help/mutual aid organizations for psychiatric consumer/survivors. *J Community.* 1998; **26**(6): 881–912.

30 Freire P. *Pedagogy of the Oppressed.* New York, NY: Seabury; 1970.

31 Lewin K. Action research and minority problems. *J Soc Issues.* 1946; **2**: 34–46.

32 Harding CM, Brooks GW, Ashikaga JS, *et al.* The Vermont longitudinal study of persons with severe mental illness, II: long-term outcome of subjects who retrospectively met DSM-III criteria for schizophrenia. *Am J Psychiatry.* 1987; **144**(6): 727–35.

33 Pratt CW, Gill KJ, Barrett NM, *et al.*, op. cit.

34 Spagnolo A, *et al.*, op. cit.

CHAPTER 10

Conclusion

This (tenth) chapter of the book addresses missing points in the literature to date about PCC for people with SMI. It proposes a principled vision, briefly summarizing and attempting to move beyond the state of the art as presented in other chapters of this book. As such, it is relevant to all the other chapters of the book, and is both a conclusion and an invitation for further research and development of PCC for people with SMI.

Section 10.1, *Making Sure the Person is Involved in Person-Centered Care*, argues that there remains a lack of clarity in relation to what is PCC for individuals with SMI and related matters. The section describes a number of overarching principles to guide the development and evaluation of person-centered approaches to care planning and service delivery for people with SMI, and a set of criteria by which to evaluate the degree to which a care plan for a person with SMI is person-centered.

10.1 Making Sure the Person is Involved in Person-Centered Care

Larry Davidson, Maria O'Connell and Janis Tondora

INTRODUCTION

The objective of this section is to identify a few essential principles for PCC planning and to derive from them a set of criteria by which to judge the degree to which a plan is truly person-centered. The outline of this section consists of an introduction, principles and proposed criteria in relation to PCC for people with SMI, and a related vision for the future. These principles and criteria are highlighted below:

Principle #1: People with SMI are first and foremost people, and therefore more specifically, citizens of their respective societies.

Principle #2: PCC for persons with SMIs is first and foremost similar to, rather than different from, PCC for other people.

Principle #3: Different aspects of personal decision-making can be supported in different ways.

Proposed Criteria: Is the care centered on an individual person and based on this person's unique life goals and informed by his or her needs, values and preferences?

Is the care based on the person's strengths and interests?

Does the plan clearly delineate the tasks and roles to be performed and the parties responsible for each? Of particular importance is, does the plan clearly identify the person's own sphere of responsibility and the tasks that he or she agrees to take on?

Does the plan and the care provided change over time with the person's evolving goals and needs?

Are the plan, and the services and supports offered, accessible to and understandable by the person?

Finally, does the plan encourage and support the person in assuming increasing control over his or her life, including the power to make his or her own decisions?

Overview of this Book

This is a well-researched and extremely useful book that circles around the issue of offering PCC to persons with SMI. It addresses this issue from a variety of perspectives, from philosophical and ethical to pragmatic, and considers the relevance of the issue for a variety of specialty populations, including people from various ethnic and cultural backgrounds, people with developmental disabilities or co-occurring SUDs, adolescents and people treated within forensic settings. It considers the origins of PCC in, and its similarities with, such historical antecedents as moral treatment, Rogerian psychotherapy, peer support and SDM models. Finally, it offers – perhaps more than anything – a comprehensive discussion of an array of complications that might be seen as barriers to the use of PCC with this particular population. Despite its comprehensive scope, we suggest that the volume "circles around" the issue of PCC though, because it stops short of landing on one coherent philosophical, conceptual and practical approach to the problem at hand.

Such a circling is perfectly appropriate, given the state of the field at this time. There are as many misunderstandings and misapplications of the term "person-centered" in mental health today as there are consistent approaches that can be described in detail for demonstration purposes. Simply stated, the field as a whole has yet to "land" on any one definition of or approach to PCC, and this book reflects that fact. The queasiness the reader may be feeling at this point in the text therefore cannot be attributed to this volume's editors; these are the same types of feelings – of being constantly bounced around within the pinball game that contemporary mental health practice has become – that thoughtful service providers experience on a day-to-day basis, being pushed and pulled hither and yon by managed care companies, state, county and provincial mental health authorities, legal and consumer advocates, service users and family members, politicians, and their institution's concerns about risk containment and liability. For the reader who is not a service provider, the editors and authors have given an internal glimpse into what many service providers are currently dealing with in their practice. For the reader who is a service provider, and who may already be familiar with these concerns, the editors and authors have done a favor nonetheless; in this case, assuring you that you are not suffering in isolation. Many of your colleagues are suffering alongside of you.

Perhaps the circling and landing metaphor suggested itself because one of the authors of this section (LD) was working on the section while sitting on an airplane that would soon be attempting to land at the John F. Kennedy International Airport in New York. We find the metaphor especially fitting, however, due to the tone of the current volume. Like most people in the field, almost all of the authors of the prior sections appear to agree that offering PCC to persons with SMI would be a good thing (like eventually landing this plane). They are just not yet sure how to do it. The questions include when (in the course of illness/recovery) and where (hospital or community) to offer what, precisely (what does person-centered entail), to whom (at what age, based on what criteria, in what kind of mental state, etc.), how (based on cultural and ethnic considerations), in relation to which conditions or interventions (medications, psychotherapy, addiction treatment, and/or rehabilitation), and to what anticipated ends (will it make care more effective or less costly, or perhaps the reverse). The discussions in this volume hop from one category of questions to another, without having the luxury of having any of these questions answered definitively, and thus without securing a solid grounding in any one area.

As a result, the book floats above the ground, with no clear, solid place yet to land. The utility of the book lies not only in familiarizing the reader with the current state of the field, which is similarly afloat, but in providing comprehensive discussions of the various factors that come into play in eventually choosing a suitable space to land. This book will be an extremely useful resource for navigating the various winds and taking into account the many possible weather conditions we all will face in attempting to do so.

Where, then, can we go from here? In this concluding section, we will not be able to answer all of the questions outlined above in any kind of satisfactory way. Rather, we would like to suggest three principles for the reader's consideration, which we hope will begin to simplify somewhat what is admittedly an exceedingly complex picture. Following a discussion of these principles, we will then be so bold as to offer some possible criteria for identifying a suitable place to land. We hope these suggestions and criteria will be of some use to the field as we all grapple with the challenges so thoroughly described in this volume, while also leaving ample latitude for innovating. As we think the editors and authors of this volume, along with most of its readers, would agree, we have yet to develop an adequately mature and holistic, as well as practical and effective, approach to providing PCC for persons with SMI. While we and many others are currently hard at work trying to do so, our hope and salvation lies in the new, creative innovations that will spring from the kinds of considerations contained within this volume.

Principle #1: People with SMIs are first and foremost people, and therefore more specifically, citizens of their respective societies.

As a first principle for simplifying (somewhat) the complicated picture that has been painted thus far, we would like to suggest, in agreement with the editors' important first article, that we accept that persons with SMI are, first and foremost, people just like ourselves. They were born with the same rights to citizenship that anyone else in their respective country was born, and any limitations placed upon those rights will have to be justified and sanctioned by law. If we begin with this assumption, then we need not argue for or try to justify offering PCC to persons with SMI as a separate population. If we assume an ideal of equity in the provision of health care within our respective societies, then persons with SMIs are "entitled" to PCC for the same reasons as are any other citizens. Like everyone else, they are to be offered PCC because it is in accord with the emphasis democratic societies place on personal sovereignty. These values apply in health care as well as in other spheres of society, and they apply equally as well to persons with SMI as they do to any other persons ... *unless, until, and then only for as long as* limitations placed on these values are justified and sanctioned by law (just as for any other persons).

In other words, we do not need to justify offering PCC to this particular population based on clinical rationales or effectiveness studies. Within democratic societies, PCC should be considered the default condition; that is, it should be provided unless there are clear and persuasive, and legally valid, reasons for not doing so. This takes a tremendous amount of pressure off the shoulders of PCC advocates, as it is not their case to argue. The onus is on those who wish to limit the applicability of this approach to any given population, whether that be persons with SMI, those with developmental disabilities, those with Alzheimer's, those knocked unconscious by a car accident, or those with any other special considerations, e.g. forensic populations.

Before we turn to the contentious issue of such limitations, let us pause to consider first what it is that we are arguing about. What is it, precisely, to which citizens of a democratic society are entitled *unless, until, and then only for as long as* others can justify otherwise? Prior to becoming an approach to health care delivery, PCC was an acknowledgment that people have the right to make decisions about their own health and care, and that people want care that is responsive to their personal values, needs and preferences. Framing the issue in this way has both an advantage and a disadvantage. The advantage is that this simple understanding of PCC is consistent with the focus on rights and personal sovereignty emphasized above and therefore is hard to refute or challenge based purely on principle. Few can argue that people do not want to make their own decisions (although some in this volume appeared to suggest so) or that people do not want care that is consistent with their personal values, needs and preferences. Persons with SMI want the same kind of care we all would want if we were in their situation (assuming we are not already in that situation ourselves). There is an elegant simplicity to this explanation that makes it hard to discount.

Unfortunately, the disadvantage of framing this issue in this way stems precisely from this same advantage. It is because it is hard to discount, that PCC comes to be equated with "motherhood and apple pie" (an American phrase for things that are undeniably good), and, as a result, everyone claims to be doing it already. At this vague and abstract a level, it is easy for people to dismiss the challenges inherent in having to change their practice by insisting that they already practice in a person-centered way. This is a frequent refrain from providers and program and system leaders to invitations to learn about PCC approaches, and is seen in this volume, for example, in Cross' statement that: "PCC is not a new approach to client care. Its fundamental tenets were articulated by humanistic psychologist Carl Rogers in the early 1940s".[1]

While Cross elaborates on the ways in which Rogers' approach to psychotherapy was, in fact, person-centered, the statement that PCC "is not a new approach" neglects those tenets of PCC that are, in fact, new – which were developed, that is, since the 1940s. These include: comprehensive and structured interests and strengths assessments, the inclusion of the person's "natural supporters" and legal advocates in the care planning process, articulation of clearly defined short- and long-term personal goals with measurable objectives, assignment of responsibility for different tasks and action steps to different members of the care "team," and use of new tools such as psychiatric advance directives, SDM aids, and SE, housing, socialization, and education coaches – not to mention the basic view of persons with SMI as full citizens of society, which was not introduced until the 1970s with the mental health consumer (service user) movement.[2]

Similarly, while it is useful for Charland to highlight Pinel and Chiarugi's insistence on respecting each person with an SMI as a person and on according him or her the dignity and sovereignty associated with personhood, the majority of the "moral treatment" that made its way over to England and eventually North America placed much more of an emphasis on the expertise of the superintendent and/or physician than on the knowledge and expertise of the person with the mental illness. Rather than being person-centered, care was driven by the Tukes and their successors, who viewed themselves as wise and well-socialized parents entrusted with correcting the "perversions" of reason, the "erroneous views" and "wayward propensities" of their charges – who were adults they viewed largely as poorly behaved children.[3] It would have made little sense to them to argue that these adults had the right to make their own decisions, as they viewed their faulty decisions, and the perverted reason upon which those decisions were based, as the cause for their internment. The vast majority of the day-to-day decisions made in Pinel and Chiarugi's asylums, and the Tukes' retreat, were made by the governor/superintendent and/or physician and his staff. While certainly more compassionate and humane than previous generations, these giants in the history of psychiatry, who were indeed responsible for many advances, had not already stumbled upon PCC.

On the other hand, we can say that PCC is consistent with – but is also presumed by – evidence-based medicine, as Mueser and Drake comment. We cannot equate the two, as evidence-based medicine simply presumes that all individuals have the right to make their own health care decisions; this therefore includes the person's role (including his or her needs, values and preferences) as one of the three or four components that the provider has to consider (the others being the scientific evidence, the provider's own accumulated knowledge base and clinical experience, and local resources).[4] The basis for this approach is that the person is free to (and in one way or another, will) ultimately make his or her own decisions, and therefore it behooves service providers to understand this fact and to communicate with the person and his or her family in as accurate, informative, culturally and personally responsive, and perhaps even persuasive, a way as possible so as to maximize outcomes. So, in this way, appealing to evidence-based medicine does not answer the array of questions raised above about PCC either. It provides a useful framework for the provider in suggesting how he or she might approach the task of collaborative or SDM (armed with evidence, clinical experience, etc.), but it does not clarify the task itself, nor suggest how to do it.

Finally, we should dispel upfront the common concern about PCC, in this volume voiced by O'Reilly, that it requires "that a service provider always acquiesce to a service user's wishes".[5] PCC for SMI no more requires such acquiescence than does PCC for any other medical condition. Ideally, PCC evolves within a collaborative relationship in which decision-making is viewed as shared between service providers and service users and their loved ones. Within the context of such a partnership, each party has its respective role to play. Providers assess, evaluate, diagnose, educate, inform and advise the service user and his or her loved ones about the possible courses of treatment and rehabilitation available for whatever ails the person, including the relative pros and cons of each. Providers then deliver whatever treatments and rehabilitation strategies they are competent in providing, based on the nature of the ailment and the person's informed consent. The person, in conjunction with his or her loved ones (to whatever degree he or she wishes) makes decisions about what treatments, services, interventions and supports make the most sense within his or her life context, given his or her values, needs, preferences and goals. It is no more appropriate for the person to assume the role of provider than it is for the provider to assume the authority to make the person's decisions for him or her. But this is the key point: while it is not appropriate for service users to tell providers what to do, it also is not appropriate for providers to tell service users what to do. It is the right, and ethical responsibility, of providers to practice medicine as best they can. But it also remains the person's right to make his or her own decisions about what services or supports he or she will use in his or her recovery.

Principle #2: PCC for persons with SMI is first and foremost similar to, rather than different from, PCC for other people.

This digression brings us to our second principle for consideration, which follows rather naturally from the first. If persons with SMI are first and foremost people, then perhaps PCC for persons with SMI is first and foremost similar to, if not exactly the same as, PCC for other people. This is not to say that certain adaptations may not need to be made, certain limitations might not be required, or, perhaps most importantly, certain tools might not need to be developed for a specific illness or condition. But these adaptations, limitations and additions do not have to fundamentally alter the nature of the approach itself. Just as persons with SMI are people too, our second principle suggests that we begin with an approach to PCC that would be relevant and applicable to anyone at all, and then make the adaptations, limitations and additions required by the nature of the specific mental illness this specific person is experiencing and its specific impact on his or her ability to participate fully in the process. While this principle may sound obvious, trite or simplistic, it actually profoundly influences how we view the challenge of PCC for persons with SMI.

One way to approach this challenge is from the perspective of psychopathology and disability, from the perspective, we could say, of the service provider – typically one who works in acute care settings – and, in this case, it appears to be a challenge of how one can possibly involve this person in deciding and planning for his or her own care. This person is depressed and actively suicidal, and so obviously cannot make decisions in his or her best interest. Or this person is paranoid and insists that all mental health care consists of efforts to poison, imprison, undermine or otherwise hurt him or her; how could this person possibly make informed choices about the costs and benefits of various interventions? Or this person's thoughts are disordered and he or she cannot carry on a coherent conversation; how can I possibly inform him or her of his or her diagnosis and the effective treatments available for it? Or this person has been hospitalized for having homicidal impulses and making threats to hurt other people, how can he or she participate actively in determining a course of treatment for these signs of his or her disorder? Or, as several of the authors of this volume suggested, this person has no insight into his or her illness, will not accept having an illness at all, appears to be oblivious to the fact that something is dreadfully wrong, and will not accept any psychiatric care voluntarily; what could PCC possibly mean for him or her?

These are very legitimate concerns, and it is not surprising that they are raised by people who usually work in acute care settings or in psychiatric residential treatment settings (hospitals and others), working with precisely the kinds of service users described above. What is important to remember, though, is that while such providers may spend the majority of their work lives and devote the majority of their professional practice in and to these settings, the same is not true for the majority of the people who use their services. The people described above, who may in acute episodes appear depressed and suicidal, paranoid, thought disordered, homicidal, or lacking awareness, do not spend the majority of their lives trapped within such episodes. In fact, estimates suggest that most people with serious and prolonged mental illnesses spend only about 5% of their adult lives in acute episodes of illness.[6] The longitudinal research carried out by Strauss, Harding, Ciompi, and others over the previous 30 years suggests that over half of these people will experience significant improvements in their functioning and recovery over time.[7] While the other half of this population may continue to experience and be impacted by the illness the remaining 95% of their adult lives, when not in acute episodes, most of these people have delimited impairments in only one or a few domains of functioning, while other domains of functioning remain relatively intact. As Philippe Pinel had already noted as early as 1794 in his address to the Society for Natural History in Paris:

> "The idea of madness should by no means imply a total abolition of the mental faculties. On the contrary, the disorder usually attacks only one partial faculty such as the perception of ideas, judgment, reasoning, imagination, memory, or psychologic sensitivity … A total upheaval of the rational faculty … is quite rare."[8]

To this, some readers may respond either: 1. That a "total upheaval of the rational faculty" is not at all that rare, because they see it every day in their practice; or 2. That it doesn't matter how rare it is, because they see it every day in their practice (or in their lives) and are concerned about the people they see and have to work (or live) with every day and not anyone else. Both of these understandable responses overlook an essential point. Whether or not you see people recovering from and/ or living well with SMI in your practice, it is important to know that they exist and that they outnumber, by a significant margin, those people who continue to struggle, in a Sisyphean way, in managing to get through, to survive, each day.

For one reason, it encourages the provider to look beyond the illness per se to see if there are other factors keeping the person stuck within a "patient" role, with many of these factors unfortunately stemming as much from the care setting as from the person's character or family and life history. To providers working in long-term care settings that do not allow much room for personal goal-setting or choice – such as mental hospitals, group homes or extended day care programs – and who believe that the institutional quality of the care setting is the result, rather than the cause, of the person's degree of disability, all that we can suggest is that the proof will have to be in the pudding, the believing in the seeing. Having now worked with numerous institutional settings in several states and countries, we have been continuously and consistently impressed by how much people will rise to the occasion of identifying their own goals and making their own decisions when offered the opportunity to do so. We return to examples of the kinds of goals and decisions such individuals may need to begin with below, but first we want to consider a second reason why it is important to know about recovery.

The second, and more important, reason that it is important to know that a majority of people with serious and prolonged mental illnesses have intact domains of functioning the majority of the time is that it suggests a reversal in our conventional clinical logic. It suggests, in other words, that the question described above of "how one can possibly involve this person in deciding and planning for his or her own care?" represents a backwards approach to the issue. Such an approach is more akin to a "guilty until proven innocent" presumption, as opposed to our well-honored presumption of "innocent until proven guilty." One need not have extensive experience with legal matters to appreciate just how different these approaches are. It can be exceedingly difficult to "prove" one's innocence, especially when innocence is interpreted as being a fully functioning, normal, rational and capable adult (many of us fail to meet such standards on a day-to-day basis). Our laws suggest, therefore, that it is incumbent upon the legal system instead to have to prove a person's guilt. While this is not always possible, and we are not always sure to prove the right person guilty of the right crime, it has nonetheless been agreed over time that this is, on the whole, the better of the two alternatives.

Our point is that such a principle is not limited to our judicial system, but does in fact extend to our current legal and statutory approach to mental illness as well, in which it is incumbent upon the psychiatrist and/or the judge to determine a person's incapacity, either for an acute period, e.g. 72 hours, or for an extended period of time, e.g. the indefinite assignment of a conservator of person. Short of meeting the criteria for these legal mechanisms, which we note are only applicable to a small percentage of individuals for a short period of time, a person is to be assumed to be competent and capable of making his or her own decisions, both in life and in treatment. A very different process results from this reversing of the direction of our approach from having to prove someone capable to assuming capacity until one can be proven *not* to have it. Such a reversal does away with all of the concerns about when, for whom, under what circumstances, etc., a person can be considered capable of participating in or receiving PCC. We begin with PCC as our point of departure and only diverge from it when it is necessary to do so. "Necessity" in this sense is not based on a clinical judgment, which would return us to where we began, but rather to a legal judgment. We begin with PCC and proceed accordingly *unless, until, and then only for as long as* we can justify departing from it based on the clear and convincing criteria required by law. We understand that this may not be a popular position to take among some providers but remain convinced nonetheless that unless we begin with this position we will make very little progress in transforming our practice to one that is truly person-centered.

Why is this so? There are several related reasons. For one, providers will always be able to identify shortcomings in the reasoning and judgment of people with SMI that would justify their making decisions for service users. This is not a personal indictment of individual providers (a category in which we proudly include ourselves), but an acknowledgment that providers have competing agendas that would inevitably come into conflict with, and often trump, the personal sovereignty of the individual being served; risk being perhaps the paradigmatic, but certainly not the only, agenda at play (genuine compassion being another). This is a result of structure and role, not of the intention of individual providers. For two, concerns about other agendas trumping a person's choice also derive from the unfortunate history of psychiatry and the discipline's track record of considering certain lifestyle choices as pathological that have since proven to be viable, e.g. gay, lesbian, bisexual and transgender, if not downright courageous, e.g. "run away" slaves.

A third, and the most basic, reason is because one person taking over responsibility for another person's decision-making capacity does little to promote, and indeed does much to impede, that person's recovery. The consumer (service user) literature is replete with people with SMI making eloquent pleas to be "allowed" to make their own mistakes so that they can be afforded the opportunity to learn from them, just like everybody else. The social science research literature is replete with studies of the learned helplessness, hopelessness and despair that results from other people stepping in to make decisions for another person, who then often comes to feel like he or she is no longer just like everybody else. The convictions in freedom and equality of democratic societies are founded on this principle, and the history of various civil rights movements has confirmed its wisdom. A core contention of the recovery movement is that this principle is just as applicable to persons with SMI as it is to people of color, women, and other minority or historically oppressed or marginalized groups.[9] It is in relation to these issues of personal sovereignty and agency that the recovery movement has most forcefully made its case as being its own civil rights movement,[10,11,12] and on this score that it promises to have the most substantive impact on transforming mental health practice.[13]

What implications does this view have for PCC? It suggests, for example, that the SMIs with which a person is struggling may be identified as one of the factors currently limiting the person's free exercise of his or her autonomy. The illness, that is, does not as much limit my ability as a provider to be person-centered as it might the person's ability to make fully free and autonomous decisions. In attempting to offer PCC, we therefore may need to accept responsibility for liberating the person as much as possible from the limitations imposed by the illness on his or her freedom. Rather than simply stepping in and making decisions for the person, we assume an active, and perhaps even proactive, role in identifying the ways in which the illness is interfering with the process of the person freely pursuing his or her unique interests and aspirations, and accept as our responsibility working closely with the person (over time) to develop and use mechanisms and tools for overcoming or compensating for these forms of interference. Rather than stepping in to take over the decision-making process, we step back from the process to see how we might need to assist the person in making his or her own decisions in an informed and thoughtful manner. Similar to the role of the provider in offering supported housing, supported education, SE and supported socialization, we actively and skillfully support the person in learning how to function as well as possible in this particular life domain; in this case, the domain being that of personal decision-making. Rather than contradicting Principle #2 above, this approach is a validation of its meaning.

Supported housing approximates as much as possible the experience of "normal," i.e. independent, housing for a person with a disabling serious mental illness. It is more like ordinary housing for everyone else rather than different, and only differs from ordinary housing to the extent that adaptations, limitations or additions are required by the nature of the person's illness. We are suggesting the same for what we might call "supported decision-making."

Principle #3: Different aspects of personal decision-making can be supported in different ways.

In order to implement this vision of supported decision-making, we will need to break down the process of decision-making into its constituent parts and examine the ways in which the illness might interfere with each aspect, developing interventions and tools on this basis. We give brief examples of a few of these below, in relation to the examples offered above. It should be noted that some of the strategies and tools to be mentioned in the following would be equally useful to many people who do not have SMI, and that this should not be surprising to us. It just reaffirms, once again, the importance of Principles #1 and #2 above.

Goal setting – Perhaps the first series of steps in implementing PCC is to identify the person's own hopes, dreams and aspirations, determine how these can be translated into achievable (and relatively short-term) goals, and then discern the ways in which a care plan can address these goals in relation to the person's condition and its effects. For many people with SMIs, this process may be just as straightforward as for anyone else, and in this case, no specific adaptations, limitations or additions may be required. There are many instances, however, in which this series of steps may be particularly challenging for persons with histories of SMI, and therefore this is an area that may require attention.

One common concern among providers is their sense that service users no longer have goals and have given up whatever hopes, dreams or aspirations they may have had earlier in life. This may be true for some individuals who have become demoralized over time due to repetitive failures and losses due to their illness, for others who have been socialized into a mental health system that has not cared in the past about their aspirations, or for yet others who are afraid of taking risks and having setbacks. It also may be true, however, that the provider has yet to earn the person's trust and/or that the person is depressed. In such cases, providers should assess the person for active or co-occurring depression and/or should consider that they have not yet gotten to know the person well enough and have not yet earned the level of trust required for the person to share this kind of intimate information.

In any of the cases above, including the person who still appears no longer to have goals despite trusting the provider and no longer being depressed, helping the person to get back in touch with what interested him or her, or what he or she enjoyed prior to becoming ill, may be a useful place to begin the process of igniting or jump starting the person's passion. There are many tools, including interests and strengths assessments, that may help the person to recall those things that he or she had found pleasurable or meaningful in the past. Finally, there can be no substitute for actual life experience in re-igniting, or eliciting for the first time, a person's interest, e.g. taking someone to a stable and helping them onto a horse as opposed to discussing horseback riding at a psychosocial club.[14] In the end, as long as the person remains alive, it becomes possible to identify those things that bring the person more or less pleasure and enjoyment and to maximize his or her opportunities to have the highest quality of life possible given the severity of his or her condition. As we have pointed out elsewhere, this is a stance that has traditionally been taken by hospice providers working with terminally ill patients, and could certainly be used more often in psychiatry.[15]

But what if the goals the person identifies are unrealistic, or are based on his or her illness rather than on his or her genuine preference, i.e. something he or she would want if he or she were not ill? The realistic nature of any specific goal may lie in part in the eyes of the beholder, with providers at times underestimating the capabilities of service users simply because they have an SMI. Service users complain of this, especially in terms of employment goals, when providers neglect the fact that they have a degree or a successful work history and suggest that they take an entry-level job in fast food or janitorial work, for example. One of the many lessons of the consumer (service user) movement has been that numerous people with SMI can accomplish incredible things given the opportunities and, at times, the supports. Much of what may be considered "unrealistic" may be more a reflection of the provider's limitations, either in knowing enough about the person or in being able to imagine the impossible becoming possible, than in the person's own limitations. This may be especially a concern among practitioners who only interact (knowingly) with persons with SMI within acute or supervised clinical settings, as they have little life experience to draw from in making more accurate assessments of a person's true capabilities. Here, too, structured assessments can be very useful.

Still, there will be people who express blatantly unrealistic aspirations, such as wanting to be a rock star (when they have no musical talent) or wanting to be the next president of the U.S. (when they have never held an elected office). Here, the PSR approach has been to accept the person's aspiration and to work with him or her to break the longer-term goal down into incremental, intermediate steps. A first step towards becoming a rock star may be to take up an instrument or to take voice lessons; a first step toward becoming the president of the U.S. might be to finish high school, etc. As long as the service provider is genuine in supporting the person's efforts toward these goals (after all, many people never reach their most ambitious aspirations but have a meaningful life in the process nonetheless), this approach can be highly effective. We were highly gratified, for example, when a person with schizophrenia with whom we had worked for many years finally became willing to let go of what had been an all-engrossing preoccupation with becoming a physician when he found that he had a talent for medical transcription. He called one of us several years after we were no longer working together to tell us the good news, and to thank us for never taking away his dream of working in the medical field.

A somewhat different approach may be required by people whose aspirations or goals appear to be based at least partially in the illness. One example mentioned above was that of the person who was paranoid and who was convinced that all mental health service providers were trying to poison, imprison or hurt him. How could his care planning be person-centered? When asked about his own goals, such a person would most likely mention being discharged from the hospital and being allowed to return home. But this presents the provider with a very workable goal, the next question being: "What do you think you need to do, or what needs to happen, for you to be discharged?" How this question is viewed, and whether or not it is asked, can lead to two very different outcomes.

In our experience consulting to inpatient and residential settings, it often happens that the staff have been convinced that the person needs to accept treatment, be compliant with staff requests and scheduled group activities, and eventually become less symptomatic in order to gain release. From this point of view, the person's own goals become relevant once he or she accepts and benefits from treatment and is doing better, and it is time to think about transition to a lower level of care. From the person's own point of view, however, he or she unfortunately may have little reason to participate in or accept treatment, as it appears to have very little, if anything, to do with his or her pursuit of his or her own interests and goals. From his or her perspective, all you need to do is to unlock the door and let me leave. How are medications and group therapy, for example, going to get these people to stop trying to hurt me? They are the problem, not me. Such a situation often leads understandably to a stalemate between service users and providers.

But what if the staff asks the person: "What do you think you need to do, or what needs to happen, for you to be discharged?" And what if the person says, for example, that I know if I want to be discharged and not have to return to this hospital I have to stop getting evicted from every apartment I move into. Then the next question would become: "And what happens that causes you to get evicted?" After more discussion, the staff learns that the person is convinced that people move into the apartment on either side of him, or above or beneath him, in order to continue to harass and torture him by shouting at him through the walls all hours of the day and night. He can only tolerate a certain amount of this noise and after a while picks up a broom and starts to bang against the wall in protest, at times punching holes into the sheetrock, thus leading to his eviction. At this point, the staff could ask if he might consider feeling safe in his own apartment to be a goal that he and the staff could work on together. Would he be interested in finding ways to feel safer when alone in his apartment, so that he would not be evicted and wind up back in the hospital? If his answer to this question is "yes," then there are many fruitful avenues for the staff to explore with the person in terms of increasing his feelings of safety.

But if the staff responds without insight into the individual's illness, this person will surely not follow through with outpatient care and will inevitably wind up back in the hospital anyway. This leads us to the second major component of person-centered care: care planning and the role of insight or awareness of illness.

Care planning – One of the major differences between PCC planning for people with SMIs and people with other medical conditions, practitioners may suggest, is the issue of insight. People with diabetes will know that they have diabetes; people with asthma will know that they have asthma, etc., but some will argue that most people with SMI (or at least those with schizophrenia) lack insight into having the illness and therefore will not participate in the treatments they need to manage their condition. This lack of insight poses a major challenge to PCC planning, does it not? With the exception of the person being too depressed and suicidal to articulate any other goals than dying, this theme runs throughout all of the examples given above that appear to challenge the PCC paradigm. Is insight, in fact, required for PCC?

This is a complicated question with several different answers. A first clarification is to ask: "Insight into what?" Is it necessary for a person to accept that he or she has an SMI that we describe as "schizophrenia" or "psychosis" in order to participate in and benefit from PCC? Or is it enough that the person is aware, and willing to acknowledge, that something has gone dreadfully wrong in his or her life and that he or she could benefit from some assistance from other people in trying to set things right?

A second clarification is to recall the points made above regarding the difference between being in and being outside of an acute episode of illness. People who are depressed may be too depressed to recognize that they are depressed, people who are in an acute manic episode may be too manic to recognize that they are manic, and people in an acute episode of schizophrenia may be too disorganized, paranoid or absorbed in their hallucinations and delusions to be able to step back and recognize that they are acutely symptomatic. This may no longer hold, however, when the person is no longer in an acute episode. Even in schizophrenia, for which lack of insight has been proposed for over a century to be a pathognomonic sign of the illness, we have yet to meet a person with this condition who was not aware that something had gone dreadfully wrong in his or her life. The person's own account of what had gone wrong may have differed significantly from our own, but the person nonetheless was painfully aware that there was a significant problem in his or her life and, more importantly, that he or she could benefit from the help of others, should those others be trustworthy and should they have proven to have the person's own interest at heart. As long as the person is willing to accept such help, PCC planning remains a possibility.

Why, then, do so many people with schizophrenia appear not to have insight? They may appear not to have insight because they are in the throes of an acute episode. They may appear not to have insight because they are being encountered within a clinical setting in which they feel scrutinized, devalued or put under a microscope, and where acknowledgement of their problems would be viewed as making things even worse for them. If you are stopped by the police for speeding, for example, you will not want them to know that you did not have your seatbelt fastened (a personal story, and an extra $37 ticket), or worse yet, that you have cocaine stashed in your glove box (not a personal story). They may appear not to have insight because no one has yet had, or taken, the time to earn their trust and to provide a context within which they can feel comfortable sharing their most intimate and painful secrets. Or more simply, they may appear not to have insight because, as suggested above, their explanation of their predicament differs significantly from that of the providers treating them. This is such a common problem that it deserves a few paragraphs of its own.

If lack of awareness of illness is not, after all, a pathognomonic sign of schizophrenia (it has yet to be accepted as such after a century of debate), why might it be so difficult for people with schizophrenia to accept that they have schizophrenia? In the first place, it is interesting to note that during the era in which lack of insight was first identified in schizophrenia, people were never told that they *had* schizophrenia, or any other mental illness for that matter. As recently as 25 years ago, in fact, it was still considered taboo to inform people with SMI that that was what we thought they had and what we thought was causing them problems. If we did not view service users as capable of digesting and utilizing such information, and therefore did not educate them, how could we then expect them to "accept" their diagnosis?

Even if we were to educate people in school, and the general public, about the nature of schizophrenia – as some particularly progressive countries are now beginning to do – this is far from a straightforward matter. In fact, the picture of what constitutes "schizophrenia" has only gotten more, rather than less, complicated since the term was first introduced by Bleuler at the beginning of the 20th century. As deliberations are underway for the drafting of DSM-V, many scientists are arguing that there simply is no unitary condition that we can call "schizophrenia." There may be a group of loosely related conditions that we might call "the schizophrenias" (as Bleuler had originally thought), or there may be independent conditions that we have mistakenly lumped together due to a Wittgensteinian "family resemblance"; with the now well-established heterogeneity in course and outcome being due to the fact that these are actually different conditions. Finally, the psychiatric community in Japan, for example, has decided to do away with the term schizophrenia altogether, having found it to add to rather than to reduce the complexities associated with diagnosing SMI. If after a century of dedicated clinical investigation the field of psychiatry cannot agree on what constitutes this condition we have described as schizophrenia, why should we be surprised that service users are so skeptical and unwilling to accept this designation? Especially when we have insisted for so long on designating them as "schizophrenics" rather than as people experiencing schizophrenia?

As the consumer (service user) movement has now made abundantly clear, no one should be expected to accept being "a schizophrenic." This is simply not the same as being "a diabetic" or "an asthmatic," given the history of the term and the stigma associated with it.[16] Providers who attempt to offer PCC to people whom they view as "schizophrenics" will be doomed from the start, not because of the deficits imposed by the illness, but because of their failure to show respect to the people they serve. In our experience, accepting a diagnosis such as schizophrenia, psychosis, or bipolar disorder is not a prerequisite to participating in PCC. The only prerequisites to participating in PCC are the desire to improve one's life and the willingness to see whether or not other people can play some useful role in assisting an individual in making his or her life better. If those conditions are in place, then we can enter into productive discussions about how to make that life better and what each party can contribute. This often applies even to those individuals who appear not to have goals, not to be motivated to make changes, and not to appear to be dissatisfied with their current situation – whether because of a deficit syndrome or negative symptoms on the one hand, or because of hallucinatory and/or delusional preoccupations on the other.

This point has been driven home to us in at least two ways: first, through an examination of the first-person accounts literature in which themes of loss, loneliness and the desire for love and companionship are common,[17] even for people who appear to others to be apathetic and under the sway of negative symptoms;[18] and second, through our clinical experience, in which persistence, patience and gentle prodding have been highly effective in enabling us to connect with the person who may be hiding behind or underneath the illness and the secondary effects of institutionalization and discrimination. In one such case, we were impressed by a 38-year-old man who had had a psychotic disorder for 20 years and who had lived almost exclusively in his bedroom in his mother's home for the duration of that period. He was occasionally hospitalized when he became incommunicative and stopped eating, but otherwise spent his days almost entirely alone, smoking in his room, except for brief, sporadic encounters with family members. We encountered him during one of his hospital stays and spent a week trying to talk with him and determine his reasons for not eating and no longer talking with his family. He was reticent to talk with the staff, sat silently through group meetings, and ignored his family when they came to visit. He appeared to be making no use of the hospital stay (except for minimal eating and drinking), and both the staff and family felt stuck. He appeared not to want anything, voiced no complaints or dissatisfaction, and refused to participate in care or discharge planning. He appeared to embody the deficit syndrome described by Carpenter and colleagues.[19]

This scenario continued until one of us facilitated a family meeting with the presumptive agenda of discharge planning. After a couple of weeks there appeared to be no reason to keep this man in the hospital any longer, but his family was concerned that he was only minimally better than when admitted and did not want to take him back only for him to resume his earlier behavior. The family reassured him that they wanted to take him back home, but expressed their concerns that he no longer ate meals and no longer even spoke to them, worrying that he was "wasting away" before their eyes. The provider asked the young man if he was aware of these changes in his behavior, and, if so, if he had any ideas about what might have happened. He did not respond. The provider asked the young man if he felt ready to return home under these circumstances, to which he again did not respond. After a brief, awkward, silence, the provider asked the service user if he felt that perhaps this was all life had to offer him. Was he resigned to spending the rest of his life alone in his bedroom? At this point, tears started to well up in his eyes and began to slide down his cheeks. After another brief silence, he said simply "No." After waiting for a further response which did not come, the provider then responded: "I'm glad. That would have been really awful. What else would you like to do?" At which point the service user begrudgingly explained that he had felt that his family had "given up" on him. His perception was that they had gradually invited him to fewer and fewer activities and events, had gradually sought him out less frequently, and had begun to leave him out, and leave him behind, as they went on with their own lives. His further withdrawal and refusal to eat was both a test of their abandonment (would they simply let him die, like the bug in Kafka's *Metamorphosis*?) and a sign that their giving up on him had led him to give up on himself. He was hurt and angry that, despite his many refusals, they had not continued to pursue him.

Rather than responding to what the family might have viewed as his childish obstinateness, the service user's mother was overwhelmed by his expression of affect (something she said she had not seen for 20 years) and readily understood his concerns about her preoccupation with other family matters, the decreased availability of his siblings (who now had families of their own), and how these changes in the family had affected him. The provider pointed out how the family's insistence on bringing him to the hospital, and their continued concern with his "wasting away," was "proof" that they would not simply allow him to die alone and suggested that perhaps they could discuss some of the ways in which the service user might like to be included in family activities and events. This one meeting did not, of course, bring about a significant shift in his pattern of withdrawal and isolation, or in the difficulties the family would face in trying to include him more in family life, but it did serve to establish an important lesson for the involved parties. As much difficulty as the service user had in participating in family relationships, activities and events, it was not to his benefit for the family to passively accept his withdrawal or to contribute to his further marginalization. An important challenge for the service user and his mother, and the mental health providers working with them, became how they could build bridges for him back into that world. In this case, it is quite conceivable that PCC planning would begin with the goal of increasing the person's contact with family members, with one measurable objective being that he and his mother would have several meals together each week (instead of him taking all of his meals alone in his bedroom).

Task and role assignment – This last vignette offers a useful entrée into a third component of PCC, which is the assignment of tasks and roles to the appropriate parties. As far as we know, this is one component of PCC that has been a rather recent development within psychiatry. Convening a care team and assigning various roles and tasks to various people, both paid providers and natural supporters, has been more common in the developmental disability and geriatric fields, where the assumption has been that the professional health care staff and person with the disability or illness cannot manage all of the responsibilities themselves. Such a distribution of responsibility is not desired or required in all instances of SMI, but in many cases it can be extremely useful. In addition, one of the more important and innovative aspects of this advance for persons with SMI is acknowledgement that they, too, have an important role to play in their own recovery. Rather than waiting passively for the medications to take effect, and simply doing what others tell them to do, people with SMI have to play an active role in initiating, pursuing and sustaining their recovery. The PCC plan concretizes and operationalizes this role, along with the roles that others need to play as well.

In the case described above, the questions that would emerge from framing a first objective as the service user and his mother will share several meals a week together would be: who decides on which meals, who chooses, prepares and cleans up the meal, and who is responsible, and how, for ensuring that they eat together. Does the service user decide that he will come out of his room on Mondays, Wednesdays and Sundays, or does his mother let him know when she can be home to share a meal with him? Does he want her to pick, prepare and clean up the meal, or is he interested in taking on some of these responsibilities himself? Alternatively, is she happy doing all of this herself and simply letting him know when dinner is ready, or would she like help? Can he decide on a day-to-day basis when he feels like having company, or does she need to be able to plan ahead so that she'll know when she needs to be home? Most crucially, is it up to him to come down to dinner on a pre-arranged basis, e.g. Mondays at 6:00, or is it up to her to come up to his bedroom, knock on the door and let him know when it is time for dinner? And who is to do what when he doesn't come down when dinner is ready? Is she to respect his wish not to eat, is she to badger him, is she to suggest rescheduling for a different time, or is he to be responsible for getting himself organized and respecting her need to manage her time wisely? Similar questions would emerge if a second objective would be for him to participate in other family activities. This is the level of specificity and detail that can be involved in PCC planning for individuals who are seriously disabled by a mental illness.

For people who are less seriously disabled, or disabled in different ways, the assignment of tasks and roles may look different. Physicians and/or nurse practitioners are responsible for medication evaluation, administration and monitoring; job coaches for providing job supports at the workplace; visiting nurses for administering medications on a daily basis; and volunteers or friends for accompanying the person to social and recreational activities. There is a tremendous amount of diversity both in terms of the tasks and in terms of the members of the team who can take on such tasks, including landlords, employers, tutors, family members, etc. Extremely important and often requiring the most creativity, though, is the person's own role. What can you do, and what *will* you do, to promote your own recovery? Once this is established, the remaining elements of the care plan should be designed to support the person in his or her own efforts to fulfill these responsibilities. If you agree to take medication, how can we ensure that you have the opportunities and supports to succeed in doing so? If you want to work, how can we support you in obtaining and keeping a job that interests you? As a primary rule of thumb, at least one of the person's goals should pertain to what he or she wants to be *doing* with his or her time, not just to what he or she wants to have; his or her roles and responsibilities, along with the various supports he or she will need, will follow naturally from that basis.

Feedback and ongoing revisions – As has been suggested by the examples given above, a person's goals, and the interventions, activities and people involved in attaining those goals, will naturally change over time. PCC planning is thus best understood as an ongoing process, and one that involves trial and error and the continuous eliciting and incorporation of feedback from all relevant parties. As goals are achieved, new ones are developed, or as one goal is pursued, it may morph into another goal (like the person who decided to become a medical transcriptionist instead of a doctor). Life is not typically lived (by most of us) through setting, pursuing and achieving clearly defined goals with measurable objectives, but by stumbling along as best one can from one experience to the next, with a vague sense of what one is ultimately looking for. PCC planning is thus an artificial framework overlaid on the person's life, and at best is a useful heuristic for helping the person get to where he or she is trying to go. As life is a process, however, and not a destination, we would fully expect the process to evolve over time until, in many cases, the person no longer requires such a framework for making the most of mental health care. As with mental health services in general, the goal of PCC is for the person eventually to no longer require it, with one principle being the replacement of formal services with informal and naturally occurring supports over time.

Proposed Criteria for PCC

Based on these deliberations, we would like to close by suggesting a set of criteria by which one should be able to judge whether or not, or to what degree, an approach to psychiatric care can be considered person-centered.

➤ **Is the care centered on an individual person and based on this person's unique life goals and informed by his or her needs, values and preferences?** PCC can only be carried out at the level of each individual, unique person within the context of his or her family and life. Each PCC plan should look different from any others and be based squarely on this particular individual's goals, needs, values and preferences. Does the plan provide a roadmap for where the person is headed and what he or she is trying to do in his or her life? Does the plan address a life outside of or beyond formal mental health services, or does it remain within the boundaries of the mental health system? Can you tell from the plan what the care team is trying to accomplish, not just what they are trying to get rid of or avoid? If medication is part of the plan, can you tell what the medication is to be used for? Is adherence an end in itself, or is it viewed as a route to some other, personally desirable end? Will the services offered lead to some worthwhile and wished for changes in the person's life? Generalizations about what all people with SMI want or need are no more accurate than are generalizations regarding what all psychiatrists want or need, and have little to do with PCC. PCC is precisely that: centered on the person, not on any given population.

➤ **Is the care based on the person's strengths and interests?** Is it clear how the plan will utilize identified strengths, both within the person and within his or her social milieu? Can you tell from the plan what the person's specific interests are, and how these interests have contributed to the formulation of goals and objectives? Does the plan help to move the person toward what interests him or her, or does it simply move him or her away from problematic behaviors or activities? If substance abuse is identified as a problem to be addressed, for example, does the plan also address what kind of sober activities the person may want to participate in instead? Are community activities and resources identified in the plan that would support the person in pursing his or her interests? Are there people identified in the plan with whom the person can share these interests?

➤ **Does the plan clearly delineate the tasks and roles to be performed and the parties responsible for each? Of particular importance is, does the plan clearly identify the person's own sphere of responsibility and the tasks that he or she agrees to take on?** As noted above, this is one of the more recent advances in PCC and one of the more salient in applying this approach to mental health care. What does the person need to do to promote or progress in his or her own recovery? And what kind of support will the person need in order to carry out these responsibilities successfully? These two questions form a focus of PCC plans for people with SMI, and require in-depth knowledge of the person, his or her capacities and needs, and the resources available in his or her social milieu. Based on this knowledge, the care team should be able to identify what might be the next one or two steps in the person's recovery and to sketch out, no matter how provisionally, what will be involved in the person taking these next few steps. This is how the plan becomes more than a piece of paper that satisfies regulatory, accrediting and/or reimbursing bodies and to be more of an organic and useful work in progress.

➤ **Does the plan and the care provided change over time with the person's evolving goals and needs?** PCC plans do not accept maintenance as a valid goal, as people do not want merely to be "maintained." It is quite possible for people to want to maintain a level of clinical stability, or to want to remain at a plateau of functioning for an extended period of time. Few people like change for the sake of change, and many people with SMI are afraid of taking risks or trying new things out of a very legitimate fear that they may suffer a setback (a fear often reinforced by caring practitioners who do not want to see people relapse). But life also does not stand still. Therefore, while containing one's illness may be a very real concern and goal for some people at some times, it is not possible to do so simply by maintaining one's life, i.e. by trying to stand still. Care plans anticipate that change is inevitable and that people will need to continue to adapt to new situations and new challenges, whether they like to or not. One important contribution PCC can make in such situations is to help the person identify those things that he or she wants to keep the same while other things are changing around them.

➤ **Are the plan and the services and supports offered accessible to and understandable by the person?** Just as the plan needs to identify the person's own role in promoting or pursuing recovery, the plan and the care offered need to be accessible to and understandable by the person. This is one area in which psychiatric PCC may need to incorporate the use of tools and aids to help the person compensate for cognitive impairments or a history of educational deprivation. Does the plan address those aspects of the person's own experiences that are of concern to him or her, and in a language that he or she will be able to understand and to use, e.g. voices as opposed to auditory hallucinations, feelings of being unsafe, vulnerable or unprotected as opposed to paranoia, etc.? Does the person know what he or she has agreed to receive or participate in? Has his or her consent been truly informed, or will things be done to him or her to which he or she has not agreed? Even in the case of individuals receiving treatment involuntarily, or individuals who have conservators or guardians, have concerted efforts been made to inform the person of the available options and to explain what he or she can expect to happen, including what needs to happen for him or her to no longer be receiving care involuntarily or no longer need a guardian?

➤ **Finally, does the plan encourage and support the person in assuming increasing control over his or her life, including the power to make his or her own decisions?** Here too, psychiatric PCC plans may need to focus specifically on these issues of control, empowerment and decision-making more than care plans in other specialty areas of medicine. This is not only because of the impact of mental illness on the person's life, but also because of the history of mental health care and its tendency to socialize people into a passive and helpless "patient" role. People may need to be encouraged to take back control of certain parts of their life, the responsibility for which may have been assumed by others. They may also need to be encouraged to view themselves as capable, and as having intact domains of functioning beyond the reach of the illness. They may need to be reminded of, or introduced to, their strengths and gifts; they may need a series of small successes and easy wins in order to rebuild their self-confidence and sense of personal efficacy. And they may need encouragement and support in taking risk and trying new things – perhaps even some gentle prodding to get unstuck, to be liberated from the inertia of chronic illness.

CONCLUSION: A VISION FOR THE FUTURE

These criteria are relevant to the present context, as we are challenged to introduce PCC into a field that has historically socialized people into a helpless and passive stance from which they will need to be liberated in order to take responsibility for their own recovery. In the future, however, this form of empowerment may no longer be needed, as having an SMI may no longer require accepting a subordinate role in relation to service providers. Within a respectful, collaborative system, PCC for SMI will come even more to represent PCC for other long-term medical conditions. As youth are educated about mental illnesses prior to onset, and as families come to view mental illnesses as illnesses like any other, people will be able to access mental health care in a more timely manner, and thereby derive more benefit from existing interventions. As stigma and discrimination subside, and as the social and economic condition of persons with SMI improves, new discoveries also will be made into the nature of the more focal impairments associated with these conditions, allowing subsequently for new and more effective interventions to be developed to address these impairments (cognitive remediation being a prominent and promising example). Two or three generations down the road, we are confident that mental illness will no longer subsume the entirety of a person's life but will prove to be a delimited condition that people will be able to manage as they pursue a full and gratifying life in the communities of their choice. In our estimation, the use of PCC appears to offer the best route to actualizing such a vision for the future.

REFERENCES

1 Cross L. *See* Section 1.2.2, *Rogerian and Related Psychotherapies in the Twentieth Century.*
2 Tondora J, Pocklington S, Gorges A, *et al. Implementation of Person-Centered Care and Planning: from policy to practice to evaluation.* Washington, DC: Substance Abuse and Mental Health Services Administration; 2005.
3 Davidson L, Rakfeldt J, Strauss JS. *The Roots of the Recovery Movement in Psychiatry: lessons learned.* London: Wiley-Blackwell; 2010.
4 Davidson L, Drake RE, Schmutte T, *et al.* Oil and water or oil and vinegar? Evidence-based medicine meets recovery. *Community Ment Health J.* 2009; **45**(5): 323–32.
5 O'Reilly R. *See* section 8 *Some Sober Reflections on Person-Centered Care.*
6 Wexler B, Davidson L, Styron T, *et al.* Severe and persistent mental illness. In: Jacobs S, Griffith EEH, editors. *40 Years of Academic Public Psychiatry.* London: Wiley; 2008. pp. 1–20.
7 Davidson L, Harding CM, Spaniol L. *Recovery from Severe Mental Illnesses: research evidence and implications for practice. Volume 1.* Boston, MA: Center for Psychiatric Rehabilitation of Boston University; 2005.
8 Weiner DB. Philippe Pinel's "Memoir on Madness" of December 11, 1794: a fundamental text of modern psychiatry. *Am J Psychiatry.* 1992; **149**(6): 725–32. p. 729.
9 Davidson L, Tondora J, O'Connell MJ, *et al. A Practical Guide to Recovery-Oriented Practice: tools for transforming mental health care.* New York, NY: Oxford University Press; 2009.
10 Chamberlin J. Speaking for ourselves: an overview of the ex-psychiatric inmates' movement. *Psych Rehab J.* 1984; **8**(2): 56–63.

11 Deegan PE. The independent living movement and people with psychiatric disabilities: taking back control over our own lives. *Psych Rehab J.* 1992; **15**(3): 3–19.

12 Davidson L. What happened to civil rights? *Psych Rehab J.* 2006; **30**(1): 11–14.

13 Davidson, Tondora, O'Connell, *et al.*, op. cit.

14 Bizub A, Joy A, Davidson L. "It's like being in another world": demonstrating the benefits of therapeutic horseback riding for individuals with psychiatric disability. *Psych Rehab J.* 2003; **26**(4): 377–84.

15 Deegan, op. cit.

16 Flanagan E, Davidson L. "Schizophrenics," "borderlines," and the lingering legacy of misplaced concreteness: an examination of the persistent misconception that the DSM classifies people instead of disorders. *Psychiatry.* 2007; **70**(2): 100–12.

17 Davidson L, Stayner D. Loss, loneliness, and the desire for love: perspectives on the social lives of people with schizophrenia. *Psych Rehab J.* 1997; **20**: 3–12.

18 Bouricius JK. Negative symptoms and emotions in schizophrenia. *Schizophr Bull.* 1989; **15**(2): 201–8.

19 Carpenter WT, Heinrichs DW, Wagman AM. Deficit and nondeficit forms of schizophrenia: the concept. *Am J Psychiatry.* 1988; **145**(5): 578–83.

Index

Tables and diagrams are given in italics.